700 Essential Neurology Checklists

T0136390

700 Essential Neurology Checklists

Ibrahim Imam, FRCP

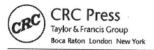

CRC Press
Taylor & Francis Group
Boca Raton London New York

CRC Press is an imprint of the
Taylor & Francis Group, an informa business

First edition published 2022
by CRC Press
6000 Broken Sound Parkway NW, Suite 300, Boca Raton, FL 33487-2742

and by CRC Press
2 Park Square, Milton Park, Abingdon, Oxon, OX14 4RN

© 2022 Taylor & Francis Group, LLC

CRC Press is an imprint of Taylor & Francis Group, LLC

This book contains information obtained from authentic and highly regarded sources. While all reasonable efforts have been made to publish reliable data and information, neither the author[s] nor the publisher can accept any legal responsibility or liability for any errors or omissions that may be made. The publishers wish to make clear that any views or opinions expressed in this book by individual editors, authors or contributors are personal to them and do not necessarily reflect the views/opinions of the publishers. The information or guidance contained in this book is intended for use by medical, scientific or health-care professionals and is provided strictly as a supplement to the medical or other professional's own judgement, their knowledge of the patient's medical history, relevant manufacturer's instructions and the appropriate best practice guidelines. Because of the rapid advances in medical science, any information or advice on dosages, procedures or diagnoses should be independently verified. The reader is strongly urged to consult the relevant national drug formulary and the drug companies' and device or material manufacturers' printed instructions, and their websites, before administering or utilizing any of the drugs, devices or materials mentioned in this book. This book does not indicate whether a particular treatment is appropriate or suitable for a particular individual. Ultimately it is the sole responsibility of the medical professional to make his or her own professional judgements, so as to advise and treat patients appropriately. The authors and publishers have also attempted to trace the copyright holders of all material reproduced in this publication and apologize to copyright holders if permission to publish in this form has not been obtained. If any copyright material has not been acknowledged please write and let us know so we may rectify in any future reprint.

Except as permitted under U.S. Copyright Law, no part of this book may be reprinted, reproduced, transmitted, or utilized in any form by any electronic, mechanical, or other means, now known or hereafter invented, including photocopying, microfilming, and recording, or in any information storage or retrieval system, without written permission from the publishers.

For permission to photocopy or use material electronically from this work, access www.copyright.com or contact the Copyright Clearance Center, Inc. (CCC), 222 Rosewood Drive, Danvers, MA 01923, 978-750-8400. For works that are not available on CCC please contact mpkbookspermissions@tandf.co.uk

Trademark notice: Product or corporate names may be trademarks or registered trademarks and are used only for identification and explanation without intent to infringe.

ISBN: 9781032117294 (hbk)
ISBN: 9781032076232 (pbk)
ISBN: 9781003221258 (ebk)

DOI: 10.1201/9781003221258

Typeset in Minion
by Newgen Publishing UK

Contents

CHAPTER 2 EPILEPSY

CHAPTER 5 NEUROINFLAMMATORY AND AUTOIMMUNE DISORDERS   89

CHAPTER 6   INFECTIONS

CHAPTER 7 HEADACHE

CHAPTER 8   VASCULAR DISORDERS 164

CHAPTER 10 SPINAL CORD DISORDERS

CHAPTER 11 ANTERIOR HORN CELL DISORDERS

CHAPTER 12   ROOT AND PLEXUS DISORDERS

CHAPTER 13   PERIPHERAL NERVE DISORDERS

CHAPTER 14 NEUROMUSCULAR JUNCTION DISORDERS

CHAPTER 15   MUSCLE DISORDERS   292

CHAPTER 16   TUMOURS   **320**

CHAPTER 17 METABOLIC AND MITOCHONDRIAL DISORDERS — 334

CHAPTER 18 DEVELOPMENTAL DISORDERS — 354

CHAPTER 19 ALLIED NEUROLOGICAL DISORDERS

Preface

This book is an extract of the online database, *Neurochecklists*, which currently consists of almost 3,500 checklists covering all aspects of neurology and its allied specialties. The 700 checklists included in this book, just under a fifth of the online database, were specifically selected for having the most general practical application. They focus on the diverse range of neurological management – history, clinical examination, investigations, and treatment, and they provide details of aetiology, epidemiology, genetics, and pathology as relevant to the topic.

The topics covered in the book, and on the online database, cover the diversity of neurological subspecialty areas such as cognitive neurology, disorders of consciousness, epilepsy, sleep disorders, movement disorders, headache, stroke, neurological infections, neuromuscular diseases, neuro-inflammation, nervous system tumours, obstetric and functional neurology. The content also provides practical information on the disorders that cross the boundaries of neurology and its allied specialties, for example neuro-ophthalmology, neurotology, psychiatry, neurosurgery, neuroradiology, and pain management. It is also relevant that many of the checklists in the book cover the intersection of neurology and general medicine, with topics on cardiovascular, respiratory, nutritional, endocrine, renal, rheumatological, haematological and gastrointestinal disorders. Other practical checklists apply to the neurological complications of operative procedures, such as cardiac and transplant surgery.

The major sources of the information in the checklists include widely regarded neurology journals such as the *Annals of Neurology*, *Brain*, the *European Journal of Neurology*, the *Journal of Neurology*, the *Journal of Neurology, Neurosurgery and Psychiatry*, *Lancet Neurology*, and *Practical Neurology*. Many standard neurology textbooks also provided valuable material. The selection of contents for the book also had a strong emphasis on evidence-based guidelines, review articles, ground-breaking studies, and relevant case reports. All the checklists on the online database are fully referenced and hyperlinked to source.

The information in this book, and the online database, is expected to be appropriate not just to neurologists and neurology trainees, but to all medical professionals requiring relevant, practical, and timely information about neurology. I therefore expect that specialists such as psychiatrists, neurosurgeons, paediatricians, general physicians, obstetricians, ophthalmologists, and specialist nurses, will find the checklists useful. Other health care professionals may also find areas of interest such as general nurses, speech therapists, physiotherapists, and occupational therapists. Medical students and researchers who also require vast amounts of neurological information, often within restricted time frames, may find many of the topics covered in the book useful. Whilst the database is not primarily intended for the non-medically trained general public, the simple and clear format may be helpful for patients who are active in the co-management of their neurological conditions, and in discussions with their physicians.

To keep the volume of the book manageable, I have not included the references, but these are freely available on the Neurochecklists website. I have also listed all the topics in the online database in the index. Purchase of this book also comes with a one-year complimentary free access to the full online database; to activate this, please email info@ neurochecklists.com with a copy of your receipt of purchase.

Like the famed Persian carpet makers who deliberately inserted errors in their products, because only God's work can be flawless, this book is by no means perfect. But unlike the legend, any mistakes in it are inadvertent for which I take full responsibility, and for which I humbly request eagle-eyed readers to point out to me.

Acknowledgements and dedication

I want to first acknowledge the constant support and selfless encouragement of my wife, Zainab, without whom this book would never have been. From conception about a decade ago, to publication, she has been there by my side, nudging and prompting, lifting me up and calming things down.

To my children Aminah, Safiyyah, Ja'far, and Maryam, I want to thank you for your cheerleading and patience, and for your wise counsel during the long road to this point.

I have only unstinting gratitude to Dr Hadi Manji to whom I owe my whole career as a neurologist in the United Kingdom. No words are sufficient to convey my eternal gratitude for his help, support, mentoring, and guidance. If this book is readable at all, it is to his invaluable advice to prune and improve the fluency. And I am also indebted to Dr Juzar Hooker for helpfully introducing me to Dr Manji, unsolicited and, as ever, considerate. And to Prof. Guy Leschziner, my thanks for his review and comments that went such a long way to make this book a reality.

There can't be a better place to acknowledge my formative training in medicine and neurology at the University College Hospital Ibadan, with special thanks to Prof. Ayodele Falase for the foresight of nudging me towards neurology; and to Prof. Adesola Ogunniyi and Dr OSA Oluwole for grounding me in the specialty under difficult infrastructural circumstances, and for guiding me towards the successful defence of my neurology dissertations. In a similar way, my appreciation goes to my trainers at the National Hospital for Neurology and Neurosurgery where I did a diploma and clinical attachment in neurology, and in the Yorkshire and South West Peninsula neurology deanery's where I retrained as a neurologist, for introducing me to the highest quality of UK neurology practice.

I must also thank Tobi Oludayomi and Stephen Bapaga of Studio 14 for the inspired creation of the neurochecklists website, and Peter Mellett for the enhancements that have made it such a powerfully handy tool.

To Miranda Bromage, Samantha Cook, and Kyle Meyer at Taylor and Francis, and to Ed Robinson at Newgen Publishing go my heartfelt appreciation for the proactive approach to getting this book published. I was expecting a hair-tearing experience, but it has been a superb and pain-free journey through which I felt supported all along the way.

Finally, this book is dedicated to my mother, Hamra Imam – the strongest influence on my development as a person and a doctor; and to the memory of Kalli Imam – a thorough gentleman and the best father anyone could ever wish for.

Introduction

The concept of checklists in Medicine was championed by the surgeon Atul Gawande whose work focused on improving surgical patient safety. His research resulted in the development, and almost universal implementation, of the World Health Organisation (WHO) Surgical Safety Checklist, a simple tool that has revolutionised surgical operating procedures globally. Narrating his personal experience of using the checklist in his book, *The Checklist Manifesto*, Gawande said "I have yet to get through a week in surgery without the checklist's leading us to catch something we would have missed", adding that, "with the checklist in place, we have caught unrecognized drug allergies, equipment problems, confusion about medications, mistakes on labels for biopsy specimens…" and "we have made better plans and been better prepared for patients".[1]

Importantly for medicine generally, Gawande noted that checklists have potential applications "beyond the operating room" when he said "…there are hundreds, perhaps thousands, of things doctors do that are as dangerous and prone to error as surgery". He gave several examples of these, such as the evaluation of headache, chest pain, lung nodules and breast lumps. He also pointed to the treatment of heart attacks, strokes, drug overdoses, pneumonias, kidney failures, seizures, and headache. Gawande's realisation that all medical activities involve risk, uncertainty, and complexity led him to recommend that all aspects of medicine be committed to checklists.

Gawande's recommendation is one driver for developing the neurology checklists in this book. Another was the need to counter the compromising effect of cognitive biases on neurological practice. These are the pervasive shortcuts or heuristics which enable quick judgments especially when making decisions when time is limited, and when facts are scarce. These heuristics and biases have been adequately described by the psychologist Daniel Kahneman in his research, and in his book, *Thinking, Fast and Slow*.[2] More specifically, the profoundly detrimental impact of cognitive biases on neurological practice was highlighted in a most revealing paper published in the *Annals of Neurology* titled "How neurologists think: a cognitive psychology perspective on missed diagnoses".[3]

The authors of the article, leading neurologists, focused on the impact on neurological practice by the biases of framing, anchoring, availability, representativeness, and obedience to authority. Another article on the same theme, published in the journal *Neurology*, was aptly titled "Recognising and reducing cognitive bias in clinical and forensic neurology"; this noted the detrimental effect of other biases such as confirmation, hindsight, base rate neglect, and the 'good old days' bias.[4] It is relevant that these human factors are all processes that are amenable to mitigation by checklists.

Checklists have been developed in all spheres of life, including in professions such as aviation and medicine, to address the consequences of the human tendency to error. The neurology checklists in this book were developed in line with this spirit of minimising error and boosting clinical safety in the care of neurological patients. They apply to all aspects of neurology, a specialty noted for its size, diversity, and complexity. It is the expectation that the use of neurology checklists will enable the quick checking-up of topics in the clinic and on ward rounds; the focused reading of specific topics for relevant information; the preparation of presentations and teachings; the revision for examinations; keeping up with the latest in the diverse neurological subspecialties; and aiding research. In essence, *700 Essential Neurology Checklists* provides handy practical, comprehensive, and evidence-based information on every aspect of neurology.

REFERENCES

1. Gawande, A. *The Checklist Manifesto*. Profile Books, London, 2011.
2. Kahneman, D. *Thinking, Fast and Slow*. Penguin Books, London, 2011
3. Vickrey BG, Samuels MA, Ropper AH. *How neurologists think: a cognitive psychology perspective on missed diagnoses*. Ann Neurol 2010; 67:425–433.
4. Satya-Murti S, Lockhart J. *Recognizing and reducing cognitive bias in clinical and forensic neurology*. Neurol Clin Pract 2015; 5:389–396.

CHAPTER 1

Disorders of cognition and consciousness

Cognitive symptoms and signs

CORTICAL RELEASE PHENOMENA

Physiological types

- [ ] Palmomental: this is the earliest and most frequent release phenomenon
- [ ] Corneomandibular: this usually occurs along with other reflexes
- [ ] Snout

Pathological types

- [ ] Asymmetrical tonic neck reflex
- [ ] Corneomandibular reflex (Wartenberg's sign)
- [ ] Glabellar tap reflex
- [ ] Grasping reflex
- [ ] Head retraction
- [ ] Jaw jerk
- [ ] Mouth open finger spread reflex (MOFS)
- [ ] Nasopalpebral reflex
- [ ] Nuchocephalic reflex
- [ ] Palmar grasp
- [ ] Palmar support
- [ ] Palmomental reflex
- [ ] Palmocervical reflex
- [ ] Paratonia
- [ ] Plantar grasp
- [ ] Plantar support
- [ ] Pollicomental reflex
- [ ] Rooting
- [ ] Snout
- [ ] Sucking
- [ ] Support
- [ ] Utilisation behaviour

Causes

- [ ] Alzheimer's disease (AD)
- [ ] Parkinson's disease (PD)
- [ ] Cerebrovascular disease
- [ ] Vascular dementia
- [ ] Frontotemporal dementia (FTD)
- [ ] Normal pressure hydrocephalus (NPH)
- [ ] Attention deficit hyperactivity disorder (ADHD)
- [ ] Schizophrenia
- [ ] Bipolar disorder
- [ ] Major depression

Clinical significance

- [ ] Physiological release phenomena are present in 50% of adults
- [ ] >3 release phenomena together are pathological
- [ ] Higher number of release phenomena correlates with poorer cognitive function
- [ ] There is better correlation with subcortical than cortical lesions
- [ ] No pathological release phenomenon is disease specific
- [ ] Snout and grasp reflexes are the best predictors of significant disease
- [ ] Suck and root reflexes are uncommon

CONFABULATION

Clinical features

- [ ] This is when false beliefs and memories are generated to fill in gaps in memory
- [ ] It is a result of deficits in memory retrieval
- [ ] It occurs involuntarily and unconsciously
- [ ] Some confabulations are partially true

Types

- [ ] Spontaneous (fantastic)
- [ ] Provoked (momentary)

Psychiatric causes

- [ ] Korsakoff's syndrome
- [ ] Split-brain syndrome
- [ ] Anosognosia for hemiplegia
- [ ] Anton's syndrome
- [ ] Capgras syndrome
- [ ] Schizophrenia

Neurological causes

- [ ] Alzheimer's disease (AD)
- [ ] Traumatic brain injury
- [ ] Hydrocephalus
- [ ] Encephalitis
- [ ] Autism
- [ ] Multiple sclerosis (MS)
- [ ] Moyamoya disease
- [ ] Cerebral aneurysms
- [ ] Brain tumours
- [ ] Frontal lobe epilepsy
- [ ] Stroke

Physiological causes

- [ ] In healthy adults and young children
- [ ] Older age
- [ ] Hypnosis

Assessment tools

- [ ] The Confabulation Battery
- [ ] The Nijmegen-Venray Confabulation List (NVCL-20)

DOI: 10.1201/9781003221258-2

PATHOLOGICAL LAUGHTER

Clinical manifestations

- [ ] This is a pseudobulbar affect
- [ ] It occurs in response to non-specific stimuli
- [ ] There is no corresponding change in affect or mood

Neoplastic causes

- [ ] Cerebellar ependymoma
- [ ] Brain metastases from lung cancer
- [ ] Meningioma
- [ ] Heralding feature of glioblastoma
- [ ] Brainstem gliomas: this causes gaze and light-induced laughter
- [ ] Trigeminal neuromas
- [ ] Trigeminal schwannoma
- [ ] Rathke cleft cyst

Neurological causes

- [ ] Motor neurone disease (MND)
- [ ] Parkinson's disease (PD)
- [ ] Alzheimer's disease (AD)
- [ ] Stroke: laughter may herald hemispheric stroke
- [ ] Basilar artery dissection and pseudoaneurysm
- [ ] Multiple sclerosis (MS): laughter occurs in 10% of cases
- [ ] Brainstem clinically isolated syndrome (CIS)
- [ ] Gelastic epilepsy: giggling or crying may precede seizures
- [ ] von Economo's disease
- [ ] Pontine tuberculoma: laughter may be a heralding sign
- [ ] Angelman syndrome
- [ ] Traumatic brain injury (TBI): this also causes pathological crying
- [ ] Tourette syndrome (TS)
- [ ] Locked-in syndrome

Treatment

- [ ] Tricyclic antidepressants
- [ ] Selective serotonin reuptake inhibitors (SSRIs)
- [ ] Dextromethorphan/quinidine sulphate (DM/Q)
- [ ] Duloxetine: a dual serotonin-norepinephrine reuptake inhibitor
- [ ] Mirtazapine: case reports

APHASIA: CLASSIFICATION

Broca's aphasia

- [ ] This is a non-fluent aphasia
- [ ] It is caused by lesions in the posterior inferior frontal lobe

Wernicke's aphasia

- [ ] This is a fluent aphasia with impaired comprehension
- [ ] It is caused by lesions in the superior posterior temporal lobe
- [ ] It presents as jargon aphasia if the supramarginal gyrus is involved

Transcortical aphasia

- [ ] Motor: this is caused by lesions in the supplementary speech area
- [ ] Sensory: this is caused by lesions in the middle and posterior cerebral artery watershed areas

Subcortical aphasia

- [ ] This is a striato-capsular aphasia
- [ ] It is associated with white matter periventricular lesions

Conduction aphasia: lesion locations

- [ ] Left posterior lateral superior temporal gyrus
- [ ] Left supramarginal gyrus
- [ ] Left posterior superior temporal sulcus

Conduction aphasia: features

- [ ] Fluent aphasia
- [ ] Impaired repetition
- [ ] Impaired phonological short-term memory
- [ ] Impaired naming

Aphemia

- [ ] Impaired articulation
- [ ] Preserved comprehension
- [ ] Preserved writing
- [ ] Preserved oropharyngeal function
- [ ] Lesions are in the left inferior premotor cortex

Pure word deafness

- [ ] Inability to comprehend spoken words
- [ ] Hearing is intact
- [ ] Lesions are in the auditory receptive areas

Other aphasia types

- [ ] Anomic aphasia
- [ ] Semantic aphasia
- [ ] Crossed aphasia
- [ ] Global aphasia
- [ ] Foreign accent syndrome (FAS)
- [ ] Thalamic aphasia

AKINETIC MUTISM

Pathology

- [ ] This is caused by disconnection of frontal-cingulate-limbic subcortical circuits
- [ ] This disrupts the frontal neuronal systems involved with executive functions
- [ ] It is usually associated with anterior cingulate lesions

Vascular causes: stroke

- [ ] Anterior cerebral artery territory
- [ ] Middle cerebral artery territory
- [ ] Posterior inferior cerebellar artery (PICA) territory
- [ ] Watershed infarction
- [ ] Paramedian thalamic stroke
- [ ] Bilateral substantia nigra stroke

Vascular causes: others

- [ ] Cerebral vein thrombosis (CVT)
- [ ] Subarachnoid haemorrhage (SAH)

Neoplastic causes

- [ ] 4th ventricle choroid plexus papilloma
- [ ] Astrocytoma infiltrating the fornix
- [ ] Pineal teratoma

Traumatic causes

- [ ] Frontal lobe damage
- [ ] Hypothalamic damage

Infective causes

- [ ] Sporadic Creutzfeldt-Jakob disease (CJD)
- [ ] Tuberculous anterior cerebral artery obliterative arteritis

Toxic and drug-induced

- [ ] Delayed post-hypoxic leukoencephalopathy (DPHL)
- [ ] Carbon monoxide poisoning
- [ ] Radiation therapy induced
- [ ] Baclofen
- [ ] Ciclosporin
- [ ] Muronomab
- [ ] Tacrolimus
- [ ] Nicotine withdrawal

Other neurological causes

- [ ] Epilepsy
- [ ] Multiple sclerosis (MS)
- [ ] Obstructive hydrocephalus
- [ ] Wernicke-Korsakoff syndrome

Treatment

- [ ] Bromocriptine
- [ ] Levodopa
- [ ] Olanzapine
- [ ] Magnesium sulphate: case report of benefit with DPHL

Delirium (acute confusional state)

DELIRIUM: RISK FACTORS

Individual risk factors

- ☐ Males
- ☐ Smoking
- ☐ Social isolation

Medical risk factors

- ☐ Dementia
- ☐ Surgery
- ☐ Infection
- ☐ Myocardial infarction (MI)
- ☐ Organ failure
- ☐ Previous delirium
- ☐ Hearing impairment
- ☐ Visual impairment
- ☐ Depression
- ☐ Electrolyte imbalance
- ☐ Dehydration
- ☐ Nutritional/vitamin deficiency
- ☐ Advanced cancer

Drug-induced risk factors

- ☐ Benzodiazepines
- ☐ Narcotics
- ☐ Anticholinergics
- ☐ Digoxin
- ☐ Theophylline
- ☐ Levodopa
- ☐ Steroids

DELIRIUM: CLINICAL FEATURES

Types of delirium

- ☐ Hyperactive
- ☐ Hypoactive
- ☐ Mixed

Cognitive and psychiatric features

- ☐ Fluctuating attention and confusion
- ☐ Clouding of consciousness
- ☐ Impaired memory
- ☐ Disorganised thinking
- ☐ Easily distracted
- ☐ Illusions
- ☐ Hallucinations: usually Lilliputian
- ☐ Emotional disturbance

Neurological features

- ☐ Myoclonus
- ☐ Ataxia
- ☐ Autonomic
- ☐ Excessive sweating
- ☐ Flushing
- ☐ Dilated pupils
- ☐ Disturbed sleep-wake cycle
- ☐ Dysarthria
- ☐ Nystagmus
- ☐ Incoherent speech

DOI: 10.1201/9781003221258-3

DELIRIUM: DIFFERENTIAL DIAGNOSIS

Neurological differentials

- ☐ Dementia
- ☐ Stroke
- ☐ Brain injury
- ☐ Migraine
- ☐ Hashimoto encephalopathy
- ☐ Transient global amnesia (TGA)
- ☐ Wernicke's aphasia
- ☐ Encephalitis
- ☐ Meningitis
- ☐ Non-convulsive status epilepsy (NCSE)

Psychiatric differentials

- ☐ Charles Bonnet syndrome (CBS)
- ☐ Depression

Medical differentials

- ☐ Acute porphyria
- ☐ Hyperviscosity syndrome

Toxic differentials

- ☐ Delirium tremens
- ☐ Neuroleptic malignant syndrome (NMS)
- ☐ Serotonin syndrome
- ☐ Drug withdrawal

DELIRIUM: MANAGEMENT

Non-drug treatments

- ☐ Reorientation
- ☐ Relaxation, e.g. massage
- ☐ Nursing in a quiet, low-lit room

Drug treatments

- ☐ Haloperidol
- ☐ Quetiapine
- ☐ Benzodiazepines

Outcome

- ☐ C-reactive protein (CRP) predicts delirium and recovery

Dementia presentations

REVERSIBLE DEMENTIA

Neurological causes

- ☐ Cerebral vasculitis
- ☐ Delirium
- ☐ Autoimmune encephalitis
- ☐ Epilepsy
- ☐ Hashimoto's encephalopathy
- ☐ Marchiafava-Bignami disease
- ☐ Normal pressure hydrocephalus (NPH)
- ☐ Pituitary insufficiency
- ☐ Post-traumatic syndromes
- ☐ Space occupying lesions (SOL)
- ☐ Subdural hematoma (SDH)

Infectious causes

- ☐ Neurosyphilis
- ☐ Meningitis
- ☐ Tuberculous meningitis
- ☐ Fungal meningitis
- ☐ Whipple's disease
- ☐ Lyme neuroborreliosis
- ☐ Intracranial empyema or abscess
- ☐ Racemose neurocysticercosis
- ☐ HIV infection
- ☐ Herpes simplex virus (HSV) encephalitis

Metabolic causes

- ☐ Alcohol abuse
- ☐ Hypo and hyperthyroidism
- ☐ Hypo and hyperparathyroidism
- ☐ Addison's disease
- ☐ Cushing's disease
- ☐ Hypoglycaemia
- ☐ Vitamin deficiencies: B1, B6, B12, and folate
- ☐ Organ failure
- ☐ Wilson's disease

Other causes

- ☐ Depression
- ☐ Drugs and toxins
- ☐ Obstructive sleep apnoea (OSA)
- ☐ Sarcoidosis
- ☐ Systemic infections
- ☐ Phaeochromocytoma

RAPIDLY PROGRESSIVE DEMENTIA

Infective causes

- ☐ Prion diseases
- ☐ Whipple's disease
- ☐ Tuberculosis
- ☐ Fungi, e.g. cryptococcus
- ☐ Bacteria
- ☐ Viruses

Neurodegenerative causes

- ☐ Corticobasal degeneration (CBD)
- ☐ Frontotemporal dementia (FTD)
- ☐ Dementia with Lewy bodies (DLB)
- ☐ Alzheimer's disease (AD)
- ☐ Progressive supranuclear palsy (PSP)
- ☐ Neuronal intranuclear inclusion disease (NIID)

Autoimmune and inflammatory causes

- ☐ Autoimmune limbic encephalitis
- ☐ Hashimoto encephalopathy
- ☐ Multiple sclerosis (MS)
- ☐ Neurosarcoidosis

Metabolic and toxic causes

- ☐ Methylmalonic academia
- ☐ Alcohol
- ☐ Methotrexate toxicity

Neoplastic causes

- ☐ Primary CNS lymphoma (PCNSL)
- ☐ Paraneoplastic
- ☐ Metastases (case report)
- ☐ Lymphomatosis cerebri
- ☐ Primary CNS lymphoma

Other causes

- ☐ Vascular
- ☐ Psychiatric
- ☐ Idiopathic: this accounts for 12% of cases

DOI: 10.1201/9781003221258-4

YOUNG-ONSET DEMENTIA: CAUSES

Neurodegenerative

- [ ] Alzheimer's disease (AD)
- [ ] Frontotemporal dementia (FTD)
- [ ] Dementia with Lewy bodies (DLB)
- [ ] Huntington's disease (HD)
- [ ] Pantethonate kinase associated neurodegeneration (PKAN)
- [ ] Neuroacanthocytosis
- [ ] Spinocerebellar ataxia (SCA)

Infective

- [ ] Creutzfeldt Jakob disease (CJD)
- [ ] HIV

Neuroinflammatory

- [ ] Multiple sclerosis (MS)
- [ ] Progressive multifocal leukoencephalopathy (PML)
- [ ] Neuropsychiatric lupus
- [ ] Autoimmune encephalitis

Metabolic

- [ ] Metabolic
- [ ] Mitochondrial diseases
- [ ] Storage diseases
- [ ] Niemann–Pick C (NPC)
- [ ] Wilson's disease

Vascular

- [ ] Vasculitis
- [ ] CADASIL
- [ ] Moyamoya disease
- [ ] Multi infarct dementia
- [ ] Amyloid

Toxic

- [ ] Manganese
- [ ] Alcohol

Other causes

- [ ] Normal pressure hydrocephalus (NPH)
- [ ] Brain tumours
- [ ] Hepatic failure

SUBACUTE ENCEPHALOPATHY: CAUSES

Neurodegenerative

- [ ] Dementia with Lewy Bodies (DLB)
- [ ] Alzheimer's disease (AD)

Infectious

- [ ] Creutzfeldt Jakob disease (CJD)
- [ ] Lyme neuroborreliosis
- [ ] HIV

Neuroinflammatory and autoimmune

- [ ] Multiple sclerosis (MS)
- [ ] Progressive multifocal leukoencephalopathy (PML)
- [ ] Sarcoidosis
- [ ] Systemic lupus erythematosus (SLE)
- [ ] Sjögren's syndrome
- [ ] Behcet's disease
- [ ] Autoimmune encephalopathy
- [ ] Vasculitis

Metabolic

- [ ] Hashimoto encephalopathy
- [ ] Vitamin B1 deficiency
- [ ] Vitamin B12 deficiency
- [ ] Uraemic encephalopathy
- [ ] Hepatic encephalopathy
- [ ] Hypo/hyperthyroidism
- [ ] Hypoglycaemia
- [ ] Hyponatraemia
- [ ] Hypercalcaemia

Malignancy-related

- [ ] Malignancies
- [ ] Malignant meningitis
- [ ] Paraneoplastic

Toxic and drug-induced

- [ ] Chemotherapy, e.g. Methotrexate
- [ ] Lithium toxicity
- [ ] Chronic carbon monoxide (CO) poisoning
- [ ] Alcohol
- [ ] Wernicke-Korsakoff syndrome
- [ ] Hydrogen sulphide exposure
- [ ] Pregabalin
- [ ] Levetiracetam

Other causes

- [ ] Radiation
- [ ] Systemic infections
- [ ] Cerebral vein thrombosis (CVT)
- [ ] Mitochondrial diseases
- [ ] Schizophrenia
- [ ] Severe depression
- [ ] Subacute encephalopathy and seizures in alcoholics (SESA)

Alzheimer's disease (AD)

ALZHEIMER'S DISEASE (AD): RISK FACTORS

Non-modifiable risk factors

- [ ] Age
- [ ] Fewer years of education
- [ ] Apolipoprotein E epsilon4 allele
- [ ] GGA3 gene deletion or variants

Lifestyle risk factors

- [ ] Smoking
- [ ] Inactivity
- [ ] Possibly dietary sugar and sweeteners

Medical risk factors

- [ ] Obesity
- [ ] Diabetes mellitus
- [ ] Hypertension
- [ ] Vitamin D deficiency
- [ ] Depression
- [ ] Hyperhomocysteine
- [ ] Rosacea
- [ ] Proton pump inhibitors (PPIs)
- [ ] Possibly polycystic kidney disease (APCKD)
- [ ] Retinal nerve fiber degeneration
- [ ] Hormone replacement therapy
- [ ] Anaemia
- [ ] Raised haemoglobin level
- [ ] Insomnia
- [ ] Cerebral microbleeds

Proposed microbial risk factors

- [ ] Escherichia Coli K99
- [ ] Fungal infections: several fungal species
- [ ] Cytomegalovirus
- [ ] Helicobacter pylori
- [ ] Herpes simplex virus type 1 (HSV1)
- [ ] Bordetalla pertussis
- [ ] Periodontitis
- [ ] Treponema pallidum
- [ ] Chlamydia pneumoniae
- [ ] Lyme neuroborreliosis

Risk factors for accelerated cognitive decline

- [ ] Increased cortical iron

Unlikely risk factors

- [ ] Traumatic brain injury (TBI)

ALZHEIMER'S DISEASE (AD): CLINICAL FEATURES

Pre-clinical features

- [ ] Difficulty learning new routes
- [ ] Forgetting where items were placed
- [ ] Forgetting new names or faces
- [ ] Language and visuospatial difficulties
- [ ] Temporal and parietal cortical thinning

Cognitive features

- [ ] Impaired naming
- [ ] Impaired praxis
- [ ] Impaired calculation
- [ ] Visuospatial dysfunction: with right parietal pathology
- [ ] Fine hand myoclonus: in familial AD

Non-cognitive features

- [ ] Seizures
- [ ] Aggression
- [ ] Delusions
- [ ] Hallucinations
- [ ] Depression
- [ ] Apathy
- [ ] Euphoria
- [ ] Anxiety
- [ ] Purposeless activities

Features of young onset AD

- [ ] More rapid brain volume loss
- [ ] Worse and more frequent electroencephalogram (EEG) changes
- [ ] More frequent non-amnestic onset
- [ ] More involvement of posterior cortical association area
- [ ] Less medial temporal involvement

DOI: 10.1201/9781003221258-5

ALZHEIMER'S DISEASE (AD): PREVENTATIVE MEASURES

Measures with very strong evidence

- ☐ Education
- ☐ Cognitive activity
- ☐ Reduction of high body mass index in late life
- ☐ Treatment of hyperhomocysteinaemia: with folic acid, vitamin B12 and vitamin B6
- ☐ Treatment of depression
- ☐ Stress reduction
- ☐ Treatment of diabetes
- ☐ Prevention of head trauma
- ☐ Controlling mid-life hypertension
- ☐ Treatment of orthostatic hypotension

Measures with weaker evidence

- ☐ Physical activity
- ☐ Treatment of mid-life obesity
- ☐ Smoking cessation
- ☐ Healthy sleeping
- ☐ Controlling cerebrovascular disease
- ☐ Improving frailty
- ☐ Controlling atrial fibrillation
- ☐ Vitamin C supplementation

Measures of uncertain benefit

- ☐ Controlling diastolic blood pressure
- ☐ Use of non-steroidal anti-inflammatory drugs (NSAIDs)
- ☐ Better social activity
- ☐ Treatment of osteoporosis
- ☐ Preventing pesticide exposure
- ☐ Preventing exposure to silicon in drinking water
- ☐ Mediterranean diet
- ☐ Neurostimulation

Measures not recommended

- ☐ Oestrogen replacement therapy: this increases the risk of dementia
- ☐ Acetylcholinesterase inhibitors

ALZHEIMER'S DISEASE (AD): NON-DRUG TREATMENTS

Give written information on clinical and social issues

- ☐ Signs and symptoms of the disease
- ☐ Course and prognosis of the disease
- ☐ Available local care and support services
- ☐ Available support groups
- ☐ Sources of financial and legal advice
- ☐ Sources for advocacy
- ☐ Medicolegal issues including driving

Discuss advanced directives

- ☐ Assess capacity for decision making
- ☐ Establish personal directives
- ☐ Discuss will
- ☐ Arrange lasting power of attorney
- ☐ Establish preferred place of care plan

Assess functional impairments

- ☐ Ability to maintain hobbies
- ☐ Ability to handle complex financial affairs
- ☐ Ability to use new equipment and tools

Non-drug interventions

- ☐ Cognitive stimulation
- ☐ Reality orientation therapy (ROT): to improve disorientation
- ☐ Recreational activities: to enhance well-being

ALZHEIMER'S DISEASE (AD): DRUG TREATMENTS

Acetylcholinesterase inhibitors (ACheI): indications

- ☐ This is indicated for mild to moderate AD
- ☐ It is also indicated for AD-associated symptoms

Acetylcholinesterase inhibitors (ACheI): types

- ☐ Donepezil 5 mg nocte: consider increasing to 10mg
- ☐ Galantamine 8mg daily
  - ○ Double the dose in 4 weeks
  - ○ Maintenance dose 16–24 mg daily
- ☐ Rivastigmine 1.5 mg bid: maximum 6mg bid

Memantine

- ☐ This is indicated for severe AD
- ☐ It is also indicated for moderate AD if intolerant of ACheI
- ☐ The dose is 5mg daily: maximum is 20mg daily
- ☐ It may be combined with ACheI

Other drug treatments

- ☐ Antidepressants
- ☐ Conventional antipsychotics with caution

Investigational drug treatments

- ☐ Masitinib
- ☐ Aducanumab
- ☐ Crenezumab
- ☐ Active AD (AADvac1) vaccine: this is against the tau protein
- ☐ Intranasal insulin

Frontotemporal dementia (FTD)

BEHAVIOURAL VARIANT FRONTOTEMPORAL DEMENTIA (BVFTLD): CLINICAL FEATURES

Features of disinhibition

- ☐ Inappropriate or offensive speech
- ☐ Public urination and masturbation
- ☐ Restlessness, impulsivity, and irritability
- ☐ Pressured speech
- ☐ Aggressiveness
- ☐ Violent outbursts
- ☐ Excessive sentimentality
- ☐ Theft and assault

Other behavioural abnormalities

- ☐ Alerted food preference/gluttony
- ☐ Change in beliefs
- ☐ Change in personality
- ☐ Hyperorality
- ☐ Wandering/pacing
- ☐ Loss of personal hygiene
- ☐ Diogenes syndrome: self-neglect and hoarding behaviour

Motor stereotypy and repetitive activities

- ☐ Rubbing
- ☐ Picking
- ☐ Pacing
- ☐ Cleaning
- ☐ Organising objects into groups
- ☐ Counting

Features associated with C9orf72 gene mutation

- ☐ Familial motor neurone disease (MND): onset is usually within 12 months of FTD diagnosis
- ☐ Familial left-hand dystonia
- ☐ Bullous pemphigoid

Neuropsychiatric features

- ☐ Lack of empathy or concern
- ☐ Emotional blunting/apathy
- ☐ Delusions: somatic, religious, and bizarre forms
- ☐ Executive dysfunction
- ☐ Poor insight
- ☐ Decreased concern about family and friends
- ☐ Impaired theory of mind
- ☐ High suicide risk

Other features

- ☐ Reduced pain response
- ☐ Self-centeredness
- ☐ Olfactory dysfunction
- ☐ Low cancer prevalence
- ☐ Food aversion: case report

Poor prognostic factors

- ☐ Neurofilament light chain (NfL): in serum and cerebrospinal fluid (CSF)

PRIMARY PROGRESSIVE APHASIA (PPA): NON-FLUENT VARIANT (NFVPPA)

Diagnostic criteria

- ☐ Language impairment
- ☐ Cognitive features
- ☐ Behavioural and psychiatric features
- ☐ Motor disturbances

Language features: relevance

- ☐ These are the most prominent features
- ☐ They are usually the only abnormalities in the first two years
- ☐ They are the main causes of impaired daily activity

Language features: manifestations

- ☐ Difficulty initiating speech
- ☐ Agrammatism
- ☐ Effortful and halting speech
- ☐ Short phrases
- ☐ Slow speech (speech apraxia)
- ☐ Impairment of naming and syntax
- ☐ Poor comprehension
- ☐ Impaired hearing
- ☐ Daily activities are normal except when on the telephone

Cognitive features

- ☐ Memory impairment
- ☐ Visuospatial difficulties
- ☐ Dyscalculia
- ☐ Disinhibition
- ☐ Constructional deficits

Behavioural and psychiatric features

- ☐ Apathy
- ☐ Depression
- ☐ Altered food preferences
- ☐ Irritability
- ☐ Stereotypic behaviour
- ☐ Disinhibition
- ☐ Reduced social awareness

Motor impairment

- ☐ Mild limb and buccofacial apraxia
- ☐ Difficulty with fine finger movements

Progression to other syndromes

- ☐ Corticobasal degeneration (CBD)
- ☐ Progressive supranuclear palsy (PSP)

Synonym

- ☐ Agrammatic variant

DOI: 10.1201/9781003221258-6

PRIMARY PROGRESSIVE APHASIA (PPA): LOGOPENIC VARIANT (LVPPA)

Pathological sites

- ☐ Left posterior superior temporal gyri
- ☐ Left middle temporal gyri
- ☐ Left inferior parietal lobule

Genetic mutations

- ☐ Progranulin (GRN)
- ☐ Microtubule-associated protein tau (MAPT)

Clinical features

- ☐ Reduced verbal output
- ☐ Low speech rate
- ☐ Word finding difficulty
- ☐ Word retrieval deficits
- ☐ Frequent pauses
- ☐ Impaired repetition
- ☐ Speech errors
- ☐ Impaired comprehension
- ☐ Impaired reading: phonological alexia
- ☐ Irritability
- ☐ Anxiety and depression
- ☐ Rapid progression to dementia

Relatively spared speech functions

- ☐ Grammar
- ☐ Single-word comprehension
- ☐ Nonverbal semantic association

Diagnostic criteria: core features

- ☐ Impaired single-word retrieval in spontaneous speech
- ☐ Impaired repetition of sentences and phrases

Diagnostic criteria: supportive features

- ☐ Phonological speech errors
- ☐ Spared single-word comprehension and object knowledge
- ☐ Preserved motor speech
- ☐ Absent agrammatic speech

Differentiating features from other PPA variants

- ☐ There are no speech-sound distortions
- ☐ There are no frank syntactic errors
- ☐ Calculation is worse affected
- ☐ The speech rate is faster than in non-fluent variant PPA
- ☐ The speech rate is slower than in semantic variant PPA

Other differentials

- ☐ Early onset Alzheimer's disease (AD)

Synonyms

- ☐ Logopenic progressive aphasia (LPA)
- ☐ Phonological variant

Amnestic syndromes

ACUTE AMNESTIC SYNDROMES

Transient amnestic syndromes

- [ ] Transient global amnesia (TGA)
- [ ] Transient epileptic amnesia (TEA)
- [ ] Transient topographical amnesia (TTA)
- [ ] Focal retrograde amnesia
- [ ] Transient semantic amnesia
- [ ] Transient autobiographical amnesia
- [ ] Transient procedural amnesia
- [ ] Transient verbal amnesia

Vascular acute amnestic syndromes

- [ ] Transient ischaemic amnesia
- [ ] Bilateral fornix stroke: subcallosal artery
  - This manifests as goblet or watch-out sign on MRI
- [ ] Bilateral hippocampal stroke
- [ ] Paramedian thalamic stroke: artery of Percheron
- [ ] Genu of internal capsule stroke
- [ ] Cerebral vein thrombosis (CVT)

Other acute amnestic syndromes

- [ ] Psychogenic amnesia
- [ ] Traumatic brain injuries (TBI): post-traumatic amnesia (PTA)
- [ ] Multiple sclerosis (MS)
- [ ] Autoimmune encephalitis
- [ ] Acute toxic metabolic disorders
- [ ] Influenza virus infection
- [ ] Opioids: especially fentanyl
- [ ] MDMA (ecstasy)
- [ ] Lorazepam

SUBACUTE AND CHRONIC AMNESTIC SYNDROMES

Neurological causes

- [ ] Korsakoff's psychosis
- [ ] Alzheimer's disease (AD)
- [ ] Spontaneous intracranial hypotension (SIH)
- [ ] Benign senescent forgetfulness
- [ ] Depression (pseudo-dementia)
- [ ] Fugue state
- [ ] Frontotemporal dementia (FTD)
- [ ] Herpes simplex virus (HSV) encephalitis
- [ ] Space occupying lesions
- [ ] Obstructive hydrocephalus

Systemic syndromes

- [ ] Alcohol excess
- [ ] Hashimoto's encephalopathy
- [ ] Cardiopulmonary arrest
- [ ] Acute respiratory failure
- [ ] Anaesthetic accidents
- [ ] Carbon monoxide poisoning
- [ ] Drowning
- [ ] Strangulation

DOI: 10.1201/9781003221258-7

TRANSIENT GLOBAL AMNESIA (TGA): RISK FACTORS AND TRIGGERS

Risk factors

- ☐ Middle or old age
- ☐ Migraine
- ☐ Cerebral vein thrombosis (CVT)
- ☐ Internal jugular vein incompetence
- ☐ Positive family history
- ☐ Stress liability personality

Triggers: medical procedures

- ☐ Cerebral angiography
- ☐ Coronary angiography
- ☐ General anaesthesia
- ☐ Spinal anaesthesia
- ☐ Gastroscopy
- ☐ Trans-oesophageal echocardiogram (TOE)
- ☐ Dobutamine stress echocardiogram
- ☐ Cardiac catheterisation
- ☐ Cardiac ablation therapy
- ☐ Photodynamic therapy
- ☐ Exercise testing on cycle ergometer
- ☐ Intracarotid amobarbital procedure
- ☐ DMSO-cryopreserved autologous peripheral blood stem cells transfusion

Triggers: others

- ☐ Stressful emotional events
- ☐ Stressful physical events
- ☐ Water contact
- ☐ Exhaustion
- ☐ Cold
- ☐ Orgasm: this may present as recurrent coital amnesia
- ☐ CNS lymphoma: case report

TRANSIENT GLOBAL AMNESIA (TGA): CLINICAL FEATURES

Clinical features

- ☐ This is characterised by an episode of abrupt onset amnesia
- ☐ The duration is usually 1–24 hours but 3% of cases last <1 hour
- ☐ The onset is usually in the morning but not on awakening
- ☐ Amnesia is anterograde and retrograde
- ☐ The period of retrograde amnesia shrinks with recovery
- ☐ There is a permanent amnesia for the event
- ☐ Repetitive questioning is a typical feature
- ☐ There is disorientation in time and place
- ☐ Personal identity is retained
- ☐ Family knowledge is retained
- ☐ Migraine may be comorbid
- ☐ TGA is recurrent in 6–30% of cases

Associated features

- ☐ Headache
- ☐ Nausea
- ☐ Vomiting
- ☐ Myocardial injury: this manifests with increased cardiac troponin level

Exclusion criteria for TGA

- ☐ Clouding of consciousness
- ☐ Loss of personal identity
- ☐ Other neurological deficits
- ☐ Focal neurological signs during or after the event
- ☐ Lack of resolution within 24 hours

Possible predictors of recurrent TGA

- ☐ Migraine
- ☐ Reversible MRI DWI abnormalities
- ☐ Familial cases

Magnetic resonance imaging (MRI) features

- ☐ MRI or diffusion weighted imaging (DWI) may show ischaemic lesions
- ☐ These are in the temporal lobes/hippocampus
- ☐ DWI lesions are most evident within 12–24 hours of onset
- ☐ The lesions may be visible up to 6 days after onset
- ☐ The MRI is however usually normal

TRANSIENT GLOBAL AMNESIA (TGA): DIFFERENTIAL DIAGNOSIS

Neurological

- ☐ Concussion
- ☐ Seizures
- ☐ Transient ischaemic attacks (TIAs)
- ☐ Migraine
- ☐ Head injury
- ☐ Pituitary tumours
- ☐ Brain tumours

Drugs

- ☐ Benzodiazepines
- ☐ Zolpidem
- ☐ Alcoholic blackouts

Psychiatric

- ☐ Hysterical fugue
- ☐ Electroconvulsive therapy (ECT)

Encephalopathy

WERNICKE'S ENCEPHALOPATHY: CLINICAL FEATURES

Nutritional risk factors

- ☐ Alcoholism: alcohol intake >20 units a day
- ☐ Gastrointestinal disease and surgery
- ☐ Hyperemesis gravidarum
- ☐ Fasting
- ☐ Starvation
- ☐ Malnutrition
- ☐ Poorly balanced diet
- ☐ Bariatric surgery
- ☐ Parenteral nutrition
- ☐ Diarrhoea and vomiting

Medical risk factors

- ☐ Infections
- ☐ Malignancy
- ☐ AIDS

Metabolic risk factors

- ☐ Renal disease
- ☐ Dialysis
- ☐ Hypoxic encephalopathy
- ☐ Thyroid disease
- ☐ Stem cell transplantation
- ☐ Bone marrow transplantation

Neurological risk factors

- ☐ Third ventricle tumours
- ☐ Herpes simplex (HSV) encephalitis
- ☐ Delirium tremens
- ☐ Peripheral neuropathy (PN)

Other risk factors

- ☐ Psychiatric diseases
- ☐ Iatrogenic
- ☐ Intravenous (IV) glucose

Clinical features

- ☐ Confusion
- ☐ Confabulation
- ☐ Ophthalmoparesis
- ☐ Nystagmus: vertical and horizontal
- ☐ Bilateral lateral rectus weakness
- ☐ Conjugate gaze paralysis
- ☐ Retrograde and anterograde amnesia
- ☐ Recent memory is worse affected (Ribot's law)
- ☐ Cerebellar ataxia
- ☐ Peripheral neuropathy (PN)
- ☐ Postural hypotension
- ☐ Impaired olfaction
- ☐ Dietary deficiency

WERNICKE'S ENCEPHALOPATHY: MRI FEATURES

Typical location of lesions

- ☐ Medial thalami
- ☐ Periventricular region
- ☐ Periaqueductal area
- ☐ Mamillary bodies
- ☐ Tectal plate

Unusual location of lesions in non-alcoholics

- ☐ Cerebellum
- ☐ Cranial nerve nuclei
- ☐ Caudate nuclei
- ☐ Splenium of corpus callosum
- ☐ Red nuclei
- ☐ Dentate nuclei
- ☐ Cerebral cortex

Diffusion weighted imaging (DWI) changes: locations

- ☐ Mammillary bodies
- ☐ Periaqueductal gray matter
- ☐ Hypothalamus
- ☐ Dorsal medial thalamus

Other MRI features

- ☐ Contrast enhancement of thalamus and mamillary bodies
- ☐ Cortical laminar necrosis and haemorrhage: on susceptibility weighted MRI

DOI: 10.1201/9781003221258-8

KORSAKOFF SYNDROME

Risk factors

- [ ] Thiamine deficiency
- [ ] Chronic alcohol misuse
- [ ] Possible genetic predisposition
- [ ] Non-alcoholic cases of thiamine deficiency
- [ ] Carbon monoxide (CO) poisoning
- [ ] Lead poisoning
- [ ] Arsenic poisoning
- [ ] Diabetes mellitus
- [ ] Infections

Clinical features

- [ ] Impaired memory and learning
  - ○ Implicit memory is preserved
- [ ] Alert and responsive
- [ ] Repeatedly asking the same questions
- [ ] Reading the same page for hours
- [ ] Inability to recognize recently met people
- [ ] It is often not preceded by Wernicke encephalopathy

Magnetic resonance imaging (MRI) lesions: locations

- [ ] Mammillary bodies
- [ ] Mammillothalamic tract
- [ ] Anterior thalamus

POSTERIOR REVERSIBLE ENCEPHALOPATHY SYNDROME (PRES): CLINICAL FEATURES

Typical PRES triad

- [ ] Seizures
- [ ] Visual disturbance
- [ ] Headache

Neurological features

- [ ] Headache
- [ ] Encephalopathy
- [ ] Seizures: including status epilepticus
- [ ] Myelopathy

Visual features

- [ ] Visual loss
- [ ] Hemianopia
- [ ] Visual neglect
- [ ] Visual hallucinations
- [ ] Cortical blindness

Blood pressure in PRES

- [ ] Blood pressure is usually normal
- [ ] It is mildly increased in 30% of cases: this is possibly reactive

Recurrent PRES

- [ ] PRES recurs in 4–14% of cases
- [ ] This is probably associated with primary hypertension

Possible PRES variants

- [ ] Generalised reversible encephalopathy syndrome
- [ ] Reversible hypertensive encephalomyelopathy
- [ ] Spinal variant
- [ ] Brainstem and cerebellar variant

Poor prognostic features

- [ ] Encephalitis
- [ ] Altered mental state
- [ ] Subarachnoid haemorrhage (SAH)
- [ ] Raised C-reactive protein (CRP)
- [ ] Impaired coagulation

POSTERIOR REVERSIBLE ENCEPHALOPATHY SYNDROME (PRES): RISK FACTORS

Vascular disorders

- ☐ Hypertension
- ☐ Pre-eclampsia
- ☐ Eclampsia

Autoimmune disorders

- ☐ Systemic lupus erythematosus (SLE)
- ☐ Systemic sclerosis (SS)
- ☐ Wegener's granulomatosis
- ☐ Polyarteritis nodosa (PAN)

Medical disorders

- ☐ Tertiary hyperparathyroidism
- ☐ Hypomagnesaemia
- ☐ Hypercalcaemia
- ☐ Malignancies
- ☐ Sepsis
- ☐ Tumour lysis syndrome
- ☐ Hypocholesterolaemia
- ☐ HIV infection
- ☐ Ephedra overdose
- ☐ Guillain–Barre syndrome (GBS)

Immunosuppressant therapy

- ☐ Ciclosporin
- ☐ Tacrolimus
- ☐ Cytarabine
- ☐ Cisplatin
- ☐ Gemcitabine
- ☐ Tiazofurin
- ☐ Bevacizumab

Other medical interventions

- ☐ Blood transfusion
- ☐ Red blood cell transfusion
- ☐ Erythropoietin
- ☐ Intravenous immunoglobulins (IVIg)
- ☐ Dialysis
- ☐ Dimethylsulphoxide stem cells
- ☐ Triple H therapy

POSTERIOR REVERSIBLE ENCEPHALOPATHY SYNDROME (PRES): DIFFERENTIALS

Encephalitic

- ☐ Infectious
- ☐ Paraneoplastic
- ☐ Autoimmune

Vascular

- ☐ Reversible cerebral vasoconstriction syndrome (RCVS)
- ☐ Primary angiitis of the central nervous system (PACNS)
- ☐ Posterior circulation stroke
- ☐ Subcortical leukoaraiosis

Demyelinating

- ☐ Progressive multifocal leukoencephalopathy (PML)
- ☐ Osmotic demyelination disorders (ODD)
- ☐ Acute disseminated encephalomyelitis (ADEM)

Other differentials

- ☐ Toxic leukoencephalopathy
- ☐ Brain tumours
- ☐ Status epilepticus

POSTERIOR REVERSIBLE ENCEPHALOPATHY SYNDROME (PRES): MANAGEMENT

Magnetic resonance imaging (MRI): FLAIR hyperintensities

- ☐ There are FLAIR hyperintensities in almost all cases
- ☐ These are mainly parieto-occipital in location
- ☐ Other brain areas and the cortex may also be affected

Magnetic resonance imaging (MRI): haemorrhage types

- ☐ Parenchymal hematoma
- ☐ Small haemorrhages
- ☐ Subarachnoid haemorrhage (SAH)

Magnetic resonance imaging (MRI): other features

- ☐ Symmetric vasogenic oedema
- ☐ Hydrocephalus
- ☐ Focal areas of restricted diffusion

Cerebrospinal fluid (CSF) features

- ☐ Albumino-cytologic dissociation
- ☐ Raised protein with very little increase in cell count

Treatment

- ☐ Stop provoking drugs
- ☐ Treat underlying disorders
- ☐ Treat hypertension: reduce blood pressure by 25% in the first few hours

OSMOTIC DEMYELINATION DISORDERS (ODD): CAUSES

Metabolic causes

- ☐ Rapid correction of hyponatraemia: but it may also occur with slow correction
- ☐ Hyponatremia
- ☐ Hypophosphatemia

Drug-withdrawal

- ☐ Desmopressin
- ☐ Carbamazepine
- ☐ Thiazide diuretics
- ☐ Selective serotonin reuptake inhibitors (SSRIs)

Gastrointestinal causes

- ☐ Liver transplantation
- ☐ Liver failure
- ☐ Acute haemorrhagic pancreatitis

Nutritional causes

- ☐ Malnutrition
- ☐ Dehydration
- ☐ Water intoxication
- ☐ Acute hypoglycaemia
- ☐ Eating disorders

Other causes

- ☐ Alcoholism
- ☐ Peritoneal dialysis
- ☐ Malignancies
- ☐ Heat stroke
- ☐ HIV infection

OSMOTIC DEMYELINATION DISORDERS (ODD): CLINICAL FEATURES

Types of ODD

- ☐ Central pontine myelinolysis (CPM): in central basis pontis
- ☐ Extrapontine myelinolysis: in the thalamus, basal ganglia, cerebellum, and spinal cord

Neurological features

- ☐ Lethargy
- ☐ Impaired consciousness
- ☐ Pseudobulbar palsy
- ☐ Dysarthria
- ☐ Dysphagia
- ☐ Flaccid quadriparesis
- ☐ Locked-in syndrome
- ☐ Cranial nerve palsies
- ☐ Cognitive dysfunction: subcortical/frontal
- ☐ Headache
- ☐ Seizures
- ☐ Man-in-the-barrel syndrome
- ☐ Bilateral vocal fold immobility (BVFI)

Movement disorders

- ☐ Cerebellar ataxia: especially with alcoholism
- ☐ Myoclonus
- ☐ Tremor
- ☐ Corticobasal syndrome (CBS)
- ☐ Parkinsonism
- ☐ Multiple system atrophy (MSA)

Psychiatric features

- ☐ Catatonia
- ☐ Mania

OSMOTIC DEMYELINATION DISORDERS (ODD): MANAGEMENT

Magnetic resonance imaging (MRI) brain

- ☐ This demonstrates the Omega (trident) sign
- ☐ This is a symmetrical central area of triangular pontine demyelination
- ☐ It is hyperintense on T2 and hypointense on T1 sequences
- ☐ The outer pontine rim is normal

Treatment of hyponatraemia

- ☐ Correct hyponatraemia slowly
- ☐ This is usually done at a rate of <6–8 mmol/L per 24-hour period
- ☐ A slower rate of 4–6 mmol/L in 24 hours is indicated in high risk individuals

Potentially beneficial treatments

- ☐ Thiamine and multivitamins: in at-risk subjects (alcoholism and malnutrition)
- ☐ Steroids
- ☐ Intravenous immunoglobulin (IVIg)
- ☐ Thyrotropin releasing hormone (TRH)
- ☐ Plasma exchange (PE)

Transient loss of consciousness (TLOC)

TRANSIENT LOSS OF CONSCIOUSNESS (TLOC): CAUSES

Cardiac causes

- ☐ Hypertrophic cardiomyopathy
- ☐ Arrhythmogenic right ventricular dysplasia
- ☐ Severe ischemic left ventricular dysfunction
- ☐ Congenital heart defect
- ☐ Left atrial myxoma
- ☐ Pulmonary embolism
- ☐ Cardiac arrhythmias

Reflex causes

- ☐ Vasovagal
- ☐ Carotid sinus hypersensitivity
- ☐ Situational, e.g. cough and micturition

Other causes

- ☐ Traumatic brain injury (TBI)
- ☐ Orthostatic hypotension
- ☐ Postural tachycardia syndrome (POTS)
- ☐ Psychogenic

Causes of nocturnal TLOC

- ☐ Epilepsy
- ☐ Sleep disorders
- ☐ Hyperventilation attacks
- ☐ Hypoglycaemia
- ☐ Vasovagal syncope
- ☐ Cardiac arrhythmias

TRANSIENT LOSS OF CONSCIOUSNESS (TLOC): CLINICAL FEATURES

Features suggestive of syncope

- ☐ Upright posture
- ☐ Prodrome of nausea or sweating: these are very unlikely in seizures
- ☐ Occurrence in syncope-provoking circumstances
- ☐ Pale appearance
- ☐ Brief duration

Features suggestive of seizures

- ☐ Age <45 years
- ☐ Prodromal deja vu/jamais vu
- ☐ Head turning to one side
- ☐ Frothing at the mouth
- ☐ Facial cyanosis: this is also seen with cardiac syncope
- ☐ Long duration of unconsciousness
- ☐ Hemi-weakness on recovery
- ☐ Lateral tongue biting
- ☐ Amnesia for event
- ☐ Unusual posturing
- ☐ Prolonged limb jerking
- ☐ Postictal disorientation or confusion: this is the best predictor of seizures

Features suggestive of cardiac TLOC

- ☐ Age >65 years
- ☐ Family history of sudden cardiac death under the age of 40 years
- ☐ Family history of inherited cardiac conditions
- ☐ Exertional TLOC
- ☐ Absence of prodromal symptoms
- ☐ New or unexplained breathlessness
- ☐ Heart failure
- ☐ Heart murmur
- ☐ Abnormal electrocardiogram (ECG)

Non-discriminatory features

- ☐ Injury
- ☐ Incontinence
- ☐ Eyewitness accounts: these are often mistaken

DOI: 10.1201/9781003221258-9

TRANSIENT LOSS OF CONSCIOUSNESS (TLOC): DIFFERENTIALS

Neurological differentials

- ☐ Carotid TIA
- ☐ Vertebrobasilar TIA
- ☐ Coma
- ☐ Intracerebral haemorrhage (ICH)
- ☐ Subarachnoid haemorrhage (SAH)
- ☐ Cataplexy
- ☐ Pseudocoma
- ☐ Falls without loss of consciousness

Medical differentials

- ☐ Hypoglycaemia
- ☐ Hypoxia
- ☐ Hyperventilation with hypocapnia
- ☐ Intoxication

Cardiovascular differentials

- ☐ Cardiac arrest
- ☐ Subclavian steal syndrome

CHAPTER 2

Epilepsy

Seizure risk factors

SEIZURES: MEDICAL RISK FACTORS

Neurological infections

- ☐ Encephalitis
- ☐ Meningitis

Human herpes virus (HHV)

- ☐ HHV predisposes to mesial temporal lobe epilepsy
- ☐ This is most frequent with HHV6B and HHV8
- ☐ HHV6B and HHV7 are associated with febrile status epilepticus (FSE)

Vascular

- ☐ Subdural haematoma (SDH)
- ☐ Brain tumours
- ☐ Ischaemic stroke
- ☐ Intracerebral haemorrhage (ICH)

Neurological disorders

- ☐ Multiple sclerosis (MS)
- ☐ Autoimmune diseases
- ☐ Cerebral dysgenesis

Traumatic

- ☐ Traumatic brain injury (TBI)
- ☐ Perinatal brain injury
- ☐ Intracranial surgery

Autoimmune

- ☐ Systemic lupus erythematosus (SLE)
- ☐ Bullous pemphigoid
- ☐ Coeliac disease

Metabolic

- ☐ Electrolyte abnormalities
- ☐ Inborn errors of metabolism
- ☐ Organ failure
- ☐ Pyridoxine deficiency
- ☐ Hypoglycaemia
- ☐ Fever
- ☐ Anoxic encephalopathy
- ☐ Eclampsia
- ☐ Alcohol use and withdrawal

SEIZURES: DRUG-INDUCED

Antibiotics

- ☐ Cephalosporins
- ☐ Imipenem
- ☐ Ciprofloxacin
- ☐ Isoniazid
- ☐ Probably not Fluoroquinolones

Antidepressants and antipsychotics

- ☐ Citalopram
- ☐ Tricyclics
- ☐ Venlafaxine
- ☐ Bupropion
- ☐ Clozapine

Anti-epileptic drugs (AEDs)

- ☐ Carbamazepine
- ☐ Lamotrigine
- ☐ Tiagabine

Chemotherapy

- ☐ Amsacrine
- ☐ Asparaginase
- ☐ Busulfan
- ☐ Carmustine
- ☐ Cisplatin
- ☐ Cytarabine
- ☐ Cyclosporine
- ☐ Dacarbazine
- ☐ Etoposide
- ☐ 5 fluorouracil (5FU)
- ☐ Fludarabine
- ☐ Gemcitabine
- ☐ Ifosfomide
- ☐ Interferonα
- ☐ Intrathecal chemotherapy
- ☐ Methotrexate
- ☐ Nelarabine
- ☐ Paclitaxel
- ☐ Vincristine

Abuse drugs

- ☐ Amphetamines
- ☐ Cocaine

Other drugs

- ☐ Tramadol
- ☐ Diphenhydramine
- ☐ Mefanemic acid
- ☐ Theophylline
- ☐ Baclofen
- ☐ Eucalyptus oil inhalation
- ☐ Ranolazine

DOI: 10.1201/9781003221258-11

SEIZURES: RISKS FOR RECURRENCE

Recurrence risk after first seizure

- [ ] The risk is <20% at 6 months
- [ ] The risk increases to 40–50% at 2 years
- [ ] Seizure recurrence after 24 hours indicates epilepsy

Subject-related risk factors

- [ ] Age ≥16 years
- [ ] Generalised anxiety
- [ ] Lifetime mood disorder

Seizure-related risk factors

- [ ] Seizures after starting AEDs
- [ ] Generalised tonic-clonic seizure
- [ ] Myoclonic seizure
- [ ] Status seizure
- [ ] Febrile seizure
- [ ] Sleep seizure at onset
- [ ] Number of all seizures at presentation

Pathology-related risk factors

- [ ] Primary neurological disorder
- [ ] Focal symptomatic cause
- [ ] Abnormal electroencephalogram (EEG)

Environmental risk factors

- [ ] Low atmospheric pressure
- [ ] High humidity

Treatment-related risk factors

- [ ] Deferred treatment of first seizure (FIRST and MESS trials)
- [ ] Requirement of >1 antiepileptic drug (AED)

Risk factors for poor seizure control at 5 years

- [ ] High number of seizures
- [ ] Poor treatment history
- [ ] History of neurological insult
- [ ] History of epilepsy in a first-degree relative

Seizures: clinical features

SEIZURES: TYPICAL FEATURES

Seizure prodrome

- ☐ Premonitory symptoms occur in 17–41% of patients
- ☐ They are more likely in older subjects
- ☐ They precede seizures by 6–12 hours

Seizure markers

- ☐ Rapid onset
- ☐ Brief duration
- ☐ Altered complexion
- ☐ Auras
- ☐ Absences
- ☐ Myoclonus
- ☐ Convulsions
- ☐ Open eyes
- ☐ Incontinence
- ☐ Lateral tongue bite
- ☐ Impaired breathing
- ☐ Post ictal confusion
- ☐ Delayed recovery
- ☐ Self-injury

Inter-ictal non-seizure features

- ☐ Aggression
- ☐ Apathy
- ☐ Depression
- ☐ Dysphoria
- ☐ Fatigue
- ☐ Generalised anxiety disorder
- ☐ Insomnia
- ☐ Irritability
- ☐ Obsessive-compulsive symptoms
- ☐ Perceived stress

SEIZURES: DIFFERENTIAL DIAGNOSIS

Transient neurological events

- ☐ Transient ischaemic attack (TIA)
- ☐ Migraine
- ☐ Transient global amnesia (TGA)
- ☐ Non-epileptic myoclonus

Sleep disorders

- ☐ Hypnic jerks
- ☐ Narcolepsy
- ☐ Parasomnias
- ☐ REM sleep behaviour disorder (RBD)
- ☐ Periodic leg movements of sleep (PLMS)

Psychiatric disorders

- ☐ Psychogenic seizures
- ☐ Panic attacks

Medical disorders

- ☐ Hypoglycaemia
- ☐ Syncope

Hyperkinetic disorders

- ☐ Hemifacial spasm
- ☐ Tics
- ☐ Paroxysmal non kinesigenic dyskinesia (PNKD)

Paediatric differential diagnosis

- ☐ Staring spells
- ☐ Shuddering attacks
- ☐ Mannerisms
- ☐ Breath holding spells
- ☐ Reflux
- ☐ Spasmus nutans
- ☐ Hyperekplexia
- ☐ Sandifer syndrome

DOI: 10.1201/9781003221258-12

FEBRILE SEIZURES (FS): CLINICAL FEATURES

Risk factors

- ☐ Dravet syndrome
- ☐ Genetic epilepsy with febrile seizures + (GEFS+)
- ☐ Conjugated pneumococcal vaccine
- ☐ Iron deficiency anaemia
- ☐ Male sex
- ☐ Preterm birth
- ☐ Perinatal brain injury
- ☐ Infections
- ☐ Low magnesium

Diagnostic criteria

- ☐ Generalised seizures
- ☐ Fever ≥100.4°F (38°C)
- ☐ Age between 6 month and 5 years
- ☐ Duration <15 minutes
- ☐ Absence of neurological deficits
- ☐ No associated acute nervous system disease
- ☐ No previous afebrile seizures

Types

- ☐ Simple FS
- ☐ Complex FS: criteria
  - ○ Episodes associated with focal post-ictal features, e.g. Todd's paralysis
  - ○ Prolonged episodes
  - ○ Episodes that recur within 24 hours in the same febrile illness
- ☐ Febrile status epilepticus (FSE): FS associated with hippocampal pathology

Recurrence: epidemiology

- ☐ Recurrence occurs in about a third of cases
- ☐ 75% of these recur within 12 months
- ☐ The age at recurrence is usually <15 months

Recurrence: risk factors

- ☐ Family history of epilepsy or febrile seizures
- ☐ Frequent febrile illnesses
- ☐ Loy body temperature at onset
- ☐ Attendance at a day nursery
- ☐ Abnormal electroencephalogram (EEG): especially pseudo-petit mal discharge (PPMD)

Risk factors for progression to epilepsy

- ☐ Male sex
- ☐ Preterm birth
- ☐ Brain injury at birth
- ☐ Bacterial infections
- ☐ Complex febrile seizures
- ☐ Onset of febrile seizures after the third year of life
- ☐ Family history of epilepsy
- ☐ Multiple episodes of febrile seizures
- ☐ Focal features in the first two episodes of recurrence

TRANSIENT EPILEPTIC AMNESIA (TEA)

Epidemiology

- ☐ This is a syndrome of mesial temporal lobe epilepsy
- ☐ Males account for a half to two-thirds of cases
- ☐ The mean onset age is 57–62 years
- ☐ It is the most salient feature of epilepsy in most cases
- ☐ It is the only feature of epilepsy in a third of cases
- ☐ There are frequent episodes: median of 12 annually
- ☐ It may develop after years of focal retrograde amnesia (FRA)

Amnesia: features

- ☐ The amnestic episodes are recurrent
- ☐ They usually last 30–60 minutes: TGA episodes last 4–12 hours
  - ○ The episodes may however last several hours
- ☐ Amnesia is often on awakening: unlike in TGA
- ☐ There is retrograde and often partial anterograde amnesia
  - ○ Patients may remember not having been able to remember
- ☐ The period of amnesia may cover days to years
- ☐ Repetitive questioning occurs in about a half of cases

Accelerated long term forgetting (ALF)

- ☐ This occurs in about half of cases
- ☐ There is rapid loss of adequately laid memories
- ☐ There is long-term forgetting of verbal material
- ☐ There is no recall after 6 weeks
- ☐ Interictal memory impairment occurs in about 80% of cases

Seizures: types

- ☐ Brief loss of responsiveness
- ☐ Complex partial
- ☐ Tonic-clonic
- ☐ Olfactory hallucinations: these occur in >50% of cases
- ☐ Automatisms

Compulsive versifying

- ☐ This is a form of hypergraphia
- ☐ It develops after treatment with Lamotrigine
- ☐ Subjects read multiple rhyming poems

Other reported features

- ☐ Loss of remote autobiographical memory for up to 40 years
- ☐ Olfactory impairment

POST-ICTAL PSYCHOSIS OF EPILEPSY

Demographic features

- ☐ The incidence is about 6%
- ☐ It is usually in people with chronic epilepsy

Onset and course

- ☐ It usually starts with a cluster of generalised tonic clonic seizures
- ☐ There is a lucid interval of 8–72 hours before onset of psychosis
  - ○ The interval may be up to a week
- ☐ Psychosis lasts a mean duration of 83 hours
- ☐ There is a tendency for psychosis to recur

Psychiatric features

- ☐ Delusions
- ☐ Hallucinations
- ☐ Strong affective features
- ☐ Preserved insight
- ☐ Increased risk of suicide

Neurological features

- ☐ Mild confusion
- ☐ Delirium
- ☐ Clouding of consciousness
- ☐ Amnesia for the event
- ☐ Increased mortality

Electroencephalogram (EEG) features

- ☐ There is usually an extra-temporal seizure focus on EEG
- ☐ There may be bilateral interictal epileptiform discharges

Treatment

- ☐ Optimise anti-epileptic drug (AED) treatment
- ☐ Antipsychotics
- ☐ Benzodiazepines for ictal and post-ictal psychosis
- ☐ Epilepsy surgery

Myoclonus

MYOCLONUS: CLASSIFICATIONS AND DIFFERENTIALS

Physiological myoclonus

- ☐ Hiccups
- ☐ Nocturnal myoclonus (hypnic jerks)
- ☐ Sleep transition myclonus
- ☐ Fear-associated myoclonus

Epileptic myoclonus

- ☐ Juvenile myoclonic epilepsy (JME)
- ☐ Progressive myoclonic epilepsy (PME)

Pathological myoclonus

- ☐ Essential myoclonus
- ☐ Symptomatic myoclonus
- ☐ Psychogenic myoclonus
- ☐ Negative myoclonus
- ☐ Post hypoxic myoclonus (PHM)

Classification by site of origin

- ☐ Cortical
- ☐ Subcortical: segmental (palatal) or non-segmental
- ☐ Spinal: segmental or propriospinal
- ☐ Peripheral: root, plexus, nerve, or anterior horn cell (AHC)

Classification by spread

- ☐ Focal
- ☐ Multifocal
- ☐ Generalised

Classification by posture

- ☐ Rest
- ☐ Postural
- ☐ Action
- ☐ Orthostatic

Differential diagnosis

- ☐ Simple partial motor seizures
- ☐ Tics
- ☐ Chorea
- ☐ Fasciculations
- ☐ Startle syndromes

MYOCLONUS: NEUROLOGICAL CAUSES

Neurodegenerative

- ☐ Lewy body disease (LBD)
- ☐ Parkinson's disease dementia (PDD)
- ☐ Multiple system atrophy (MSA)
- ☐ Progressive supranuclear palsy (PSP)
- ☐ Corticobasal degeneration (CBD)
- ☐ Alzheimer's disease (AD)
- ☐ Young onset Huntington's disease (HD)
- ☐ Dentatorubral pallidolyusian atrophy (DRPLA)

Infectious

- ☐ Creutzfeldt Jakob disease (CJD)
- ☐ Subacute sclerosing pan-encephalitis (SSPE)
- ☐ Whipple's disease
- ☐ AIDS dementia
- ☐ Encephalitis
- ☐ Tetanus

Hereditary

- ☐ Familial progressive poliodystrophy
- ☐ Myoclonus dystonia

Late onset asymmetric myoclonus

- ☐ This is primary progressive myoclonus of aging
- ☐ It is of cortical origin
- ☐ There is no associated dementia or alternative causes
- ☐ It may mimic epilepsia partialis continua (EPC)

Other causes

- ☐ Hypoxic brain injury

DOI: 10.1201/9781003221258-13

MYOCLONUS: DRUG-INDUCED

Antidepressants and antipsychotics

- ☐ Nortriptyline
- ☐ Selective serotonin reuptake inhibitors (SSRIs)
- ☐ Lithium
- ☐ Venlafaxine
- ☐ Typical antipsychotics
- ☐ Atypical antipsychotics, e.g. Clozapine

Anti-epileptic drugs (AEDs)

- ☐ Carbamazepine
- ☐ Clobazam
- ☐ Gabapentin
- ☐ Lamotrigine
- ☐ Phenobarbitone
- ☐ Phenytoin
- ☐ Pregabalin
- ☐ Topiramate
- ☐ Valproate
- ☐ Vigabatrin

Antimicrobials

- ☐ Quinolone antibiotics
- ☐ Cephalosporins
- ☐ Sulphonamides
- ☐ Aminoglycosides
- ☐ Mefloquine
- ☐ Aciclovir

Anti-Parkinsonian drugs

- ☐ Levodopa and dopamine agonists
- ☐ Amantadine
- ☐ COMT inhibitors
- ☐ MAO inhibitors

Chemotherapy

- ☐ Ifosfamide
- ☐ Chlorambucil
- ☐ Prednimustine

Anti-arrhythmics

- ☐ Verapamil
- ☐ Flecainide

Other drugs

- ☐ Benzodiazepines
- ☐ Bismuth salts
- ☐ Contrast agents
- ☐ Hydrocodone
- ☐ Metoclopramide
- ☐ Propofol
- ☐ Salbutamol inhaler
- ☐ Tranexamic acid
- ☐ Vitamin B12

MYOCLONUS: SYSTEMIC CAUSES

Organ failure

- ☐ Uraemic encephalopathy
- ☐ Hepatic encephalopathy
- ☐ Pulmonary failure

Metabolic abnormalities

- ☐ Hyponatraemia
- ☐ Hypoglycaemia
- ☐ Hyperglycaemia
- ☐ Hyperosmolar non-ketotic coma (HONK)
- ☐ Hypophosphatemia

Mitochondrial disorders

- ☐ MERRF
- ☐ MELAS
- ☐ Leigh syndrome
- ☐ Alpers syndrome
- ☐ Leber hereditary optic neuropathy (LHON)
- ☐ POLG (polymerase gamma) disorders

Thyroid disorders

- ☐ Hashimoto thyroiditis
- ☐ Hyperthyroidism
- ☐ Steroid-responsive encephalopathy with autoimmune thyroid disease (SREAT)

Miscellaneous causes

- ☐ Paraneoplastic
- ☐ Nicotinic acid deficiency encephalopathy

Acronyms

- ☐ MERRF: Myoclonus epilepsy with ragged red fibers
- ☐ MELAS: Mitochondrial encephalopathy, lactate acidosis and stroke-like episodes

Major epilepsy types

CHILDHOOD ABSENCE EPILEPSY (CAE)

Epidemiology

- ☐ This is possibly a channelopathy
- ☐ The onset is before 10 years of age: usually between 3–8 years
- ☐ The onset is <4 years in subjects with glucose transporter type 1 deficiency
- ☐ Females are at a higher risk
- ☐ There is a positive family history in 16–45% of cases
- ☐ There is a history of febrile seizures in about 30% (FS+)

Clinical features of absences

- ☐ Absences are the only seizure type
- ☐ There is brief loss of consciousness: this is not induced or triggered
- ☐ The events occur frequently: up to 200 a day
- ☐ There is spontaneous remission in about 70%: this is usually in adolescence
- ☐ Remission is usually 2–5 years from onset
- ☐ Generalised tonic-clonic seizures develop in most of those who do not remit

Electroencephalography (EEG)

- ☐ Generalised bilateral 2.5–4 Hz spike
- ☐ Slow-wave discharges (SWD)

Treatment

- ☐ Ethosuximide (ESM): this has a better effect on attention
- ☐ Valproate: this has a better side effect profile and controls myoclonus
- ☐ Lamotrigine

Contraindicated medications

- ☐ Carbamazepine
- ☐ Vigabatrin
- ☐ Tiagabine

EYELID MYOCLONIA WITH ABSENCES (JEAVON'S SYNDROME)

Types

- ☐ Idiopathic form
- ☐ Secondary forms: associated with cryptogenic or symptomatic epilepsy

Epidemiology

- ☐ There is frequently a family history of epilepsy and febrile seizures
- ☐ It starts between the ages of 3 to 7 years
- ☐ It persists into adulthood
- ☐ It may be precipitated by Carbamazepine therapy

Features of eyelid myoclonia

- ☐ Fluttering, jerking eyelid movements: provoked by eye closure
- ☐ Rapid blinking

Other clinical features

- ☐ Eyeball rolling
- ☐ Upward eye deviation
- ☐ Retropulsive eyeball movements
- ☐ Head retroflexion
- ☐ Limb myoclonus may occur
- ☐ Tonic-clonic seizures: very rarely
- ☐ Photosensitivity

Differential diagnosis

- ☐ Facial tics
- ☐ Non-epileptic paroxysmal eyelid movements
- ☐ Random rhythmic eye closure in other idiopathic epilepsies
- ☐ Eye blinking in childhood and juvenile absence epilepsy
- ☐ Symptomatic absence epilepsy
- ☐ Fixation-off sensitive epilepsy
- ☐ Benign myoclonic epilepsy of infancy
- ☐ Eyelid flickering or fluttering
- ☐ Mannerisms
- ☐ Self-induced seizures

Electroencephalogram (EEG): features

- ☐ 3–6 Hz generalised polyspike and wave complexes
- ☐ Paroxysmal occipital bursts
- ☐ Photosensitivity with improvement in the dark
- ☐ Spontaneous absences after eye closure: with 3 Hz spike and wave discharges

Treatment

- ☐ Valproate
- ☐ Ethosuximide
- ☐ Benzodiazepines, e.g. Clonazepam

Contraindicated medications

- ☐ Carbamazepine
- ☐ Vigabatrin
- ☐ Tiagabine

DOI: 10.1201/9781003221258-14

JUVENILE ABSENCE EPILEPSY (JAE)

Clinical features

- [ ] The onset age is 10–17 years
- [ ] There is less severe impairment of consciousness than in childhood absences
- [ ] There are fewer absences a day
- [ ] Generalised tonic clonic seizures (GTCS) occur in about 80% of cases
- [ ] There are associated myoclonic jerks

Treatment

- [ ] Valproate
- [ ] Lamotrigine
- [ ] Ethosuximide: this is third line

Contraindicated medications

- [ ] Carbamazepine
- [ ] Vigabatrin
- [ ] Tiagabine

IDIOPATHIC GENERALISED EPILEPSY (IGE)

Types

- [ ] Childhood absence epilepsy (CAE): the onset age is 4–8 years
- [ ] Juvenile absence epilepsy (JAE): the onset age is >10 years
- [ ] Juvenile myoclonic epilepsy (JME): the onset age is in adolescence
- [ ] Generalised tonic-clonic seizures (GTCS): alone or on awakening (GTCSA)
- [ ] Idiopathic generalised epilepsy of late onset: the onset age is >20 years

Genetic mutations

- [ ] SLC2A1: causing GLUT 1 deficiency
- [ ] GABRG2
- [ ] GABRA1
- [ ] Copy number variants (CNV)

Seizure types

- [ ] Typical absence seizures
- [ ] Myoclonic seizures
- [ ] Generalised tonic-clonic seizures (GTCS)

Differential diagnosis

- [ ] Epileptic encephalopathy with neuronal migration disorders
  - Especially with DCX gene mutations
- [ ] Progressive myoclonic epilepsy (PME)

Electroencephalogram (EEG): features

- [ ] Generalised spike and wave discharges at >2.5 Hz
- [ ] Spike or poly-spike wave discharges
- [ ] Bursts of regular spike and waves
- [ ] Epileptiform K complexes

Synonym

- [ ] Genetic generalised epilepsy (GGE)

JUVENILE MYOCLONIC EPILEPSY (JME): CLINICAL FEATURES

Epidemiology

- ☐ The onset age is typically 12–18 years
  - ○ But it is after the age of 30 years in about 5% of cases
- ☐ It may start as late as the 8th decade
- ☐ There is a positive family history in about 50% of cases

Myoclonic features

- ☐ Myoclonic jerks occur on or after awakening (chronosensitivity)
- ☐ They usually appear in the upper limbs
- ☐ They are often photosensitive
- ☐ They may provoke falls

Reflex features

- ☐ Photosensitivity
- ☐ Eye-closure sensitivity
- ☐ Praxis induction: seizures triggered by cognitive tasks
- ☐ Language-induced orofacial reflex myoclonus

Other seizure types

- ☐ Generalised tonic-clonic seizures
- ☐ Absence seizures

Triggers for seizures

- ☐ Alcohol
- ☐ Sleep deprivation

Cognitive features

- ☐ Executive dysfunction is common
- ☐ This correlates with praxis induction and eye-closure/ photosensitivity

Adult onset JME

- ☐ Febrile seizures are less frequent than in classic JME
- ☐ There are fewer absence seizures than in classic JME

Risk factors for refractory JME

- ☐ Co-occurrence of three seizure types
- ☐ Absence seizures
- ☐ Psychiatric features
- ☐ Early onset age of seizures
- ☐ History of childhood absence epilepsy
- ☐ Praxis-induced seizures

GENERALISED EPILEPSY WITH FEBRILE SEIZURES PLUS (GEFS+)

Genetic transmission

- ☐ This is a subset of familial febrile seizures
- ☐ It is autosomal dominant with incomplete penetrance
- ☐ The mutation may arise de novo
- ☐ There are recognised mutations in 10% of families

Genetic mutations

- ☐ SCN1A
- ☐ SCN1B
- ☐ GABRG2
- ☐ SCN8A

Genetic subtypes

- ☐ GEFS+ type 1: SCN1B gene mutation on chromosome 19
- ☐ GEFS+ type 2: SCN1A gene mutation on chromosome 2
- ☐ GEFS+ type 3: GABRG2 gene mutation on chromosome 5

Phenotypes

- ☐ Classical GEFS+
- ☐ Borderline GEFS+
- ☐ Unclassified epilepsy
- ☐ Alternative syndromic diagnoses
- ☐ Dravet syndrome
- ☐ Panayiotopoulos syndrome
- ☐ Atypical benign epilepsy with centrotemporal spikes (BECTS)
- ☐ Epilepsy with auditory features

Clinical features

- ☐ It is childhood onset
- ☐ It progresses beyond 6 years
- ☐ There are multiple febrile seizures
- ☐ It stops by mid-childhood
- ☐ It may overlap with idiopathic generalised epilepsy (IGE)

Possible associated features

- ☐ Absence seizures
- ☐ Myoclonic seizures
- ☐ Atonic seizures
- ☐ Myoclonic-astatic epilepsy (MAE)
- ☐ Febrile seizures (FS)
- ☐ Complex partial seizures
- ☐ Focal seizures

Treatment

- ☐ Drug prophylaxis is often not helpful
- ☐ Rescue benzodiazepines may be effective in some cases
- ☐ Vagus nerve stimulation (VNS) or surgery may help in refractory cases

Synonym

- ☐ Genetic epilepsy with febrile seizures plus

TEMPORAL LOBE EPILEPSY WITH HIPPOCAMPAL SCLEROSIS (TLE-HS): FEATURES

Motor symptoms

- ☐ Lip smacking
- ☐ Chewing
- ☐ Swallowing
- ☐ Fumbling
- ☐ Feet shuffling
- ☐ Violence
- ☐ Aggression
- ☐ Laughter: gelastic epilepsy
- ☐ Running: epilepsy procursiva
- ☐ Going around in circles: volvular epilepsy
- ☐ Aimless wandering: poriomania

Visual symptoms

- ☐ Micropsia
- ☐ Macropsia
- ☐ Palinopsia
- ☐ Tilting of environment

Auditory and gustatory symptoms

- ☐ Buzzing
- ☐ Roaring
- ☐ Repeated words
- ☐ Music
- ☐ Salivation
- ☐ Thirst sensation
- ☐ Visceral sensation

Dyscognitive and affective symptoms

- ☐ Déjà vu
- ☐ Jamais vu
- ☐ Depersonalisation
- ☐ Recurring memory fragments/scenes
- ☐ Memory interruption
- ☐ Sadness
- ☐ Anger
- ☐ Happiness
- ☐ Sexual excitement
- ☐ Fear
- ☐ Anxiety
- ☐ Impaired verbal learning
- ☐ Impaired visual memory

Other symptoms

- ☐ Vertiginous sensations
- ☐ Epigastric rising sensations
- ☐ Hallucinations
- ☐ Olfactory symptoms
- ☐ Hypergraphia
- ☐ Post ictal features: aphasia, nose-wiping, paralysis

FRONTAL LOBE EPILEPSY: CLINICAL FEATURES

Epidemiology

- ☐ The onset age ranges from infancy to adolescence
  - ○ But it is usually between 14–20 years of age
- ☐ There is a family history of epilepsy in 25% of cases

Pathogenesis

- ☐ Seizures often arise from non-REM sleep
- ☐ They are related to sleep rather than to nighttime
- ☐ They are called nocturnal frontal lobe epilepsy (NFLE) if they occur exclusively in sleep
- ☐ The seizure focus may be extra-frontal

Typical seizures

- ☐ The seizures have an abrupt onset and termination
- ☐ The seizures last <2 minutes
- ☐ There is often a somatosensory aura
- ☐ Subjects often awaken from sleep with a cry
- ☐ The seizures tend to cluster

Motor movements

- ☐ Adversive head movements: these are usually away from the seizure focus
- ☐ Cycling movements
- ☐ Clapping
- ☐ Genital manipulation
- ☐ Hand rubbing
- ☐ Kicking
- ☐ Limb posturing
- ☐ Rocking
- ☐ Running
- ☐ Paroxysmal dystonia
- ☐ Pelvic thrusting
- ☐ Screaming
- ☐ Tonic posturing

Vocal features

- ☐ Ictal aphasia
- ☐ Ictal pouting: chapeau de gendarme sign
- ☐ Vocalisation
- ☐ Ictal speech: with elevated pitch

Sleep associated features

- ☐ Paroxysmal arousals: these occur several times at night
- ☐ Excessive daytime sleepiness (EDS)
- ☐ Nocturnal enuresis
- ☐ Sleep-related violent behaviour
- ☐ Nocturnal wanderings

Prognosis

- ☐ The long-term outcome is poor
- ☐ Terminal remission occurs in about a quarter of patients

Synonyms

- ☐ Paroxysmal hypnogenic dyskinesia
- ☐ Paroxysmal nocturnal dyskinesia
- ☐ Sleep related hypermotor epilepsy (SHE)

OCCIPITAL LOBE EPILEPSY

Causes

- ☐ Idiopathic occipital epilepsies
- ☐ Childhood epilepsy syndromes
- ☐ Malformations of cortical development
- ☐ Progressive myoclonic epilepsies
- ☐ Mitochondrial disorders
- ☐ Epilepsy with bilateral occipital calcifications

Visual hallucinations

- ☐ The onset is abrupt
- ☐ They start in the contralateral visual field
- ☐ They are coloured and circular
- ☐ There may be flashes of colour or light
- ☐ There may be associated scotomas, hemianopia, or amaurosis

Illusionary distortions

- ☐ Size
- ☐ Shape
- ☐ Illumination
- ☐ Colour
- ☐ Clarity
- ☐ Loss of colour

Other symptoms

- ☐ Sensation of ocular movement
- ☐ Tinnitus
- ☐ Vertigo
- ☐ Ictal vomiting
- ☐ Eye deviation
- ☐ Autonomic features
- ☐ Forced eye closure
- ☐ Palpebral jerks
- ☐ Post ictal blindness
- ☐ Migraine-like headache
- ☐ Symptoms of spread to other lobes

Differential diagnosis

- ☐ Migraine
- ☐ Glaucoma
- ☐ Retinal detachment
- ☐ Charles Bonnet syndrome (CBS)
- ☐ Peduncular hallucinosis
- ☐ Narcolepsy
- ☐ Delirium
- ☐ Psychoses

Status epilepticus

CONVULSIVE STATUS EPILEPTICUS: CLINICAL FEATURES

Definitions
- ☐ Recurrent generalised convulsions with no complete recovery of consciousness
- ☐ One prolonged convulsion

Types
- ☐ Tonic–clonic
- ☐ Tonic
- ☐ Clonic
- ☐ Myoclonic

Stages
- ☐ Impending
- ☐ Established
- ☐ Subtle
- ☐ Refractory

Motor features
- ☐ Muscle contractions: tonic and then alternating tonic and clonic
- ☐ Nystagmus
- ☐ Facial twitching
- ☐ Postictal Todd's paralysis

Autonomic features
- ☐ Tachycardia
- ☐ Cardiac arrhythmias
- ☐ Hypertension
- ☐ Fever
- ☐ Salivation
- ☐ Vomiting
- ☐ Incontinence

Predictors of poor prognosis
- ☐ Older age: ≥65 years
- ☐ Potentially fatal aetiologies
- ☐ De novo onset in hospitalised patients
- ☐ Impairment of consciousness
- ☐ Prolonged seizure duration
- ☐ Focal neurological signs at onset
- ☐ Medical complications
- ☐ Inadequate Benzodiazepine dosing

Outcome prediction scales
- ☐ Status epilepticus severity score (STESS)
- ☐ Epidemiology-based mortality score in status epilepticus (EMSE)
- ☐ Modified Rankin Scale (mRS) score

CONVULSIVE STATUS EPILEPTICUS: MANAGEMENT

Initial treatment options
- ☐ Intravenous Lorazepam 0.1mg/kg or 4mg: repeatable after 10mins
- ☐ Intravenous Diazepam: 10mg and repeatable
- ☐ Intramuscular Midazolam

Alternative initial treatment options
- ☐ Intravenous Phenobarbitone
- ☐ Rectal Diazepam
- ☐ Buccal Midazolam
- ☐ Midazolam nasal spray: for seizure clusters

Second line treatment: intravenous after 20 minutes
- ☐ Fosphenytoin
- ☐ Phenytoin
- ☐ Valproate
- ☐ Levetiracetam
- ☐ Phenobarbitone: if the other options are not available

Third line treatment: after 40 minutes
- ☐ Repeat second-line treatments
- ☐ Thiopental
- ☐ Midazolam
- ☐ Pentobarbital
- ☐ Propofol

Emerging treatments
- ☐ Intranasal Diazepam
- ☐ Intravenous Clonazepam

DOI: 10.1201/9781003221258-15

NON-CONVULSIVE STATUS EPILEPTICUS (NCSE): CLINICAL FEATURES

Impaired higher brain function

- [ ] Amnesia
- [ ] Confusion and delirium
- [ ] Confabulation
- [ ] Neglect
- [ ] Impaired body schema
- [ ] Cortical blindness
- [ ] Fluctuating mental state
- [ ] Coma
- [ ] Dementia

Impaired speech and language

- [ ] Alexia
- [ ] Aphasia and aphasic status epilepticus
- [ ] Perseveration
- [ ] Reduced verbal fluency
- [ ] Muteness
- [ ] Echolalia
- [ ] Stuttering

Psychiatric features

- [ ] Hallucinations: olfactory, gustatory, auditory, and visual
- [ ] Delusions
- [ ] Psychosis
- [ ] Mood disturbance
- [ ] Fear
- [ ] Agitation

Movement disorders

- [ ] Gaze deviation
- [ ] Spontaneous nystagmus
- [ ] Catatonia
- [ ] Myoclonus: face and limbs
- [ ] Paralysis
- [ ] Tonic and clonic movements
- [ ] Orofacial movements: chewing, swallowing, and lip movements
- [ ] Staring

Automatisms and autonomic features

- [ ] Repetitive blinking
- [ ] Nose wiping
- [ ] Facial pantomime
- [ ] Persisting laughter: status gelasticus
- [ ] Flatulence and belching
- [ ] Borborygmi
- [ ] Prolonged apnea
- [ ] Cardiac arrest

Other neurological features

- [ ] Vertigo and dizziness
- [ ] Headache
- [ ] Sensory disturbance and pain
- [ ] Strictly electroencephalographic NCSE: with no clinical features

REFRACTORY STATUS EPILEPTICUS (RSE): CLASSIFICATION

Refractory status epilepticus (RSE)

- [ ] This is status epilepticus which is resistant to two anti-epileptic drugs (AEDs)
- [ ] One of the AEDs should be a Benzodiazepine
- [ ] Older age is a risk factor

Super refractory status epilepticus (SRSE)

- [ ] This is status epilepticus persisting after general anaesthesia
  - ○ Or recurring ≥24 hours after anaesthesia
- [ ] Younger age is a risk factor

New onset refractory status epilepticus (NORSE)

- [ ] This is persistent status epilepticus with no identifiable cause

Febrile infection-related epilepsy syndrome (FIRES)

- [ ] This is a form of NORSE
- [ ] There is a preceding febrile infection within 2 weeks of onset

SUPER REFRACTORY STATUS EPILEPTICUS (SRSE)

Definitions
- ☐ Status epilepticus persisting after general anaesthesia
- ☐ Status epilepticus recurring ≥24 hours after anaesthesia

Complication
- ☐ Brain atrophy: this may progress even after treatment

Non-drug treatment options
- ☐ Identify and treat focal lesions
- ☐ Hypothermia at 32–35°C
- ☐ Ketogenic diet

Drug treatment options
- ☐ Steroids with or without intravenous immunoglobulins (IVIg)
- ☐ Steroids with or without plasma exchange (PE)
- ☐ Paraldehyde
- ☐ Rufinamide
- ☐ Stiripentol
- ☐ Ketamine: this is an emerging drug option
- ☐ Intravenous (IV) Magnesium: with IV Pyridoxine in children

Interventional treatment options
- ☐ Electroconvulsive therapy (ECT)
- ☐ Cerebrospinal fluid (CSF) drainage
- ☐ Vagus nerve stimulation (VNS)
- ☐ Deep brain stimulation (DBS)
- ☐ Transcranial magnetic stimulation (TMS)

General care and monitoring
- ☐ Daily electroencephalogram (EEG)
- ☐ Intensive therapy unit care
- ☐ Fluid balance
- ☐ Anti-thrombotic therapy
- ☐ Skin care

Sudden unexpected death in epilepsy (SUDEP)

SUDDEN UNEXPECTED DEATH IN EPILEPSY (SUDEP): SUBJECT-RELATED RISK FACTORS

Individual risk factors

- ☐ Adult age
- ☐ Male gender
- ☐ Duration of epilepsy >15 years
- ☐ Onset age of epilepsy <16 years
- ☐ Learning difficulty
- ☐ Obstructive sleep apnoea (OSA)

Behavioural risk factors

- ☐ History of alcohol abuse
- ☐ Sleeping alone
- ☐ Sleeping in the prone position
- ☐ Absence of nocturnal surveillance
- ☐ Lack of contact with health care in the previous year
- ☐ Use of antidepressants or anxiolytics

Possible genetic risk mutations

- ☐ SCN5A
- ☐ KIF6
- ☐ TBX18
- ☐ DEPDC5
- ☐ SCN8A
- ☐ TBC1D24

SUDDEN UNEXPECTED DEATH IN EPILEPSY (SUDEP): RISK FACTORS

Pathological risk factors

- ☐ Dentate gyrus abnormalities
- ☐ Neuropeptide depletion in the amygdala
  - ○ Galanin, neuropeptide Y (NPY), and somatostatin (SST)
- ☐ Reduced cortical adenosine receptors
- ☐ Increased neuronal adenosine receptors

Seizure-related risk factors

- ☐ Uncontrolled generalised tonic-clonic convulsions (GTCs)
- ☐ Symptomatic epilepsy
- ☐ Early onset refractory epilepsy
- ☐ Epileptic encephalopathy
- ☐ Nocturnal seizures
- ☐ Untreated epilepsy
- ☐ Long duration seizures
- ☐ Terminal seizure: this occurs in 90% of SUDEP cases
- ☐ Primary generalised epilepsy in men
- ☐ Failed assessment for epilepsy surgery
- ☐ Post convulsive central apnoea (PCCA)

Prolonged post-ictal generalised EEG suppression (PGES)

- ☐ PGES duration >50 seconds may indicate SUDEP risk
- ☐ Shorter duration PGES have also been reported in SUDEP
- ☐ One study however doubts the significance of PGES as a risk for SUDEP

Antiepileptic drug (AED) related risk factors

- ☐ Sub-therapeutic AED levels
- ☐ Valproate level >100mg/L
- ☐ Unclear treatment history
- ☐ Frequent AED prescribing changes
- ☐ AED withdrawal

Doubtful risk factors

- ☐ Polytherapy: an unlikely risk factor if seizures are controlled
- ☐ Carbamazepine in females
- ☐ Lamotrigine in females

DOI: 10.1201/9781003221258-16

SUDDEN UNEXPECTED DEATH IN EPILEPSY (SUDEP): CLINICAL INDICATORS

Pre-ictal respiratory features

- ☐ Respiratory dysfunction
- ☐ Hypoventilation

Pre-ictal cardiac features

- ☐ Abnormal heart rate variability (HRV)
  - ○ This indicates severe autonomic dysregulation
  - ○ It is worse with sodium channel (SCN) mutations
- ☐ Sympathetic hyperactivity

Ictal features

- ☐ ≥2 generalised seizures in the preceding day
- ☐ Generalised tonic clonic seizure at onset
- ☐ Ictal central apnoea (ICA)

Post-ictal (terminal) cardiorespiratory features

- ☐ Tachycardia
- ☐ Tachypnoea
- ☐ Asystole
- ☐ Post convulsive central apnoea (PCCA)

Differential diagnosis

- ☐ Sudden cardiac death (SCD)
- ☐ Sudden infant death syndrome (SIDS)
- ☐ Sudden unexplained death in childhood (SUDC)

SUDDEN UNEXPECTED DEATH IN EPILEPSY (SUDEP): MANAGEMENT

Improve night-time conditions

- ☐ Sleep supine
- ☐ Use seizure alarms
- ☐ Use anti-suffocation pillows
- ☐ Improve night-time supervision and precautions
- ☐ Use nocturnal checking/listening devices
- ☐ Share rooms
- ☐ Treat obstructive sleep apnoea

Optimise seizure control

- ☐ Encourage compliance
- ☐ Limit number of antiepileptic drugs (AEDs)
- ☐ Rapid seizure identification
- ☐ Identify surgically remediable cases early

Consider alternative epilepsy interventions

- ☐ New drug combinations
- ☐ Dietary therapy
- ☐ Vagal nerve stimulation (VNS)
- ☐ Palliative surgery

Preventative measures

- ☐ Simple resuscitation
- ☐ Clearing airway obstruction
- ☐ Patient repositioning from prone to lateral
- ☐ Use of lattice pillows
- ☐ Post-ictal stimulation
- ☐ Postictal oxygen therapy

Proposed preventative measures

- ☐ Selective serotonin reuptake inhibitors (SSRIs)
  - ○ They may improve respiratory drive and reduce ictal hypoxaemia
- ☐ Opiate receptor inhibitors
- ☐ Adenosine receptor inhibitors
- ☐ Cardiac pacemakers
- ☐ Implantable cardioverter defibrillators

SUDEP discussion points with patient

- ☐ Do not discuss SUDEP until the diagnosis is established
- ☐ Individualize SUDEP risk in discussions
  - ○ Determine patient's preferred learning style and expectations
- ☐ Discuss SUDEP as part of a comprehensive education programme
- ☐ Explore patient's readiness to learn about SUDEP
- ☐ Emphasise risk of SUDEP to encourage compliance
- ☐ Describe research going on into SUDEP

CHAPTER **3**

Sleep disorders

Narcolepsy

NARCOLEPSY: CLINICAL FEATURES

Demographic features

- ☐ Narcolepsy usually starts in adolescence
- ☐ The onset age is 15–40 years
- ☐ It is slightly more frequent in males
- ☐ It may be triggered by H1N1 influenza virus infection and immunisation

Excessive sleepiness: features

- ☐ A background feeling of sleepiness
- ☐ Episodes of irresistible urge to sleep
- ☐ Naps occurring at inappropriate times
- ☐ Naps occurring several times a day and lasting minutes to hours

Cataplexy

- ☐ These are episodes of partial or generalised loss of muscle tone
- ☐ They last <1 minute during which awareness is maintained
- ☐ These follow emotional arousal: amusement, anger, elation
- ☐ They may be triggered by anticipation of emotion
- ☐ There may be associated limb twitching

Sleep paralysis

- ☐ This is the inability to move for 1–2 minutes
- ☐ It occurs at sleep onset or at awakening

Hypnagogic hallucinations

- ☐ These are vivid dream-like states occurring at sleep onset

Sleepiness-related daytime symptoms

- ☐ Blurred vision
- ☐ Diplopia
- ☐ Poor memory
- ☐ Impaired concentration
- ☐ Impact on relationships and employment

Complex sleep-onset movements

- ☐ Stereotypies
- ☐ Perioral movements
- ☐ Dyskinetic-dystonic movements

Associated sleep disorders

- ☐ Sleep disordered breathing (SDB)
- ☐ Periodic limb movements of sleep (PLMS)
- ☐ Disturbed night sleep
- ☐ Sleep walking
- ☐ Automatic behaviour
- ☐ Sweet cravings especially at night
- ☐ Micro sleeps
- ☐ Vivid dreams

Other clinical features

- ☐ Chronic pain
- ☐ Obesity: this is usually in narcolepsy with cataplexy
- ☐ Increased creative thinking

NARCOLEPSY: DIFFERENTIAL DIAGNOSIS

Causes of secondary narcolepsy

- ☐ Brainstem stroke
- ☐ Cranial radiation
- ☐ Encephalomyelitis
- ☐ Hypothalamic-pituitary disorders
  - ○ Arteriovenous malformations (AVMs)
  - ○ Craniopharyngiomas
  - ○ Hypothalamic sarcoidosis
  - ○ Pituitary adenomas
- ☐ Hypoxic ischaemic injury
- ☐ Influenza H1N1 vaccination: in Europe but not in America
- ☐ Niemann–Pick type C (NPC)
- ☐ Tumours: of the brainstem or the third ventricle
- ☐ Traumatic brain injury (TBI)
- ☐ Multiple sclerosis (MS)
- ☐ Neurodegenerative diseases

Differential diagnosis of excessive sleepiness

- ☐ Poor night sleep
- ☐ Obstructive sleep apnoea (OSA)
- ☐ Circadian rhythm disorder
- ☐ Idiopathic hypersomnolence
- ☐ Periodic limb movements of sleep (PLMS)
- ☐ Depression
- ☐ Head injury
- ☐ Night-time pain
- ☐ Hypnotics
- ☐ Antiepileptic drugs (AEDs)
- ☐ Syncope
- ☐ Epilepsy

Differential diagnosis of cataplexy

- ☐ Niemann–Pick C disease (NPC)
- ☐ Gelastic atonic seizures
- ☐ Functional: pseudocataplexy
- ☐ Stimulus induced drop episodes (SIDEs): in Coffin-Lowry syndrome (CLS)

DOI: 10.1201/9781003221258-18

NARCOLEPSY: INVESTIGATIONS

HLA associations

- [ ] HLA-DR2
- [ ] HLA-DQB1*0602

Cerebrospinal fluid (CSF) hypocretin: values

- [ ] Normal values are >200 pg/ml
- [ ] Narcolepsy values are <110 pg/ml: this is seen in >95% of cases
- [ ] Most cases with low levels are positive for HLA-DQB1*0602
- [ ] Low levels are also seen in primary hypersomnia

Cerebrospinal fluid (CSF) hypocretin: causes of intermediate low levels

- [ ] HLA negative narcolepsy: often without cataplexy
- [ ] Periodic hypersomnia
- [ ] Guillain–Barre syndrome (GBS)
- [ ] Traumatic brain injury (TBI)
- [ ] Encephalitis
- [ ] Hashimoto thyroiditis

Multiple sleep latency test (MSLT)

- [ ] Mean sleep latency ≤8 min
- [ ] ≥2 SOREMPs (sleep onset rapid eye movement periods)

Aquaporin 4 antibodies

- [ ] Neuromyelitis optica (NMO) may present with narcolepsy
- [ ] Aquaporin 4 antibodies may be positive

NARCOLEPSY: TREATMENT OF HYPERSOMNIA

First line treatments

- [ ] Modafinil
- [ ] Sodium oxybate
- [ ] Modafinil and Sodium oxybate combination in severe cases

Other treatments

- [ ] Methylphenidate
- [ ] Amphetamine
- [ ] Methamphetamine
- [ ] Dexamphetamine
- [ ] Selegiline
- [ ] Mazindol
- [ ] Solriamfetol: this is a selective dopamine and norepinephrine reuptake inhibitor
- [ ] Pitolisant: this is a histamine H3 receptor inverse agonist

Treatment of disturbed night sleep

- [ ] Clonazepam
- [ ] Sodium oxybate
- [ ] Planned daytime naps

NARCOLEPSY: TREATMENT OF CATAPLEXY

Sodium oxybate

- ☐ This is the first line treatment
- ☐ The dose is 4.5–9g daily in two equal doses
- ☐ It may cause weight loss

Tricyclics

- ☐ Clomipramine 20–75 mg daily
- ☐ Protriptyline 2.5–10 mg daily

Selective serotonin receptor inhibitors (SSRIs)

- ☐ Femoxetine 600 mg daily
- ☐ Fluoxetine 20–60 mg daily
- ☐ Fluvoxamine 25–200 mg daily

Serotonin norepinephrine reuptake inhibitors (SNRIs)

- ☐ Venlafaxine 75–225 mg daily
- ☐ SNRIs are not evidence-based for narcolepsy

Histamine H3 receptor inverse agonist

- ☐ Pitolisant

Insomnia

INSOMNIA: CAUSES

Primary insomnia: types

- ☐ Idiopathic
- ☐ Paradoxical: this is subjective insomnia
- ☐ Psycho-physiologic: this is heightened arousal with caffeine, alcohol, jet lag, or shift work

Medical causes

- ☐ Anxiety
- ☐ Depression
- ☐ Systemic medical conditions
- ☐ Pain
- ☐ Hypnotic withdrawal

Drug-induced

- ☐ Amphetamines
- ☐ Beta blockers
- ☐ Bupropion
- ☐ Cocaine
- ☐ Fluoxetine
- ☐ Lamotrigine
- ☐ Methylphenidate
- ☐ Modafinil
- ☐ Prednisolone
- ☐ Pemoline
- ☐ Pseudoephedrine
- ☐ Theophylline
- ☐ Venlafaxine

INSOMNIA: CLINICAL FEATURES

Diagnostic criteria

- ☐ There is a disturbance of sleep onset or maintenance, or poor sleep quality
- ☐ It occurs ≥3 times a week for 1 month in non-organic insomnia
- ☐ It occurs ≥3 a week for 3 months for chronic insomnia
- ☐ There is extreme focus and worry over the sleep disorder
- ☐ There is associated impairment of daily activities and suffering
- ☐ There is a higher incidence in women and older age
- ☐ Symptoms often start with a life event

Sleep-related impairments

- ☐ Difficulty initiating sleep
- ☐ Difficulty maintaining sleep
- ☐ Early waking
- ☐ Non-restorative sleep
- ☐ Resistance to going to bed on schedule

Daytime impairments

- ☐ Daytime sleepiness
- ☐ Fatigue
- ☐ Malaise
- ☐ Poor energy and motivation
- ☐ Impaired attention and concentration
- ☐ Memory impairment
- ☐ Hyperactivity
- ☐ Impulsivity
- ☐ Aggression
- ☐ Ruminations

Complications

- ☐ Headaches
- ☐ Gastrointestinal disturbances
- ☐ Hypertension
- ☐ Delusions
- ☐ Mood disorders
- ☐ Irritability
- ☐ Error proneness
- ☐ Accidents
- ☐ Poor social and occupational performance

DOI: 10.1201/9781003221258-19

INSOMNIA: NON-DRUG TREATMENTS

Cognitive behaviour therapy (CBT)

- ☐ This is first line treatment for chronic insomnia
- ☐ It changes beliefs and attitudes to insomnia and sleep hygiene

Sleep hygiene: helpful habits

- ☐ Have a regular morning arousal time
- ☐ Take regular exercise but not within 3 hours of sleep
- ☐ Practice positive thinking and relaxation before bed
- ☐ Have fixed bed and wake times
- ☐ Sleep in a comfortable environment
- ☐ Avoid clock watching and daytime naps
- ☐ Adopt the 20-minute toss and turn rule: this is getting up after 20 minutes of failed attempted sleep

Sleep hygiene: factors to avoid at bedtime

- ☐ Caffeine
- ☐ Alcohol
- ☐ Nicotine
- ☐ Hunger
- ☐ Loud noises
- ☐ Brightness

Stimulus control therapy

- ☐ This is learning to associate the bed and bedroom with sleep
- ☐ It helps to establish a consistent sleep-wake cycle

Paradoxical intention

- ☐ This is avoiding effortful attempts to fall asleep
- ☐ Remaining passively awake helps to reduce the anxiety of trying to fall asleep

Other psychological therapies

- ☐ Biofeedback therapy: this helps to control physiologic parameters
- ☐ Relaxation therapy: to reduce bedtime somatic tension and intrusive thoughts
- ☐ Sleep restriction therapy: restrict bedtime only for sleeping

INSOMNIA: DRUG TREATMENTS

Indication for drug treatments

- ☐ Failure of cognitive behaviour therapy (CBT)

Drug treatments indicated for short-term use: ≤4 weeks

- ☐ Benzodiazepines
- ☐ Benzodiazepine receptor agonists
- ☐ Antidepressants

Benzodiazepine receptor agonists: Z drugs

- ☐ Zaleplon: for sleep onset insomnia
- ☐ Eszoplicone: for sleep onset and sleep maintenance insomnia
- ☐ Zolpidem: for sleep onset and sleep maintenance insomnia
- ☐ Zoplicone

Sedating antidepressants: if there is co-existing mood disorder

- ☐ Doxepin: for sleep maintenance insomnia
- ☐ Triazolam: for sleep onset insomnia
- ☐ Trazodone: for sleep onset or sleep maintenance insomnia
- ☐ Amitriptyline
- ☐ Mirtazapine

Dual orexin receptor antagonists (DORA)

- ☐ Suvorexant
- ☐ Daridorexant
- ☐ Lemborexant

Other drug treatments

- ☐ Temazepam: a short/intermediate acting benzodiazepine
  - ○ For sleep onset and sleep maintenance insomnia
- ☐ Ramelteon: a melatonin receptor agonist
  - ○ For sleep onset insomnia
- ☐ Tiagabine: for sleep onset or sleep maintenance insomnia
- ☐ Gabapentin

Treatments not recommended

- ☐ Antihistamines, e.g. diphenhydramine
- ☐ Antipsychotics
- ☐ Melatonin
- ☐ Tryptophan
- ☐ Phyto-therapeutics
- ☐ Homeopathy
- ☐ Acupuncture
- ☐ Valerian

Hypersomnia

CENTRAL HYPERSOMNIAS: CLASSIFICATION

Narcolepsy

- ☐ Narcolepsy
- ☐ Narcolepsy with cataplexy

Recurrent hypersomnia

- ☐ Kleine-Levin syndrome (KLS)
- ☐ Kleine-Levin syndrome (KLS) without compulsive eating
- ☐ Menstrual related hypersomnia (MRH)
- ☐ Recurrent hypersomnia with comorbidity (RHC)

Medical conditions causing hypersomnia and narcolepsy

- ☐ Parkinson's disease (PD)
- ☐ Multiple sclerosis (MS)
- ☐ Stroke
- ☐ Traumatic brain injury (TBI)
- ☐ Brain tumours
- ☐ Trypanosomiasis
- ☐ Limbic encephalitis
- ☐ Encephalitis lethargica
- ☐ Myotonic dystrophy
- ☐ Niemann–Pick type C (NPC) disease
- ☐ Substance intake, e.g. dopaminergic drugs

Idiopathic hypersomnia

- ☐ Idiopathic hypersomnia with long sleep time
- ☐ Idiopathic hypersomnia without long sleep time

CENTRAL HYPERSOMNIA: DRUG TREATMENTS

Amphetamines and derivatives

- ☐ Methylphenidate
- ☐ Dextroamphetamine
- ☐ Pemoline

Non-amphetamine CNS stimulants

- ☐ Modafinil
- ☐ Armodafinil

Other drugs

- ☐ Sodium oxybate
- ☐ Caffeine
- ☐ Atomoxetine: an antidepressant with stimulant properties
- ☐ Selegiline
- ☐ Mazindol: a dopamine norepinephrine uptake inhibitor

DOI: 10.1201/9781003221258-20

IDIOPATHIC HYPERSOMNIA: CLINICAL FEATURES

Types

- ☐ Idiopathic hypersomnia with prolonged night sleep: sleep lasting >10 hours
- ☐ Idiopathic hypersomnia without prolonged night sleep

Background

- ☐ This is possibly the same as narcolepsy type 2
- ☐ The mean onset age is 16–19 years

Classical features

- ☐ Family history of sleep disorder: this is present in about 35% of cases
- ☐ Excessive daytime sleep (EDS): this is long and unrefreshing in most cases
- ☐ Prolonged night-time sleep
- ☐ Disturbed sleep: with restlessness and frequent arousals
- ☐ Difficulty waking
- ☐ Vivid dreams
- ☐ Sleep drunkenness
- ☐ Habitual dreaming
- ☐ Brain fog
- ☐ Memory impairment

Associated disorders

- ☐ Mood disturbance
- ☐ Headaches
- ☐ Orthostatic symptoms
- ☐ Obesity
- ☐ Hypothyroidism
- ☐ Raynaud's phenomenon
- ☐ Sleep paralysis and hypnagogic hallucinations

Possible triggers

- ☐ Viral infection
- ☐ Head injury
- ☐ Primary mood disorder
- ☐ Weight gain

Possible aggravating factors

- ☐ Alcohol
- ☐ Heavy meals
- ☐ Winter
- ☐ Increased physical activity
- ☐ Psychological stress
- ☐ Menses

Course

- ☐ The course may fluctuate
- ☐ 10% of cases progress over the years
- ☐ 11% of cases experience spontaneous remission

IDIOPATHIC HYPERSOMNIA: MANAGEMENT

HLA studies

- ☐ It is not associated with HLA DR2 or DQ1

Multiple sleep latency test (MSLT)

- ☐ Sleep latency is prolonged: longer than in narcolepsy
- ☐ Slow wave sleep is increased

Polysomnography

- ☐ This is performed over 6 hours for short sleep latency type
- ☐ The test duration is over 10 hours for long sleep latency type

Cerebrospinal fluid (CSF)

- ☐ Hypocretin level is usually normal

Stimulant therapy

- ☐ Modafinil
- ☐ Methylphenidate
- ☐ Dextroamphetamine

Investigational treatments

- ☐ Clarithromycin
- ☐ Flumazenil
- ☐ Pitolisant

REM sleep parasomnias

REM SLEEP BEHAVIOUR DISORDER (RBD): RISK FACTORS

Synucleinopathies

- ☐ Parkinson's disease (PD)
- ☐ Lewy body disease (LBD)
- ☐ Multiple system atrophy (MSA)
- ☐ Primary autonomic failure (PAF)

Tauopathies

- ☐ Alzheimer's disease (AD)
- ☐ Corticobasal degeneration (CBD)
- ☐ Progressive supranuclear palsy (PSP)
- ☐ Frontotemporal dementia (FTD)

Other neurodegenerative diseases

- ☐ Spinocerebeller ataxia 3 (SCA 3)
- ☐ Motor neurone disease MND)
- ☐ Narcolepsy
- ☐ Huntington's disease (HD)

Drug-induced

- ☐ Sertraline
- ☐ Venlafaxine
- ☐ Mirtazapine
- ☐ Bisoprolol
- ☐ Tramadol
- ☐ Clomipramine
- ☐ Selegiline
- ☐ Tricyclics
- ☐ Cholinergic cognitive enhancers

Other causes

- ☐ Chiari malformation
- ☐ Autoimmune limbic encephalitis
- ☐ Focal vascular lesions
- ☐ Tumours
- ☐ Multiple sclerosis (MS)
- ☐ Guillain–Barre syndrome (GBS)
- ☐ Tourette's syndrome
- ☐ Autism
- ☐ Epilepsy
- ☐ Post-traumatic stress disorder (PTSD)
- ☐ Pontine stroke
- ☐ GBA (glucocerebrosidase) gene mutations

Potential risk factors

- ☐ Smoking
- ☐ Head injury
- ☐ Pesticide exposure
- ☐ Farming
- ☐ Welding

REM SLEEP BEHAVIOUR DISORDER (RBD): CLINICAL FEATURES

Epidemiology

- ☐ The mean onset age is about 60 years
- ☐ Males account for >80% of cases

Physical features

- ☐ Limb jerking
- ☐ Jumping out of bed
- ☐ Flailing
- ☐ Running
- ☐ Grabbing
- ☐ Punching
- ☐ Strangulating
- ☐ Aggressiveness

Language features

- ☐ Talking
- ☐ Shouting
- ☐ Screaming
- ☐ Swearing
- ☐ Singing

Emotional features

- ☐ Annoyance
- ☐ Fear
- ☐ Joy

Semi-purposeful actions

- ☐ Giving a speech
- ☐ Eating
- ☐ Reaching
- ☐ Riding

Dream-related symptoms

- ☐ Unpleasant dreams: insects, animals, being chased
- ☐ Defensive dreams: in about 90% of cases
- ☐ Vivid recollection of dreams

Associated symptoms

- ☐ Higher olfactory threshold
- ☐ Impaired colour discrimination
- ☐ Apathy and anxiety
- ☐ Autonomic dysfunction: urinary, bowel, and erectile dysfunction
- ☐ Sleep bruxism
- ☐ Falling out of bed
- ☐ Progressive cognitive impairment

Complications

- ☐ Injuries occur in about a third of cases
- ☐ Spouse assault occurs in about two-thirds of cases

DOI: 10.1201/9781003221258-21

REM SLEEP BEHAVIOUR DISORDER (RBD): MANAGEMENT

Main recommended drug treatments

- ☐ Clonazepam <2 mg nocte
  - ○ Use with caution in dementia and obstructive sleep apnoea (OSA)
- ☐ Melatonin 3–12 mg taken 30 minutes before sleep
  - ○ It may be combined with Clonazepam

Drug treatments which may also worsen RBD

- ☐ Dopamine agonists
- ☐ Levodopa
- ☐ Cholinesterases: especially with concomitant synucleinopathy

Poorly evidenced drug treatments

- ☐ Sodium oxybate
- ☐ Zoplicone
- ☐ Other benzodiazepines
- ☐ Desipramine
- ☐ Clozapine
- ☐ Clonidine
- ☐ Carbamazepine
- ☐ Quetiapine

Environmental treatments

- ☐ Keep sharp objects away
- ☐ Put a mattress or cushions on the floor
- ☐ Use bedside protective barriers

Pressurised bed alarm

- ☐ This delivers a calming message
- ☐ It is customised with a familiar voice

ANTI-IGLON5 ANTIBODY SYNDROME: CLINICAL FEATURES

Phenotypes

- ☐ Sleep disorder: parasomnia and sleep-related breathing difficulty
- ☐ Bulbar syndrome
- ☐ Progressive supranuclear palsy (PSP-like) syndrome
- ☐ Cognitive decline: with or without chorea

Sleep related features

- ☐ Sleep disordered breathing
- ☐ Sleep apnoea
- ☐ Sleep vocalisations
- ☐ Snoring
- ☐ Excessive daytime sleepiness (EDS)
- ☐ Sleep-related abnormal behaviours: such as threading a needle, salting food, dabbing perfume

Bulbar features

- ☐ Dysarthria
- ☐ Dysphagia: this may be the initial presentation
- ☐ Facial palsy
- ☐ Ptosis

Respiratory features

- ☐ Central hypoventilation
- ☐ Obstructive sleep apnoea
- ☐ Respiratory failure
- ☐ Stridor: from vocal cord paralysis

Movement disorders

- ☐ Chorea
- ☐ Parkinsonism
- ☐ Ataxia
- ☐ Cranio-cervical dystonia
- ☐ Facial myokymia
- ☐ Mandibular myorhythmia

Dysautonomia

- ☐ Bladder dysfunction
- ☐ Gastrointestinal dysmotility
- ☐ Impaired thermoregulation
- ☐ Orthostatic intolerance

Hyperexcitability

- ☐ Cramps
- ☐ Fasciculations
- ☐ Myoclonus
- ☐ Exaggerated startle

Other features

- ☐ Subacute encephalitis
- ☐ Depression
- ☐ Cognitive impairment
- ☐ Seizures
- ☐ Gait instability
- ☐ Eye movement disorders

ANTI-IGLON5 ANTIBODY SYNDROME: MANAGEMENT

Pathogenesis

- ☐ This is a tauopathy
- ☐ It is caused by IgG4 or IgG1 antibodies to IgLON5
- ☐ IgLON5 is a neuronal cell adhesion protein

HLA allele risk factors

- ☐ HLA-DRB1*1001
- ☐ HLA-DQB1*0501

Pathology

- ☐ There are hyperphosphorylated tau deposits in the neurones
- ☐ These are particularly seen in the hypothalamus and brainstem tegmentum
- ☐ The deposits are however not always present

Investigations

- ☐ Anti IgLON5 antibody titer: in the serum and cerebrospinal fluid (CSF)
- ☐ Brain magnetic resonance imaging (MRI): this is usually non-specific
- ☐ Cerebrospinal fluid (CSF): this may show mild pleocytosis
- ☐ Polysomnography
- ☐ Videofluoroscopy

Treatment

- ☐ Methylprednisolone
- ☐ Plasma exchange (PE)
- ☐ Rituximab
- ☐ Adjunctive cyclophosphamide: case report

Predictors of treatment response

- ☐ Cognitive impairment
- ☐ Non-classical phenotypes
- ☐ HLA-DQB1*05:01 without HLA-DRB1*10:01
- ☐ Cerebrospinal fluid inflammation
- ☐ Combination immunotherapy
- ☐ Azathioprine or Mycophenolate therapy

EXPLODING HEAD SYNDROME (EHS)

Demographic features

- ☐ This often occurs in middle to old age
- ☐ It usually affects women

Clinical features

- ☐ It is a paroxysmal sensory parasomnia
- ☐ It occurs at transition to sleep or on waking
- ☐ Subject awakens with an exploding noise in the head
- ☐ There is an associated with flash of light in 10% of cases
- ☐ There may be up to 7 episodes per night
- ☐ There is usually no associated headache
- ☐ It has been reported as a brainstem aura of migraine
- ☐ Daytime attacks may occur

Potential triggers

- ☐ Sleep deprivation
- ☐ Stress

Differential diagnosis

- ☐ Epilepsy
- ☐ Stroke

Treatment

- ☐ Clomipramine
- ☐ Topiramate

Synonym

- ☐ Episodic cranial sensory shock

Non-REM sleep parasomnias

CONFUSIONAL AROUSALS

Defining features

- ☐ These are brief episodes of arousal from sleep
- ☐ They are frequently associated with other sleep disorders

Types

- ☐ Sleep drunkenness: severe morning sleep inertia
- ☐ Sexsomnia: sleep-related sexual behaviours

Predisposing factors

- ☐ Young age: <35 years
- ☐ Shift or night work
- ☐ Drugs: especially antidepressants
- ☐ Smoking
- ☐ Obstructive sleep apnoea

Motor features

- ☐ Hypnic jerks
- ☐ Trembling
- ☐ Shivering
- ☐ Eye opening
- ☐ Head elevation
- ☐ Staring
- ☐ Face rubbing
- ☐ Yawning
- ☐ Scratching
- ☐ Moaning
- ☐ Mumbling
- ☐ Hypnic jerks

Associated psychiatric disorders

- ☐ Bipolar disorder
- ☐ Panic disorder
- ☐ Anxiety
- ☐ Adjustment disorder

Associated sleep disorders

- ☐ Narcolepsy
- ☐ Periodic limb movements of sleep (PLMS)
- ☐ Sleep talking
- ☐ Hypnagogic or hypnopompic hallucinations
- ☐ Hypersomnia or deep sleep
- ☐ Excessive daytime sleepiness (EDS)

Treatment

- ☐ Benzodiazepines
- ☐ Selective serotonin reuptake inhibitors (SSRIs)
- ☐ Scheduled awakenings

SLEEP WALKING (SOMNAMBULISM)

Defining features

- ☐ This is partial arousal during slow wave sleep
- ☐ It may be preceded by sleep terrors in younger age

Clinical features

- ☐ Subjects abruptly sit forward and walk
- ☐ There are no facial expressions
- ☐ The eyes are usually open: they are shut in REM parasomnias
- ☐ They may handle nearby objects
- ☐ They may perform searching acts
- ☐ They may carry out coherent interactive speech
- ☐ They may be agitated ambulation: especially in older subjects
- ☐ There may be associated violence

Associated pain disorders

- ☐ Headache
- ☐ Migraine
- ☐ Chronic pain

Predisposing genetic susceptibility

- ☐ There is a strong familial history of somnambulism
- ☐ There is an association with HLA DQB1*05:01

Predisposing medications

- ☐ Zolpidem
- ☐ Sodium oxybate
- ☐ Neuroleptics
- ☐ Lithium
- ☐ Amitriptyline
- ☐ Beta-blockers
- ☐ Topiramate

Other predisposing factors

- ☐ Sleep deprivation
- ☐ Stress
- ☐ Alcohol
- ☐ Fever
- ☐ Parkinson's disease (PD)
- ☐ Hyperthyroidism

Differential diagnosis: nocturnal frontal lobe epilepsy

- ☐ This is distinguished by the frontal lobe epilepsy and parasomnias scale (FLEP)

Non-drug treatments

- ☐ Scheduled awakenings
- ☐ Relaxation exercises
- ☐ Hypnosis

Drug treatments

- ☐ Clonazepam
- ☐ Imipramine
- ☐ Paroxetine
- ☐ Melatonin

DOI: 10.1201/9781003221258-22

SLEEP TALKING (SOMNILOQUY)

Epidemiology and pathology

- ☐ This usually occurs in childhood
- ☐ There may be a familial predisposition
- ☐ It arises from both REM and non-REM sleep

Content of speech

- ☐ Isolated words or sentences
- ☐ Speech
- ☐ Conversations

Associated features

- ☐ It is occasionally associated with body movements
- ☐ There is amnesia for the event
- ☐ There is usually no associated emotion

Associated disorders

- ☐ Obstructive sleep apnoea
- ☐ Other arousal disorders
- ☐ Other REM sleep parasomnias
- ☐ Dementia: especially dementia with Lewy bodies (DLB)

CHAPTER **4**

Movement disorders

Parkinsonism

PARKINSON'S DISEASE (PD): NEUROLOGICAL RISK FACTORS

Strong risk factors

- ☐ Depression
- ☐ Traumatic brain injury (TBI)
- ☐ REM sleep behaviour disorder (RBD)
- ☐ Family history of neurological disease

Genetic risk factors

- ☐ PD specific genes: especially LRRK2
- ☐ Glucocerebrosidase (GBA) mutation
- ☐ 22q11.2 chromosomal deletion
- ☐ Monogenic genes: these are found in 30% of familial and 3–5% of sporadic PD

Brain structural risk factors

- ☐ Hyperechogenic substantia nigra on transcranial ultrasound
- ☐ Giant Virchow-Robin spaces (VRSs)

Other possible PD risk factors

- ☐ Brain organochlorines
- ☐ Bipolar disorder

PARKINSON'S DISEASE (PD): SYSTEMIC RISK FACTORS

Strong risk factors

- ☐ Pesticides, e.g. organophosphates and carbamate
- ☐ Constipation

Risk occupations: possibly

- ☐ Welding: because of exposure to manganese fumes
- ☐ Computer programmers
- ☐ High stress jobs

Infections

- ☐ Prion-like particles
- ☐ Hepatitis C virus (HCV)
- ☐ Helicobacter pylori

Dietary and intestinal

- ☐ Dairy products
- ☐ Inflammatory bowel disease (IBD): the risk is reduced by anti TNF therapy
- ☐ Immunosuppressants

Other reported PD risk factors

- ☐ Rosacea
- ☐ Melanoma
- ☐ Smoking
- ☐ Multiple sexual partners
- ☐ Diabetes
- ☐ Renal dysfunction and proteinuria
- ☐ Hypothyroidism
- ☐ Low lymphocyte counts

Controversial risk factor: appendectomy

- ☐ Some studies report appendectomy increases PD risk
- ☐ The risk is supposedly due to inflammation or the release of α synuclein from the appendix
- ☐ The increased risk is however not confirmed in some studies

Controversial risk factor: Statin use

- ☐ Statins are reported as risk factors in a few studies
- ☐ But most reports do not identify statins as PD risk factors
- ☐ Some reports suggest that statins are protective against PD

DOI: 10.1201/9781003221258-24

PARKINSON'S DISEASE (PD) GENETICS: CLASSIFICATION

Autosomal dominant

- [ ] PARK1 (SNCA)
- [ ] PARK3
- [ ] PARK4 (SNCA)
- [ ] PARK5 (UCHL1)
- [ ] PARK8 (LRRK2)
- [ ] PARK11 (GIGYF2)
- [ ] PARK13 (HTRA2)
- [ ] PARK17 (VPS35)
- [ ] PARK18 (EIF4G1)
- [ ] PARK21 (TMEM230 or DNAJC13)
- [ ] PARK22 (CHCHD2)
- [ ] DCTN1: Perry syndrome
- [ ] NOTCH2NLC GCC repeat expansion

Autosomal recessive

- [ ] PARK2 (Parkin)
- [ ] PARK6 (PINK1)
- [ ] PARK7 (DJ1)
- [ ] PARK9 (ATP13A2): Kufor Rakeb
- [ ] PARK14 (PLA2G6)
- [ ] PARK15 (FBXO7)
- [ ] PARK19A and PARK19B (DNAJC6)
- [ ] PARK20 (SYNJ1)
- [ ] PARK23 (CPS13C)
- [ ] PTRHD1 (C2orf79): Parkinsonism with intellectual disability

X-linked

- [ ] PARK12
- [ ] RAB39B: X-linked parkinsonism with intellectual disability

Unclassified

- [ ] PARK10
- [ ] PARK16

Lysosomal storage disorders genes

- [ ] GBA1: Gaucher's disease
- [ ] SMPD1
- [ ] ATP13A2
- [ ] GALC

PARKINSON'S DISEASE (PD): BRADYKINESIA

Manifestations of bradykinesia

- [ ] Shuffling or festinant gait
- [ ] Reduced arm swing
- [ ] PD dysgraphia: this is slow handwriting with micrographia
- [ ] Difficulty turning over in bed
- [ ] Postural instability
- [ ] The Rolex sign: self-winding wrist watches stop working because of reduced arm movements

Facial bradykinesia

- [ ] Reduced spontaneous and voluntary facial expression (hypomimia)
- [ ] Wide palpebral fissures with a staring look
- [ ] Reduced blinking
- [ ] Reduced wrinkles around the eyes
- [ ] Open mouth
- [ ] Unable to make incongruous facial expressions
- [ ] Flattened nasolabial folds: they are deep in progressive supranuclear palsy (PSP)
- [ ] Dopamine responsive
- [ ] Symptoms improve in sleep

PARKINSON'S DISEASE (PD): RESTING TREMOR

Clinical types

- [ ] Pill rolling tremor
- [ ] Finger flexion-extension
- [ ] Finger abduction-adduction

Clinical features

- [ ] The tremor is rhythmic and alternating
- [ ] It is 'wrong-sided' in 4% of cases: contralateral to the more rigid side
- [ ] It may be voluntarily suppressed
- [ ] It is best examined with the hands completely prone and hanging down
- [ ] It may be dopamine responsive or resistant

Functional MRI features

- [ ] There is increased thalamic activity in dopamine-responsive tremor
- [ ] There is increased cerebellar activity in dopamine-resistant tremor

Differential diagnosis

- [ ] Scans without evidence of dopaminergic deficits (SWEDDS)
- [ ] Essential tremor (ET) with rest tremor
- [ ] Dystonic tremor
- [ ] Holmes tremor

Progression

- [ ] Tremor usually indicates a benign disease course
- [ ] It is less treatment-responsive than other PD motor symptoms
- [ ] It diminishes with disease progression

Other PD tremor types

- [ ] Pure or isolated postural tremor: this is not dopaminergic
- [ ] Re-emergent postural tremor
- [ ] Combined rest and postural/kinetic tremor
- [ ] Orthostatic tremor (OT)

PARKINSON'S DISEASE (PD): FREEZING OF GAIT

Types

- [ ] Start hesitation
- [ ] Turn hesitation
- [ ] Hesitation in tight corners
- [ ] Destination hesitation
- [ ] Open space hesitation
- [ ] Increased head-pelvis coupling during turning

Clinical patterns

- [ ] Tumbling in place
- [ ] Shuffling forward
- [ ] Total akinesia

Clinical features

- [ ] It is a sudden and brief inability to move forward
- [ ] This usually occurs during gait initiation or turning
- [ ] It is a late feature in idiopathic PD
- [ ] It is a risk factor for falling
- [ ] Walking improves at night if freezing is dopamine-induced
  - ( ) This is the sleep-benefit effect

Clinical assessment

- [ ] Observing the subject walking with quick, short steps
- [ ] Observing the subject turning rapidly

Strategies to treat freezing

- [ ] Paying attention to gait
- [ ] Increasing step amplitude
- [ ] Maintaining stepping rhythm
- [ ] Using lateral weight shifts
- [ ] Making wide turning arcs
- [ ] Using walking aids
- [ ] Using visual cues
- [ ] Exercise
- [ ] Adaptations to improve safety

Drug-treatments

- [ ] Rasagiline: this may reduce the risk of developing freezing of gait
- [ ] High-dose Levodopa: up to 1000 mg/day
- [ ] Consider addition of Amantadine: up to 600 mg/day

Treatment of co-morbidities

- [ ] Anxiety
- [ ] Depression
- [ ] Cognitive impairment

Other treatments

- [ ] Deep brain stimulation (DBS): it improves the speed of gait
- [ ] Intraduodenal Levodopa gel
- [ ] Apomorphine
- [ ] Electroconvulsive therapy (ECT)
- [ ] Transcranial magnetic stimulation (TMS)

PARKINSON'S DISEASE (PD): DIFFERENTIAL DIAGNOSIS

Parkinsonian differentials

- ☐ Vascular Parkinsonism
- ☐ Drug-induced Parkinsonism
- ☐ Dementia with Lewy bodies (DLB)
- ☐ Multiple system trophy (MSA)
- ☐ Progressive supranuclear palsy (PSP)

Tremor differentials

- ☐ Fragile X tremor ataxia syndrome (FXTAS)
- ☐ Scans without evidence of dopamine deficiency (SWEDDS)
- ☐ Essential tremor
- ☐ Adult onset dystonia: this may present with resting tremor

Structural differentials

- ☐ Giant midbrain or hemispheric perivascular spaces
- ☐ Sphenoid ridge meningiomas
- ☐ Frontoparietal meningiomas

Red flags against PD diagnosis

- ☐ Early falls
- ☐ Poor levodopa response
- ☐ Symmetry
- ☐ Lack of tremor
- ☐ Early autonomic dysfunction
- ☐ Preserved olfactory testing

Tests to differentiate PD from MSA: more impaired in MSA

- ☐ The bulbocavernosus reflex (BCR)
- ☐ Sphincter electromyogram (sphincter EMG)
- ☐ Post-void residual volume

Emerging differentiating tests of PD

- ☐ 3 Tesla diffusion tensor imaging (DTI)
  - ○ It may distinguish PD from MSA, PSP and essential tremor (ET)
- ☐ Submandibular gland biopsy: it shows α-synuclein
- ☐ Skin biopsy: it shows α-synuclein

PARKINSON'S DISEASE (PD): TREATMENT OF MOTOR FEATURES

Treatments to reduce off-time

- ☐ Levodopa
- ☐ Dopamine agonists (DA): Pramipexole, Ropinirole, Cabergoline
- ☐ Monoamine oxidase-B (MAO-B) inhibitors: Rasagiline, Selegiline, Safinamide
- ☐ Catechol-O-methyl transferase (COMT) inhibitors: Entacapone, Tolcapone, Opicapone
- ☐ Amantadine
- ☐ Apomorphine: intermittent or continuous subcutaneous injections
- ☐ Anticholinergics
- ☐ Continuous intestinal infusion of levodopa/Carbidopa (CIILC)
- ☐ Deep brain stimulation (DBS)

Treatment of tremor

- ☐ Exhaust routine motor treatment
- ☐ Rasagiline
- ☐ Beta blockers
- ☐ Gabapentin
- ☐ Clozapine
- ☐ Subcutaneous Apomorphine
- ☐ Surgery
- ☐ MRI-guided focused ultrasound thalamotomy

Treatment of postural deformities

- ☐ Levodopa
- ☐ Anticholinergics
- ☐ Baclofen
- ☐ Benzodiazepines
- ☐ Botulinum toxin
- ☐ Orthopaedic surgery
- ☐ Dystonia neurosurgery
- ☐ Istradefylline: it may also reduce off-time

Treatment of freezing of gait (FOG)

- ☐ Cueing training: auditory, visual, and somatosensory
- ☐ Cycling
- ☐ Laser equipment as cueing aids: shoes and rolling walkers
- ☐ Istradefylline

Acute alternatives to oral treatments

- ☐ Dispersible Levodopa
- ☐ Inhaled Levodopa
- ☐ Crushed immediate release dopamine agonists: Pramipexole, Ropinirole
- ☐ Nasogastric tube
- ☐ Gastrostomy
- ☐ Transdermal Rotigotine
- ☐ Subcutaneous Apomorphine

MULTIPLE SYSTEM ATROPHY (MSA): CLINICAL FEATURES

Motor subtypes

- ☐ MSA-C: Cerebellar predominant
- ☐ MSA-P: Parkinsonism predominant

Non-motor variants

- ☐ Isolated stridor
- ☐ REM sleep behaviour disorder (RBD)
- ☐ Early autonomic features
- ☐ Sudden death

Premotor symptoms

- ☐ Urgency and nocturia
- ☐ Erectile dysfunction (ED)
- ☐ Postural dizziness
- ☐ REM sleep behaviour disorder (RBD)
- ☐ Stridor

Motor features

- ☐ Pyramidal signs
- ☐ Jerky tremor
- ☐ Oculomotor abnormalities
- ☐ Rapid progression: wheelchair sign within 10 years
- ☐ Severe dysphonia and dysarthria
- ☐ Sighing

Dystonia

- ☐ Orofacial
- ☐ Laryngeal
- ☐ Antecollis: cervical dystonia
- ☐ Focal limb dystonia
- ☐ Writer's cramp
- ☐ Equinovarus foot
- ☐ Hand/feet contractures
- ☐ Camptocormia
- ☐ Pisa syndrome
- ☐ Levodopa-induced dystonia

Autonomic features

- ☐ Erectile dysfunction
- ☐ Orthostatic hypotension

Sleep-related features

- ☐ REM sleep behaviour disorder (RBD)
- ☐ Snoring
- ☐ Sleep apnoea
- ☐ Insomnia
- ☐ Daytime sleepiness

Other features

- ☐ Pathologic laughter and crying
- ☐ Cold hands and feet
- ☐ Restless legs syndrome (RLS)
- ☐ Cognitive impairment: possibly related to corpus callosum atrophy

MULTIPLE SYSTEM ATROPHY (MSA): INVESTIGATIONS

Magnetic resonance imaging (MRI)

- ☐ Hot cross bun sign
- ☐ Increased putaminal DWI ADC coefficient in MSA-P
- ☐ Increased putaminal iron in MSA-P
- ☐ MRI features may predate clinical diagnosis by up to 2 years

Transcranial ultrasound

- ☐ Hyperechogenic lenticular nuclei in Parkinson's plus
- ☐ Hyperechogenic substantia nigra in Parkinson's disease (PD)

Other brain imaging

- ☐ Dopamine receptor SPECT: reduced striatal binding in MSA and PSP
- ☐ Positron emission tomography (PET)
  - ○ Hypometabolism in basal ganglia (BG), brainstem, and cerebellum
- ☐ Brain perfusion SPECT: striatal hyperperfusion in MSA-P

Cardiac MIBG scintigraphy scan

- ☐ There is cardiac sympathetic denervation in PD
- ☐ This may however occasionally be seen in MSA

Sphincter electromyogram (EMG)

- ☐ This distinguishes MSA from PD in the first 5 years
- ☐ It does not distinguish MSA from progressive supranuclear palsy (PSP)

Bulbocavernosus reflex (BCR)

- ☐ This shows prolonged latency and low amplitude
- ☐ It may distinguish MSA from Parkinson's disease in the early stages

Optical coherence tomography (OCT): features

- ☐ Peripapillary retinal nerve fiber layer (RNFL) atrophy
  - ○ With relative preservation of the temporal sector of the RNFL
- ☐ Macular ganglion cell layer (GCL) complex atrophy: less severe than in PD

Other investigations

- ☐ Post void residual volume: this may be more appropriate than sphincter EMG
- ☐ COQ2 mutation: this may increase the risk of MSA-C
- ☐ Uric acid levels: high levels may limit MSA progression
- ☐ Positron emission tomography (PET): there is early and widespread microglial activation

PROGRESSIVE SUPRANUCLEAR PALSY (PSP): CLINICAL FEATURES

Domains clinically predictive of PSP

- ☐ Oculomotor dysfunction
- ☐ Postural instability
- ☐ Akinesia
- ☐ Cognitive dysfunction

Facial features

- ☐ Frontalis over-activity
- ☐ Staring, surprised, worried, or astonished appearance
- ☐ Procerus sign: vertical wrinkling of the forehead
  - ○ This is due to dystonia of the corrugator and orbicularis oculi muscles

Ophthalmic features

- ☐ Apraxia of eyelid opening
- ☐ Involuntary eyelid closure
- ☐ Loss of Bell's phenomenon
- ☐ Slow and infrequent blinking
- ☐ Blurred vision
- ☐ Dry eyes
- ☐ Slow vertical saccades
- ☐ Saccadic intrusions
- ☐ Vertical gaze palsy with 'round the houses' sign
- ☐ Photophobia

Postural and gait abnormalities

- ☐ The gait is lurching, stiff, and broad-based
- ☐ There is prominent postural instability and falls within the first year
- ☐ Falls are often backward: due to abnormal otolith reflexes and thalamic postural control
- ☐ There is associated retrocollis
- ☐ There may be associated orthostatic tremor

Bulbar features

- ☐ Dysphagia
- ☐ Low pitched dysarthria
- ☐ Freezing of swallowing (FOS)
- ☐ Central hypoventilation (Ondine's curse)
- ☐ Absent auditory blink and acoustic startle reflexes

Applause sign

- ☐ This is the inability to refrain from repeating an action: it is a sign of impaired motor control
- ☐ It is assessed by the three-clap test
- ☐ Reports are conflicting whether it distinguishes PSP from PD

Other features

- ☐ Early cognitive impairment: this occurs in 50% of cases
  - ○ It is present in 22% of early multiple system atrophy (MSA)
- ☐ Dirty tie phenomenon: due to sloppy eating
  - ○ This is a result of gaze palsy, poor hand coordination, and difficulty chewing
- ☐ Speech impairment: groaning, moaning, grunting, humming, growling speech
- ☐ Arm levitation

Poor prognostic markers

- ☐ Sleep disturbance
- ☐ Hallucinations

PROGRESSIVE SUPRANUCLEAR PALSY (PSP): DIFFERENTIAL DIAGNOSIS

Parkinson's disease (PD)

- ☐ Micrographia is decremental in PD: this is unlike in PSP

Corticobasal degeneration (CBD)

- ☐ Features are asymmetrical in CBD
- ☐ Apraxia is frequent in CBD
- ☐ There is associated alien limb phenomenon in CBD

Other Parkinsonian disorders

- ☐ Dementia with Lewy bodies (DLB): delusions are prominent
- ☐ Multiple system atrophy (MSA): the onset age is younger than in PSP
- ☐ Post encephalitic parkinsonism: oculogyric crises are characteristic
- ☐ Perry syndrome
- ☐ Kufor-Rakeb
- ☐ Gaucher's disease

Cognitive disorders

- ☐ Alzheimer's disease (AD)
- ☐ Frontotemporal lobar degeneration (FTLD)
- ☐ Prion disease

Mokri syndrome

- ☐ This is a PSP-like phenotype following aortic bypass surgery with deep hypothermia
- ☐ It presents with supranuclear gaze palsy in all cases
- ☐ There is dysarthria in 96% of cases
- ☐ About 80% have gait imbalance
- ☐ There are delayed seizures in 30% of cases
- ☐ The course is biphasic: initial latent and later progressive phases
- ☐ MRI may show mild atrophy of the midbrain tegmentum and frontal lobes

Other differentials

- ☐ Whipple's disease
- ☐ Niemann–Pick C (NPC) disease
- ☐ Subcortical gliosis
- ☐ Cerebrovascular disease (CVD)
- ☐ Pineal region tumours: they may present with a PSP phenotype

DEMENTIA WITH LEWY BODIES (DLB): CLINICAL FEATURES

Essential and core clinical features of DLB

- ☐ Dementia
- ☐ Fluctuating cognition
- ☐ Recurrent well-formed visual hallucinations
- ☐ REM sleep behaviour disorder (RBD) without atonia: in ¾ of confirmed cases
- ☐ Spontaneous Parkinsonism

Autonomic features

- ☐ Orthostatic hypotension
- ☐ Constipation
- ☐ Urinary incontinence

Psychiatric features

- ☐ Depression
- ☐ Complex systematised delusions
- ☐ Apathy
- ☐ Anxiety
- ☐ Hallucinations other than visual
- ☐ Complex illusions: reproducible by the pareidolia test
- ☐ Severe neuroleptic sensitivity

Corticobasal syndrome (CBS) presentation

- ☐ DLB with either progressive supranuclear palsy (PSP) or Alzheimer disease (AD)
- ☐ The age of onset is younger than in typical DLB
- ☐ There are more Lewy bodies in the motor cortex

Other supportive features

- ☐ Postural instability: causing repeated falls
- ☐ Syncope
- ☐ Transient loss of consciousness (TLOC)
- ☐ Hypersomnia
- ☐ Hyposmia
- ☐ Impaired colour discrimination: this predicts visual hallucinations
- ☐ Fluctuating level of daytime functioning
- ☐ Excessive daytime drowsiness
- ☐ Difficulty with daytime arousal and attention

Other features

- ☐ Supranuclear gaze palsy
- ☐ Akinetic crisis
- ☐ Rhinorrhoea: this is the runny nose sign

Old synonyms

- ☐ Diffuse Lewy body disease (DLBD)
- ☐ Lewy body dementia (LBD)
- ☐ Dementia associated with cortical Lewy bodies (DCLB)
- ☐ Lewy body variant of Alzheimer's disease (LBVAD)
- ☐ Senile dementia of Lewy body type (SDLT)

DEMENTIA WITH LEWY BODIES (DLB): INVESTIGATIONS

Indicative biomarkers of DLB

- ☐ Dopamine transporter (DaT) scan: this shows reduced caudate and posterior putamen binding
- ☐ MIBG myocardial scintigraphy: this shows low uptake
- ☐ Polysomnography: this shows REM sleep without atonia

Magnetic resonance imaging (MRI) brain: atrophic areas

- ☐ Amygdala
- ☐ Striatum
- ☐ Hypothalamus
- ☐ Dorsal midbrain
- ☐ Relatively preserved hippocampus and medial temporal lobes

Magnetic resonance imaging (MRI) brain: loss of swallow tail sign

- ☐ This is caused by loss of the nigrosome hyperintensity of the substantia nigra
- ☐ It is seen on MRI susceptibility weighted imaging (SWI)
- ☐ It is also seen in Parkinson's disease (PD)

Diffusion tensor imaging (DTI): increased diffusion areas

- ☐ Pericallosal
- ☐ Frontoparietal
- ☐ Occipital

Single photon emission and positron emission tomography (FP-CIT SPECT)

- ☐ This shows generalised low uptake
- ☐ There is decreased perfusion and glucose metabolism in parietal and occipital areas
- ☐ It has a sensitivity of 78% and a specificity of 90%

Electroencephalogram (EEG): features

- ☐ Prominent posterior slow-wave activity
- ☐ Early slowing of background activity
- ☐ Temporal lobe transient spikes
- ☐ Intermittent frontal delta activity

Other investigations

- ☐ Polysomnography

Emerging investigations

- ☐ Skin biopsy: this shows α-synuclein deposits
- ☐ GBA mutations: this is a risk factor for DLB in Spanish populations

CORTICOBASAL DEGENERATION (CBD): CLINICAL FEATURES

CBD phenotypes

- ☐ Corticobasal syndrome (CBS)
- ☐ Frontotemporal dementia (FTD)
- ☐ Progressive supranuclear palsy (PSP)
- ☐ Posterior cortical atrophy (PCA)
- ☐ Frontal behavioural-spatial syndrome (FBS)
- ☐ Nonfluent/agrammatic variant of primary progressive aphasia (naPPA)
- ☐ Progressive supranuclear palsy (PSP)

Parkinsonian features

- ☐ Asymmetric onset
- ☐ Akinetic rigidity
- ☐ Tremor
- ☐ Mild and transient Levodopa-responsiveness

Other movement disorders

- ☐ Unilateral clumsy, stiff, or jerky arm
- ☐ Fixed dystonic posturing of the arm
- ☐ Apraxia
- ☐ Myoclonus
- ☐ Gait instability: falls occur in about a third of cases

Cortical features

- ☐ Hemineglect
- ☐ Frontal release signs
- ☐ Alien limb
- ☐ Cortical sensory loss

Behavioural features

- ☐ Apathy
- ☐ Antisocial behaviour
- ☐ Irritability
- ☐ Disinhibition
- ☐ Hypersexuality

Speech and language features

- ☐ Aphasia
- ☐ Apraxia of speech
- ☐ Dysarthria

Fulminant or rapidly progressive CBD (RP-CBD)

- ☐ This manifests with rapid progression over a mean of 2.5 years
- ☐ There is severe nigral cell loss and heavy tau load
- ☐ There is mild TDP-43 pathology in some cases

Other features

- ☐ Cognitive impairment
- ☐ Supranuclear ophthalmoplegia
- ☐ Pyramidal features
- ☐ Agrypnia excitata: insomnia and autonomic overactivity

CORTICOBASAL DEGENERATION (CBD): DIAGNOSIS

Atypical presentations of CBD

- [ ] Rapid progression
- [ ] Asymmetrical tremulous-parkinsonism with early postural instability
- [ ] Progressive non-fluent aphasia
- [ ] Behavioural variant frontotemporal dementia

Differential diagnoses

- [ ] Progressive supranuclear palsy (PSP): vertical gaze palsy
- [ ] Multiple system atrophy (MSA): severe autonomic dysfunction
- [ ] Parkinson's disease (PD): rest tremor and levodopa responsiveness
- [ ] Alzheimer's disease (AD): early dementia
- [ ] Frontotemporal degeneration (FTD)
- [ ] Cerebrotendinous xanthomatosis (CTX)
- [ ] Gaucher's disease

Diagnostic criteria for probable CBD

- [ ] Insidious onset of typical phenotypes
- [ ] Gradual progression for at least 1 year
- [ ] Onset age ≥50 years
- [ ] Absent family history
- [ ] No known tau mutations, e.g. MAPT

Diagnostic criteria for possible CBD

- [ ] These are the same as for probable CBD but additionally:
- [ ] There is no age or family history limitation to the criteria
- [ ] Tau mutations are permitted by the criteria
- [ ] The criteria allow for a PSP phenotype

Pathology

- [ ] It is a tauopathy
- [ ] Astrogliopathy is the earliest stage

Levodopa responsiveness

- [ ] This is positive in some patients
- [ ] Use 50/200 mg of Carbidopa/Levodopa three times a day for ≥2 months
- [ ] The response should last ≥1 year

Dystonia

DYT1: EARLY ONSET PRIMARY DYSTONIA

Genetics

- ☐ This is caused by mutations in the DYT1 (TOR1A) gene on chromosome 9
- ☐ It is a GAG deletion
- ☐ The transmission is autosomal dominant with reduced penetrance
- ☐ The gene product is Torsin A

Demographic features

- ☐ It is most prevalent in Ashkenazi Jews
- ☐ The mean onset age is 12 years
- ☐ Late onset cases may present: after the age of 26 years

Dystonia phenotypes

- ☐ Limb onset
- ☐ Cervical dystonia
- ☐ Cranial dystonia
- ☐ Spasmodic dysphonia
- ☐ Writer's cramp

Dystonia features

- ☐ It usually presents as pure dystonia
- ☐ Subsequent generalisation occurs in about 50% of cases
  - ○ This is unlike adult onset idiopathic dystonia
- ☐ There may be associated increased risky behaviour

Differential diagnosis

- ☐ Parkinson's disease (PD)

Treatment

- ☐ Anti-cholinergics
- ☐ Levodopa
- ☐ Benzodiazepines
- ☐ Botulinum toxin
- ☐ Pallidal deep brain stimulation (DBS)

Synonyms

- ☐ Early onset torsion dystonia
- ☐ Oppenheim's dystonia

DYT5: DOPA-RESPONSIVE DYSTONIA (DRD): CLINICAL FEATURES

Genetics

- ☐ This is caused by mutations in the GTP cyclohydrolase 1 (GTPCH1) gene on chromosome 14
- ☐ More than 100 mutations have been described
- ☐ Point mutations occur in 54% of cases and deletions in 8%
- ☐ The transmission is autosomal dominant

Pathology

- ☐ GTPCH1 is required for synthesis of tetrahydrobiopterin (BH4)
- ☐ The pathology results from partial deficiency of tetrahydrobiopterin (BH4)
- ☐ BH4 deficiency causes tyrosine hydroxylase deficiency at dopamine neuron terminals

Epidemiology

- ☐ Onset is usually in the first decade: it typically starts around the age of 6 years
- ☐ There is a female preponderance but adult onset cases are more often males

Features of limb dystonia

- ☐ Asymmetric postural limb dystonia is often the first presentation
- ☐ It manifests as pes equinovarus
- ☐ It spreads to other limbs over 10–15 years
- ☐ It becomes less progressive with age
- ☐ There is diurnal variation: dystonic gait develops in the afternoon
- ☐ Diurnal fluctuation diminishes with age

Features of postural tremor

- ☐ Postural tremor is often the first feature of adult onset cases
- ☐ It worsens and spreads
- ☐ Levodopa may prevent tremor developing

Other dystonic features

- ☐ Writer's cramp
- ☐ Spasmodic dysphonia

DOI: 10.1201/9781003221258-25

Associated clinical features

- ☐ Short stature with early onset cases
- ☐ Psychomotor delay
- ☐ Parkinsonism
- ☐ Tremor
- ☐ Restless legs syndrome (RLS)
- ☐ Gait instability
- ☐ Ptosis
- ☐ Hypotonia
- ☐ Incoordination
- ☐ Obsessive compulsive disorder (OCD)
- ☐ Recurrent depression
- ☐ Recurrent tendonitis
- ☐ Sleep disorders: excessive sleep, nightmares, and difficult sleep onset

Synonym

- ☐ Segawa syndrome

DYT8: PAROXYSMAL NON-KINESIGENIC DYSKINESIA 1 (PNKD1)

Genetics and epidemiology

- ☐ This is caused by mutations in the myofibrillo-genesis regulator 1 (MR1) gene on chromosome 2
- ☐ The transmission is autosomal dominant
- ☐ Onset may be in infancy, childhood, or adult age

Major features

- ☐ Premonitory sensation of muscle tightening
- ☐ Attacks of dystonia and chorea
- ☐ Dystonic posturing of the limbs
- ☐ Improvement of symptoms in pregnancy

Characteristics of dystonic episodes

- ☐ They affect the limbs, face, jaw, tongue, and trunk
- ☐ They may be spontaneous or triggered
- ☐ They occur weekly or more often
- ☐ They usually last 10–60 minutes but they may go on for several hours
- ☐ They may cause dysarthria and dysphagia
- ☐ They may be followed by brief periods of sleep

Triggers for episodes

- ☐ Fatigue
- ☐ Coffee
- ☐ Alcohol
- ☐ Stress
- ☐ Nicotine
- ☐ Excitement
- ☐ Hunger
- ☐ Spontaneous
- ☐ They are not triggered by exercise: unlike in DYT9

Associated features

- ☐ Migraine: this is present in about 50% of cases
- ☐ Spastic paraparesis
- ☐ Myokymia

Treatment

- ☐ Clonazepam
- ☐ Diazepam
- ☐ Haloperidol
- ☐ Anticholinergics

Synonym

- ☐ Paroxysmal dystonic choreoathetosis (PDC)

DYT11: MYOCLONUS DYSTONIA: CLINICAL FEATURES

Clinical patterns

- ☐ Early childhood onset myoclonus/dystonia involving the upper body
- ☐ Early childhood onset dystonia involving the lower limbs
  - ○ This progresses to myoclonus and upper body involvement
- ☐ Later childhood onset myoclonus/dystonia involving the upper body with cervical involvement

Demographic features

- ☐ The onset age is from childhood to early adolescence
- ☐ It usually starts before the age of 26 years: the age range is 1–16 years
- ☐ It has a progressive course before stabilisation

Features of myoclonus

- ☐ Myoclonus is usually in the proximal limbs and upper body
- ☐ It is lightening-like
- ☐ It may occur at rest
- ☐ It may be provoked by writing and drawing
- ☐ There is alcohol responsiveness in some cases
- ☐ Laryngeal myoclonus is occasionally associated

Features of dystonia

- ☐ Torticollis
- ☐ Laterocollis
- ☐ Axial dystonia
- ☐ Writer's cramp
- ☐ Foot dystonia
- ☐ Falls
- ☐ Alcohol-induced dystonia
- ☐ Facial tics

Psychiatric features

- ☐ Generalised anxiety disorder
- ☐ Depression
- ☐ Phobias
- ☐ Obsessive-compulsive disorder
- ☐ Psychosis
- ☐ Alcohol dependence
- ☐ Substance abuse
- ☐ Cognitive dysfunction

Other features

- ☐ Short stature
- ☐ Joint laxity
- ☐ Microcephaly
- ☐ Association with Russell Silver dwarfism

Differential diagnosis

- ☐ Parkinson's disease (PD)
- ☐ Opsoclonus myoclonus syndrome (OMS)

Synonym

- ☐ Myoclonic dystonia-11

DYT12: RAPID ONSET DYSTONIA-PARKINSONISM (RDP)

Genetics

- ☐ This is caused by mutations in the ATP1A3 (alpha 3 subunit of Na/K ATPase) gene
- ☐ This is on chromosome 19
- ☐ The transmission is autosomal dominant

Other ATP1A3 spectrum disorders

- ☐ Alternating hemiplegia of childhood (AHC)
- ☐ CAPOS syndrome
- ☐ Early infantile epileptic encephalopathy (EIEE)
- ☐ Fever-induced paroxysmal weakness and encephalopathy
- ☐ Paroxysmal asymmetric dystonic arm posturing

RPD overlap syndromes

- ☐ RPD-AHC
- ☐ AHC-CAPOS
- ☐ RPD-AHC-CAPOS

Onset age features

- ☐ The onset is from childhood to early adult age
- ☐ The onset age range is 8–55 years
- ☐ Infantile onset cases present with developmental delay, hypotonia, and ataxia
- ☐ The onset may be slow

Clinical features

- ☐ There is a vague prodrome of limb dystonia, dysphonia, and dysarthria
- ☐ Onset of generalised dystonia is within minutes to days
- ☐ Severe disability develops within days to weeks
- ☐ Symptoms spread rostro-caudally: face to arms to legs
- ☐ The clinical course subsequently stabilizes but later exacerbations may occur
- ☐ Bulbar symptoms may be prominent: dysarthria, dysphagia, and dysphonia

Triggers

- ☐ Psychological/emotional stress
- ☐ Fever
- ☐ Childbirth
- ☐ Exercise
- ☐ Alcohol

Other features

- ☐ Parkinsonism without tremor at onset
- ☐ Seizures
- ☐ Depression
- ☐ Social phobia
- ☐ Poor levodopa-responsiveness
- ☐ Electrocardiogram abnormalities

Acronym

- ☐ CAPOS: cerebellar ataxia, areflexia, pes cavus, optic atrophy, and sensorineural hearing loss

CERVICAL DYSTONIA: CLINICAL FEATURES

General features

- [ ] This may be isolated or part of a generalised dystonia
- [ ] The dystonia may be tonic, clonic, or tremulous

Postural cervical deformities

- [ ] Rotatory torticollis (rotatocollis) in about 80% of cases
- [ ] Anterocollis
- [ ] Retrocollis
- [ ] Laterocollis
- [ ] Combinations: these occur in more than two-thirds of cases

Associated dystonias

- [ ] Oromandibular dystonia
- [ ] Blepharospasm
- [ ] Writer's cramp
- [ ] Upper limb dystonias

Associated features

- [ ] Scoliosis
- [ ] Head tremor
- [ ] Laryngeal dystonia

Geste antagoniste (alleviating manouevres)

- [ ] These are sensory tricks that resolve the dystonia
- [ ] These include touching the chin, lower face, the back, or the top of the head
- [ ] Voluntary tonic eye deviation may also serve as a sensory trick
- [ ] It does not work if someone else touches these parts
- [ ] It will however work if the subject uses someone else's limb to touch the chin
  - ○ This is 'closing the loop' sign

Complications

- [ ] Local pain
- [ ] Cervical radiculopathy: in about a third of cases
- [ ] Contractures
- [ ] Myelopathy
- [ ] Anxiety and depression

Differential diagnosis

- [ ] Atlanto-axial dislocation
- [ ] C2-C3 rotatory dislocation
- [ ] Tics
- [ ] Psychogenic
- [ ] Tardive dyskinesia
- [ ] Parkinson's disease (PD)
- [ ] Wilson's disease
- [ ] Abnormal neck anatomy

Outcome

- [ ] Rapid deterioration occurs in most cases in the first 5 years
- [ ] A period of stabilisation follows
- [ ] Spontaneous remission occurs in about 25% of cases
  - ○ This is especially in younger patients in the first year
- [ ] Symptoms often recur within 5 years of remission

CERVICAL DYSTONIA: MANAGEMENT

Palliative manoeuvres

- [ ] Sensory tricks (geste antagoniste)
- [ ] Leaning against high backed chair
- [ ] Putting something in the mouth
- [ ] Pulling the hair
- [ ] Relaxation
- [ ] Avoiding fatigue and stress

Oral treatment

- [ ] Clonazepam
- [ ] Diazepam
- [ ] Baclofen
- [ ] Anticholinergic drugs: Diphenhydramine
- [ ] Tetrabenazine ± Lithium

Chemo-denervation

- [ ] Botulinum toxin
- [ ] Phenol
- [ ] Alcohol

Deep brain stimulation (DBS)

- [ ] This targets the globus pallidus internus (GPi) or subthalamic nucleus (STN)
- [ ] It is usually done bilaterally
- [ ] It is safe and effective
- [ ] It may rarely cause akinesia and freezing of gait
- [ ] There is a risk of speech and swallowing difficulties

Surgical treatment

- [ ] Intrathecal Baclofen
- [ ] Selective peripheral denervation: upper cervical dorsal ramisectomy
- [ ] Microvascular decompression: of the posterior inferior cerebellar artery (PICA)

Other treatments

- [ ] Supportive therapy
- [ ] Counselling
- [ ] Physical therapy

WILSON'S DISEASE: NEUROLOGICAL FEATURES

Dystonic features

- ☐ Fixed forced smile (risus sardonicus)
- ☐ Excessive grinning to mild stimuli
- ☐ Sustained open-mouth smile (vacuous smile)
- ☐ Tremor
- ☐ Wing-beating or flapping tremor

Associated movement disorders

- ☐ Action tremor
- ☐ Parkinsonism
- ☐ Ataxia
- ☐ Choreoathetosis
- ☐ Myoclonus: this may be the first presentation
- ☐ Stereotypies
- ☐ Tics
- ☐ Restless legs syndrome (RLS)

Associated neurological features

- ☐ Dysarthria
- ☐ Drooling
- ☐ Pyramidal signs: this is usually without weakness
- ☐ Pseudobulbar palsy
- ☐ Seizures: this is usually after starting treatment
- ☐ Migraine
- ☐ Dysautonomia
- ☐ Acute stroke-like presentation
- ☐ Myopathy with cramps
- ☐ Neuroleptic hypersensitivity
- ☐ Cognitive impairment

Ophthalmic features

- ☐ Kayser-Fleischer (KF) rings
- ☐ Sunflower cataracts
- ☐ Slow saccades
- ☐ Impaired up-gaze
- ☐ Impaired vertical pursuits
- ☐ Strabismus without nystagmus

Psychiatric features

- ☐ Personality change
- ☐ Irritability and emotionality
- ☐ Anxiety and depression
- ☐ Impulsivity and disinhibition
- ☐ Reckless behaviour
- ☐ Substance abuse
- ☐ Catatonia
- ☐ Mania
- ☐ Acute psychosis

Clinical features related to Zinc therapy

- ☐ Peripheral neuropathy (PN)
- ☐ Myelodysplastic syndrome

WILSON'S DISEASE: MANAGEMENT

Treatment phases

- ☐ Initial therapy
- ☐ Maintenance therapy
- ☐ Pre-symptomatic treatment

Penicillamine: dosing

- ☐ The starting dose is 250 mg four times a day or 500 mg twice a day
- ☐ It is used with Pyridoxine
- ☐ Paradoxical neurological worsening may occur: this is usually within 4 weeks
- ☐ This may be prevented with a low starting dose

Penicillamine: complications

- ☐ Nephrotoxicity
- ☐ Systemic lupus erythematosus (SLE)
- ☐ Pancytopaenia
- ☐ Acute hypersensitivity reaction
- ☐ Elastosis perforans serpiginosa (skin rash)

Trientine

- ☐ 750–1500 mg in two or three divided doses daily
- ☐ 750 mg to 1000 mg for maintenance therapy
- ☐ This is taken 1 hour before or 2 hours after meals
- ☐ There is a risk of paradoxical neurological worsening on initiation
  - ○ Possibly due to toxic effect of mobilised free copper
- ☐ There is a risk of bone marrow toxicity

Zinc acetate

- ☐ This is usually indicated for maintenance therapy
- ☐ It induces intestinal cell metallothionein
- ☐ The dose is 50 mg three times a day
- ☐ It takes 4–8 months for response
- ☐ It may cause gastric discomfort
- ☐ It is less effective than Trientene but it has a safer side effect profile
- ☐ It is safe in pregnancy
- ☐ It does not cause neurological worsening
- ☐ Urinary copper is accurate for monitoring: Zinc does not induce urinary excretion

Liver transplantation: indications

- ☐ Decompensated liver disease
- ☐ Acute liver failure (fulminant Wilson's disease)

Other treatments

- ☐ Adjunctive vitamin E
- ☐ Avoid high copper foods: liver, shellfish
- ☐ Ammonium tetrathiomolybdate: this is an experimental therapy

Precautions in pregnancy and surgery

- ☐ Reduce the doses of Penicillamine and Trientine
- ☐ This is to promote wound healing

Tremor

TREMORS: MEDICAL CAUSES

Dystonic tremor: causes

- ☐ Wilson's disease
- ☐ Fragile X tremor ataxia syndrome (FXTAS)
- ☐ Task-specific tremor

Other primary tremor disorders

- ☐ Essential tremor
- ☐ Orthostatic tremor
- ☐ Oculopalatal tremor
- ☐ Palatal tremor

Tremors with neurological disorders

- ☐ Parkinsonian tremor
- ☐ Neuropathic tremor
- ☐ Holmes tremor
- ☐ Cerebellar tremor
- ☐ Spinocerebellar ataxia (SCA)
- ☐ Post-encephalitic tremor
- ☐ Familial cortical-myoclonic tremor with epilepsy (FCMTE)
- ☐ Kennedy disease (X-linked bulbar and spinal muscular atrophy; SBMA)

Metabolic tremors

- ☐ Thyrotoxicosis: it may present with abdominal tremor
- ☐ Hyperparathyroidism
- ☐ Hypocalcaemia
- ☐ Hypomagnesaemia
- ☐ Hyponatraemia
- ☐ Hypoglycaemia

Toxin-induced tremors

- ☐ Mercury
- ☐ Lead
- ☐ Arsenic
- ☐ Bismuth

Other tremors

- ☐ Physiological tremor
- ☐ Psychogenic tremor

ESSENTIAL TREMOR (ET): TREMOR FEATURES

Demographic features

- ☐ The median onset age is 15 years
- ☐ It has an equal sex distribution
- ☐ A family history is absent in >50% of cases
- ☐ Family history is less likely in childhood and late-onset ET

Postural limb tremor features

- ☐ Bilateral action tremor
- ☐ Flexion-extension
- ☐ Asymmetrical

Head tremor features

- ☐ Most cases are 'no-no' type
- ☐ This is more likely to develop in females
- ☐ It does not spread caudally from the head

Alcohol sensitivity

- ☐ The tremor-relieving effect of alcohol lasts about 3 hours
- ☐ It is more likely with early-onset ET[5]
- ☐ The tremor rebounds afterwards

Other tremor features

- ☐ Intention tremor
- ☐ Facial tremor
- ☐ Jaw tremor
- ☐ Voice tremor
- ☐ Tongue tremor
- ☐ Impaired tandem walk

Red flags against essential tremor diagnosis

- ☐ Gait disturbance
- ☐ Focal tremor
- ☐ Sudden or rapid onset
- ☐ Isolated head tremor with dystonic posturing
- ☐ Leg tremor
- ☐ Unilateral rest tremor
- ☐ Bradykinesia
- ☐ Use of tremor-inducing drugs
- ☐ Re-emergent tremor

Predictors of fast progression

- ☐ Older onset age
- ☐ Older age
- ☐ Isolated limb tremor without associated head tremor

DOI: 10.1201/9781003221258-26

ESSENTIAL TREMOR (ET): NON-TREMOR FEATURES

Non-motor features

- [ ] Cognitive impairment
- [ ] Anxiety
- [ ] Depression
- [ ] Social phobias
- [ ] Olfactory deficits
- [ ] Hearing loss
- [ ] High frailty scores in elderly patients
- [ ] Enfeeblement: being prematurely old, helpless, or debilitated

Parkinsonian features

- [ ] Parkinsonism may develop subsequent to the diagnosis of essential tremor
- [ ] This relationship is more than would be expected by chance
- [ ] This is usually as Parkinson's disease (PD)
- [ ] It may manifest as progressive supranuclear palsy (PSP)
- [ ] Essential tremor may also present with resting tremor

Magnetic resonance imaging (MRI) brain: features

- [ ] There are white matter ultrastructural abnormalities on diffusion tensor images (DTI)
- [ ] These are especially in the cerebellar peduncles
- [ ] They are also prominent in the thalamo-cortical visual pathways

ESSENTIAL TREMOR (ET): DRUG TREATMENT

Level A: established effective

- [ ] Propranolol
- [ ] Primidone

Level B: probably effective

- [ ] Topiramate: this is as effective as Propranolol and Primidone at doses >200 mg daily
- [ ] Alprazolam
- [ ] Atenolol
- [ ] Gabapentin
- [ ] Sotalol

Level C: possibly effective

- [ ] Nadolol
- [ ] Nimodipine
- [ ] Clonazepam

Level U: insufficient evidence

- [ ] Pregabalin
- [ ] Zonisamide
- [ ] Clozapine
- [ ] Clonidine

Ineffective

- [ ] Levetiracetam
- [ ] Flunarizine
- [ ] Amantadine
- [ ] Mirtazapine

Absolute contraindications to beta blockers

- [ ] Moderate to severe asthma
- [ ] Significant bradykinesia or heart block
- [ ] Symptomatic hypotension
- [ ] End stage heart failure
- [ ] Concurrent calcium channel blockers: Diltiazem or Verapamil

Relative contraindications to beta blockers

- [ ] Chronic obstructive pulmonary disease (COPD)
- [ ] Depression
- [ ] Diabetes mellitus
- [ ] Erectile dysfunction

Ataxia

FRIEDREICH'S ATAXIA (FA): CLINICAL FEATURES

Genetics

- [ ] This is caused by mutations in the FRDA gene on chromosome 9q13
- [ ] The transmission is autosomal recessive
- [ ] It is a GAA trinucleotide repeat expansion disease
- [ ] The repeat size correlates with disease severity
- [ ] There is reduced frataxin expression

Sites of pathology

- [ ] Dorsal root ganglia (DRG)
- [ ] Posterior columns
- [ ] Corticospinal tracts
- [ ] Heart

Onset age and types

- [ ] Classical onset age is <20 years: the range is 2–51 years
- [ ] Very young onset age: this is associated with p.C282Y heterozygosity
- [ ] Late-onset Friedreich's ataxia (LOFA): onset age is >25 years
- [ ] Very late onset Friedreich's ataxia (VLOFA): onset age is >40 years

Neurological features

- [ ] Progressive ataxia
- [ ] Dysarthria
- [ ] Spastic paraparesis
- [ ] Sensory peripheral neuropathy (PN)
- [ ] Reduced reflexes with extensor plantar responses
- [ ] Acardian variant: slow progression with no diabetes or cardiac involvement

Ophthalmic features

- [ ] Reduced visual acuity
- [ ] Optic atrophy occasionally
- [ ] Nystagmus
- [ ] Abnormal saccades
- [ ] Vestibular dysfunction
- [ ] Deafness rarely

Systemic features

- [ ] Diabetes mellitus
- [ ] Hypertrophic cardiomyopathy: this is the main determinant of prognosis
- [ ] Pes cavus
- [ ] Scoliosis
- [ ] Sudomotor dysfunction: reduced sweating
- [ ] Lower urinary tract symptoms (LUTS)
- [ ] Urinary sphincter disturbance
- [ ] Bladder dysfunction
- [ ] Sexual dysfunction

Magnetic resonance imaging (MRI)

- [ ] Atrophy: spinal cord, superior cerebellar peduncles, and cerebral grey and white matter
- [ ] Increased iron in the dentate nuclei

DOI: 10.1201/9781003221258-27

FRIEDREICH'S ATAXIA (FA): MONITORING

Annual surveillance

- ☐ Electrocardiogram (ECG)
- ☐ 24-hour ECG: if there are palpitations
- ☐ Echocardiogram
- ☐ Blood glucose
- ☐ Oral glucose tolerance test
  - ○ HbA1C is not sensitive as diabetes may present acutely
- ☐ Audiology assessment
- ☐ Epworth Sleepiness Scale (ESS): for sleep disordered breathing

Scoliosis screening

- ☐ This is carried out between the ages of 10 and 16 years
- ☐ It is also indicated if there is spinal curvature of 20–40 degrees

Friedreich's ataxia monitoring scales

- ☐ International Cooperative Ataxia Rating Scale (ICARS)
- ☐ Friedreich Ataxia Rating Scale (FARS)
- ☐ Scale for the Assessment and Rating of Ataxia (SARA)

Indications for cardiology referral

- ☐ Cardiac symptoms
- ☐ Abnormal cardiac tests
- ☐ Before major surgery
- ☐ Pregnancy

FRIEDREICH'S ATAXIA (FA): TREATMENT

Treatment of spasticity

- ☐ Baclofen
- ☐ Tizanidine
- ☐ Benzodiazepines
- ☐ Dantrolene
- ☐ Gabapentin
- ☐ Botulinum toxin

Treatment of neuropathic pain

- ☐ Gabapentin
- ☐ Pregabalin
- ☐ Lamotrigine
- ☐ Amitriptyline
- ☐ Duloxetine

Treatment of square wave jerks and ocular flutter

- ☐ Memantine
- ☐ Acetazolamide
- ☐ Aminopyridine
- ☐ Clonazepam
- ☐ Gabapentin
- ☐ Ondansetron

Treatment of cardiomyopathy

- ☐ Cardiac transplantation

Management in pregnancy

- ☐ Glucose tolerance test between 24–28 weeks
- ☐ Heparin for deep vein thrombosis (not Warfarin)

Multidisciplinary care

- ☐ Physical therapy: for balance and strength maintenance
- ☐ Occupational therapy
- ☐ Speech and language therapy: for dysarthria and dysphagia
- ☐ Orthotics for protective foot care
- ☐ Ankle foot orthotic devices (AFOs)

Potential and investigational treatments

- ☐ Coenzyme Q10 (CoQ10) with vitamin E
- ☐ Idebenone
- ☐ Mitoquinone (MitoQ)
- ☐ Erythropoietin (EPO)
- ☐ Chelation therapy: Deferiprone
- ☐ EPI-A0001: RAID program
- ☐ HDAC inhibitors
- ☐ PPAR gamma agonists
- ☐ Varenicline
- ☐ Omaveloxolone

SPINOCEREBELLAR ATAXIA TYPE 1 (SCA 1)

Genetics

- [ ] This is caused by mutations in the ataxin 1 (ATXN1) gene on chromosome 6p
- [ ] It is a CAG trinucleotide repeat expansion disease
- [ ] >39 repeats are pathogenic
- [ ] Juvenile onset occurs with >70 repeats
- [ ] The transmission is autosomal dominant
- [ ] Onset age is in the fourth decade

Central features

- [ ] Limb ataxia
- [ ] Dysarthria
- [ ] Dysphagia
- [ ] Nystagmus
- [ ] Hypometric saccades
- [ ] Ophthalmoplegia
- [ ] Cognitive impairment in later stages
- [ ] Bulbar dysfunction terminally
- [ ] Mild optic neuropathy

Dystonic features

- [ ] Blepharospasm
- [ ] Oromandibular dystonia
- [ ] Retrocollis
- [ ] Writer's cramp

Peripheral features

- [ ] Peripheral neuropathy (PN)
- [ ] Hyporeflexia
- [ ] Proprioceptive loss

Pathology

- [ ] Ubiquitin inclusions
- [ ] Purkinje cell atrophy
- [ ] Degeneration of dentate nucleus, inferior olive, pons, and red nucleus
- [ ] Degeneration of oculomotor, vagus, and hypoglossal nuclei

Magnetic resonance imaging (MRI) brain

- [ ] Olivopontocerebellar atrophy: but this is less severe than in SCA2
- [ ] Preserved putamen and caudate: unlike in SCA3
- [ ] The hot cross bun sign has been reported

SPINOCEREBELLAR ATAXIA TYPE 2 (SCA2)

Genetics

- [ ] This is caused by mutations in the Ataxin 2 (ATXN2) gene on chromosome 12
- [ ] It is a polyQ CAG repeat disorder
- [ ] Normal repeat number is between 15–24
- [ ] >35 repeats are pathogenic but a case with 31 repeats has been reported
- [ ] The transmission is autosomal dominant
- [ ] Onset is in the third to fourth decades

Ataxic features

- [ ] Ataxia
- [ ] Ophthalmoplegia
- [ ] Slow saccades
- [ ] Dysarthria

Other movement disorders

- [ ] Parkinsonism: with shorter repeat expansions
  - ( ) This may be the presenting feature
- [ ] Dystonia: lower cranial, jaw, and tongue
- [ ] Chorea

Peripheral nerve features

- [ ] Sensory neuronopathy
- [ ] Axonal peripheral neuropathy (PN)

Magnetic resonance imaging (MRI) brain

- [ ] Severe olivopontocerebellar atrophy

SPINOCEREBELLAR ATAXIA TYPE 3 (SCA3): CLINICAL FEATURES

Genetics

- ☐ This is caused by mutations in the ataxin 3 (ATXN3, MDJ1) gene on chromosome 14q
- ☐ It is a CAG polyglutamine repeat expansion disease
- ☐ The mutation causes a toxic gain of function
- ☐ The transmission is autosomal dominant
- ☐ SCA3 may also be associated with C9orf72 gene mutations
- ☐ The APOE ε2 allele may reduce the age of onset of SCA3

Types

- ☐ Type 1: Early onset with spasticity and dystonia
- ☐ Type 2: Pure cerebellar ataxia
- ☐ Type 3: Late onset with peripheral neuropathy

Ophthalmic features

- ☐ Ophthalmoplegia
- ☐ Bulging eyes
- ☐ Gaze-evoked nystagmus
- ☐ Upward gaze palsy
- ☐ Saccadic intrusions and oscillations: including pinball intrusions
- ☐ Square wave jerks
- ☐ Impaired vestibulo-ocular reflex: this is related to repeat length
- ☐ Optic atrophy

Central neurological features

- ☐ Limb and gait ataxia
- ☐ Postural instability
- ☐ Tremor
- ☐ Dystonia
- ☐ Spasticity
- ☐ Parkinsonism
- ☐ Cognitive dysfunction
- ☐ Palatal myoclonus
- ☐ Writer's cramps: this may be isolated without ataxia

Peripheral neurological features

- ☐ Peripheral neuropathy (PN)
- ☐ Widespread fasciculations
- ☐ Areflexia
- ☐ Distal atrophy
- ☐ Flexion contractures
- ☐ Chronic pain
- ☐ Autonomic dysfunction
- ☐ Weight loss
- ☐ Premature death

Differential diagnosis

- ☐ Spinocerebellar ataxia type 2 (SCA2)
- ☐ Hereditary spastic paraparesis (HSP)

Synonym

- ☐ Machado Joseph disease

SPINOCEREBELLAR ATAXIA TYPE 6 (SCA6)

Genetics

- ☐ This is caused by CAG repeat expansions on chromosome 19
- ☐ Normal repeat size is 4–15 CAG repeats: 21–28 repeats are pathogenic
- ☐ The transmission is autosomal dominant
- ☐ The mean onset age is 50 years

CACNA1A mutation associated disorders

- ☐ Familial hemiplegic migraine type 1 (FHM1)
- ☐ Episodic ataxia type 2 (EA2)

Cerebellar features

- ☐ Gait ataxia
- ☐ Dysarthria
- ☐ Dysmetria
- ☐ Perverted head shaking nystagmus
- ☐ Hypotonia

Other features

- ☐ Episodic headache and nausea
- ☐ Dysphagia
- ☐ Spasticity
- ☐ Peripheral neuropathy (PN)
- ☐ Parkinsonism
- ☐ Dystonic posturing
- ☐ Involuntary movements
- ☐ Co-existence with EA2

Investigations

- ☐ Magnetic resonance imaging (MRI) brain: this shows isolated cerebellar atrophy
- ☐ Pathology: this shows neuronal loss and aggregates in the neocortex and basal ganglia

SPINOCEREBELLAR ATAXIA TYPE 7 (SCA7)

Genetics

- ☐ This is caused by mutations in the ATXN7 (Ataxin 7) gene on chromosome 3p
- ☐ There are CAG repeat expansions with prominent anticipation
- ☐ 44–85 repeats are pathogenic
- ☐ The transmission is autosomal dominant
- ☐ The phenotypes range from asymptomatic to severe

Clinical features

- ☐ Ataxia
- ☐ Explosive speech
- ☐ Spasticity
- ☐ Impaired colour vision
- ☐ Central scotoma
- ☐ Macular visual loss
- ☐ Pigmentary retinopathy
- ☐ Cranio-cervical dystonia
- ☐ Unstable sustained vowel phonation

Magnetic resonance imaging (MRI) brain

- ☐ Cerebellar and pontine atrophy
- ☐ White matter degeneration: this is seen on tract-based studies

EPISODIC ATAXIA TYPE 1 (EA1)

Genetic mutations

- ☐ KCNA1 gene mutations: there are >10 different point mutations
- ☐ CACNA1 and SCN2A gene mutations: these possibly contribute
- ☐ The onset is under the age of 20 years in most cases

Features of ataxia

- ☐ The ataxia occurs in episodes which last seconds to minutes
- ☐ Their frequency ranges from once a month to several a day
- ☐ Ataxia is absent in some KCNA1 mutations

Associated features

- ☐ Inter-ictal myokymia
- ☐ Cerebellar features: these may become persistent
- ☐ Vertigo
- ☐ Blurred vision
- ☐ Diplopia
- ☐ Nausea
- ☐ Headache
- ☐ Sweating
- ☐ Tremor
- ☐ Dysarthria
- ☐ Shortness of breath
- ☐ Carpal spasm
- ☐ Fist clenching
- ☐ Apnoea and cyanosis

Triggers for attacks

- ☐ Rapid movements
- ☐ Physical exertion
- ☐ Trauma
- ☐ Anxiety and emotional stress
- ☐ Fever and environmental temperature
- ☐ Startle
- ☐ Repeated knee bending
- ☐ Caffeine
- ☐ Going on playground rides
- ☐ Caloric stimulation

Associated disorders

- ☐ Neuromyotonia
- ☐ Epilepsy
- ☐ Malignant hyperthermia
- ☐ Cataplexy
- ☐ Developmental delay and cognitive dysfunction
- ☐ Choreoathetosis
- ☐ Short sleep phenotype
- ☐ Muscle hypertrophy
- ☐ Skeletal deformities

Treatment

- ☐ Acetazolamide
- ☐ Carbamazepine
- ☐ Valproate

EPISODIC ATAXIA TYPE 2 (EA2)

Genetics and clinical features

- ☐ This is caused by mutations in the CACNA1A gene
- ☐ CACNA1A is also associated with FHM1 and SCA6
- ☐ The onset age is 5–20 years
- ☐ Ataxic episodes may last hours to days

Triggers

- ☐ Exercise
- ☐ Emotional stress
- ☐ Alcohol
- ☐ Caffeine

Associated features in attacks

- ☐ Vertigo
- ☐ Dysarthria
- ☐ Diplopia
- ☐ Nystagmus
- ☐ Tonic upward gaze
- ☐ Downward vertical gaze
- ☐ Migraine headache
- ☐ Seizures
- ☐ Dystonia
- ☐ Cognitive impairment
- ☐ Generalised weakness
- ☐ Hemiparesis

Associated conditions

- ☐ Inter-ictal nystagmus
- ☐ Secondary progressive ataxia
- ☐ Co-existence with SCA6
- ☐ Cognitive dysfunction
- ☐ Autism
- ☐ Childhood-onset epileptic encephalopathy

Differential diagnosis

- ☐ Epilepsy
- ☐ Stroke

Investigations

- ☐ MRI brain is usually normal: but it may show atrophy of the vermis
- ☐ Electroencephalogram (EEG): this may show inter-ictal epileptiform activity

Treatment

- ☐ Acetazolamide 250 mg to 1000 mg daily: the response is usually dramatic
- ☐ 4 aminopyridine 5 mg three times daily
- ☐ Flunarizine
- ☐ Valproate or Zonisamide: for seizures

Acronyms

- ☐ FHM1: familial hemiplegic migraine type 1
- ☐ SCA6: spinocerebellar ataxia type 6

EPISODIC ATAXIA (EA): DIFFERENTIAL DIAGNOSIS

Neurological differentials

- ☐ Basilar migraine
- ☐ Familial hemiplegic migraine (FHM)
- ☐ Paroxysmal dyskinesia
- ☐ Post-ictal state
- ☐ Spinocerebellar ataxia: especially SCA 6
- ☐ Periodic vestibulo-cerebellar ataxia

Metabolic differentials

- ☐ Hypoglycaemia
- ☐ Hyperammonaemia
- ☐ Organic acid disorders
- ☐ Hartnup disease
- ☐ Hyperpyruvic academia
- ☐ Pyruvate decarboxylase deficiency
- ☐ Pyruvate dehydrogenase deficiency
- ☐ Refsum's disease
- ☐ Porphyria
- ☐ Leigh syndrome
- ☐ Maple syrup urine disease
- ☐ Congenital lactic acidosis

SPORADIC ADULT ONSET ATAXIA: NEUROLOGICAL CAUSES

Chronic infections

- ☐ Neurosyphilis
- ☐ Creutzfeldt Jakob disease (CJD)
- ☐ Lyme neuroborreliosis
- ☐ Whipple's disease

Sporadic degenerative

- ☐ Multiple system atrophy-cerebellar (MSA-C)
- ☐ Cortical cerebellar atrophy
- ☐ Idiopathic

Hereditary

- ☐ Friedreich's ataxia (FA)
- ☐ Spinocerebellar ataxia (SCA): especially SCA6, SCA7, and SCA14
- ☐ Fragile X tremor ataxia syndrome (FXTAS)
- ☐ Hereditary spastic ataxia 7 (SPG7)
- ☐ Mitochondrial disease
- ☐ Autosomal recessive spastic ataxia of Charlevoix-Saguenay (ARSACS)
- ☐ Cockayne syndrome
- ☐ Ataxia telangiectasia (AT)
- ☐ Episodic ataxia types 1 and 2 (EA1, EA2)
- ☐ Cerebrotendinous xanthomatosis (CTX)
- ☐ Neiman Pick C (NPC)
- ☐ Ataxia with oculomotor apraxia (AOA)

Synonyms for idiopathic types

- ☐ Sporadic adult onset ataxia of unknown aetiology (SAOA)
- ☐ Idiopathic late-onset cerebellar ataxia (ILOCA)
- ☐ Idiopathic cerebellar ataxia (IDCA)

SPORADIC ADULT ONSET ATAXIA: SYSTEMIC CAUSES

Heavy metals

- ☐ Lead
- ☐ Mercury
- ☐ Thallium

Autoimmune

- ☐ Anti-GAD
- ☐ SREAT
- ☐ Anti-gliadin
- ☐ Anti-transglutaminase 6 (TG6)
- ☐ Anti-Purkinje cell antibodies
- ☐ Anti-MAG
- ☐ Anti-ARHGAP26

Paraneoplastic

- ☐ ANNA1
- ☐ CV2/CRMP5
- ☐ Ma2
- ☐ Inositol 1,4,5-trisphosphate receptor type 1 (ITPR1)
- ☐ Microtubule associated protein1B (MAP1B)
- ☐ mGluR1
- ☐ Tr (PCA-Tr)
- ☐ Yo (PCA1)
- ☐ Zic1, Zic4

Drug-induced

- ☐ Lithium
- ☐ Valproate
- ☐ Phenytoin
- ☐ Amiodarone
- ☐ Metronidazole
- ☐ Procainamide
- ☐ Calcineurin inhibitors
- ☐ Mefloquine
- ☐ Isoniazid
- ☐ 5 Fluorouracil (5FU)

Other causes

- ☐ Alcohol
- ☐ Acquired vitamin E deficiency
- ☐ Superficial siderosis
- ☐ Light chain myeloma
- ☐ Hypothyroidism
- ☐ Hypomagnesaemia: this is associated with cerebral oedema
- ☐ Hepatitis B virus (HBV) related liver cirrhosis: case report

Synonyms for idiopathic types

- ☐ Sporadic adult onset ataxia of unknown aetiology (SAOA)
- ☐ Idiopathic late-onset cerebellar ataxia (ILOCA)
- ☐ Idiopathic cerebellar ataxia (IDCA)

Acronym

- ☐ SREAT: Steroid responsive encephalopathy associated with autoimmune thyroiditis

Chorea

CHOREA: NEUROLOGICAL CAUSES

Genetic

- ☐ Huntington's disease (HD)
- ☐ Huntington's disease like 2 (HD like-2)
- ☐ Dentatorubral-pallidolyusian atrophy (DRPLA)
- ☐ Spinocerebellar ataxia (SCA): SCA2, SCA3, SCA7
- ☐ Neuroacanthocytosis
- ☐ Neuroferritinopathy
- ☐ Ataxia telangiectasia
- ☐ Benign hereditary chorea
- ☐ Paroxysmal kinesigenic choreoathetosis
- ☐ Ataxia with oculomotor apraxia (AOA)
- ☐ Pantothenate kinase-associated neurodegeneration (PKAN)
- ☐ Wilson's disease
- ☐ Niemann–Pick type C (NPC)
- ☐ Dopa-responsive dystonia (DRD)
- ☐ Mitochondrial disease

Infective

- ☐ HIV
- ☐ Toxoplasmosis
- ☐ Tuberculous meningitis (TBM)
- ☐ Creutzfeldt Jakob disease (CJD)

Focal brain lesions

- ☐ Arteriovenous malformations (AVMs)
- ☐ Multiple sclerosis (MS)
- ☐ Space occupying lesions
- ☐ Stroke
- ☐ Cerebral hypoperfusion without infarction
- ☐ Sarcoidosis
- ☐ Giant tumefactive perivascular (Virchow-Robin) spaces
- ☐ Chronic subdural haematoma (SDH)

Other causes

- ☐ Senile chorea
- ☐ Psychogenic chorea

CHOREA: SYSTEMIC CAUSES

Genetic

- ☐ Lesch–Nyhan syndrome
- ☐ Glucose transporter type 1(GLUT 1) deficiency
- ☐ Beta ketothiolase deficiency
- ☐ Propionic aciduria
- ☐ Methylmalonic aciduria
- ☐ Type 1 glutaric aciduria

Autoimmune

- ☐ Sydenham's chorea: group A streptococcal infection and rheumatic fever
- ☐ PANDAS
- ☐ Systemic lupus (SLE)
- ☐ Sjogren's syndrome
- ☐ Antiphospholipid antibody syndrome
- ☐ Behcet's disease
- ☐ Vasculitis
- ☐ Hashimoto encephalopathy

Diabetic

- ☐ Diabetic striatopathy: chorea-hyperglycaemia-basal ganglia (C-H-BG) syndrome
- ☐ Hyperosmolar non-ketotic coma (HONK)
- ☐ Non-ketotic hyperglycaemia
- ☐ Diabetic hypoglycaemia

Metabolic

- ☐ Thyrotoxicosis (hyperthyroidism)
- ☐ Hypoparathyroidism
- ☐ Hyperparathyroidism
- ☐ Hyper and hyponatraemia
- ☐ Hyper and hypocalcemia
- ☐ Hypomagnesemia
- ☐ Heavy metal poisoning: especially manganese
- ☐ Polycythaemia rubra vera
- ☐ Carbon monoxide poisoning
- ☐ Pregnancy (chorea gravidarum)

Drug-induced

- ☐ Oral contraceptives
- ☐ Anti-Parkinsonian drugs: Levodopa and Dopamine agonists
- ☐ Antiepileptic drugs (AEDs): Valproate and Carbamazepine
- ☐ Antipsychotic drugs: Neuroleptics and Lithium
- ☐ Memantine
- ☐ Steroids
- ☐ Opioid neurotoxicity: Hydromorphone
- ☐ Abuse drugs: Amphetamines and Cocaine

Other causes

- ☐ Renal cancer
- ☐ Small cell lung cancer
- ☐ Lymphoma: Hodgkin's and non-Hodgkin's
- ☐ Cardiopulmonary by-pass (post-pump chorea)
- ☐ CHAP syndrome: choreoathetosis, orofacial dyskinesia, hypotonia, pseudobulbar palsy

DOI: 10.1201/9781003221258-28

CHOREA: MANAGEMENT

Investigations

- ☐ Full blood count
- ☐ Blood film
- ☐ Serum caeruloplasmin/urine copper
- ☐ Antinuclear antibody (ANA)
- ☐ Anti dsDNA
- ☐ Lupus anticoagulant
- ☐ Anti-cardiolipin antibody
- ☐ Anti-streptolysin O (ASO) titre
- ☐ Anti-basal ganglia antibody (ABGA)
- ☐ Thyroid function test (TFT)
- ☐ Magnetic resonance imaging (MRI) brain
- ☐ Cerebrospinal fluid (CSF) analysis

Good-evidenced drug treatments

- ☐ Amantadine: Level B evidence
- ☐ Riluzole: Level B evidence
- ☐ Nabilone: Level C evidence

Neuroleptics

- ☐ Olanzapine
- ☐ Risperidone
- ☐ Quetiapine
- ☐ Sulpiride
- ☐ Haloperidol

Vesicular monoamine transporter 2 (VMAT2) blockers

- ☐ Tetrabenazine
- ☐ Deutetrabenazine
- ☐ Valbenazine
- ☐ Deep brain stimulation (DBS)

Other drug treatments

- ☐ Donepezil

HUNTINGTON'S DISEASE (HD): CLINICAL FEATURES

Psychiatric features

- ☐ Personality change
- ☐ Apathy
- ☐ Anxiety and depression
- ☐ Irritability and aggressiveness
- ☐ Obsessive-compulsive behaviour
- ☐ Dysphoria
- ☐ Agitation
- ☐ Disinhibition
- ☐ Delusions
- ☐ Psychosis

Cognitive features

- ☐ Executive dysfunction
- ☐ Perseveration
- ☐ Impulsivity and distractibility
- ☐ Perceptual distortions
- ☐ Lack of insight
- ☐ Difficulty learning new information
- ☐ Impaired recognition of negative emotions

Movement disorders

- ☐ Chorea: limb and facial
- ☐ Myoclonus
- ☐ Dystonia
- ☐ Rigidity and bradykinesia
- ☐ Spasticity
- ☐ Bruxism
- ☐ Head drop
- ☐ Balance difficulties and falls

Oculomotor disorders

- ☐ Increased saccade latency: delayed initiation of saccades
- ☐ Increased variability of saccade latency
- ☐ Distractibility: difficultly suppressing saccades to new but irrelevant visual stimuli
- ☐ Difficulty in sustaining fixation
- ☐ Slow saccades: develop later

Other neurological features

- ☐ Impaired theory of mind
- ☐ Sleep disturbance
- ☐ Dysphasia and dysphagia
- ☐ Hypersexuality
- ☐ Speech delay: this may be the first feature
- ☐ Purely cognitive onset
- ☐ Pain
- ☐ Hung-up knee jerk (HUKJ)

Systemic features

- ☐ Constipation
- ☐ Tenesmus
- ☐ Incontinence
- ☐ Weight loss: related to CAG repeat length
- ☐ Dysfunctional platelets

HUNTINGTON'S DISEASE (HD): DIFFERENTIAL DIAGNOSIS

Huntington's disease-like 1 (HDL1)

- ☐ This is caused by a prion protein gene mutation
- ☐ It presents with personality change in early to mid-childhood
- ☐ It may also manifest with chorea, myoclonus, and seizures

Huntington's disease-like 2 (HDL2)

- ☐ This is caused by mutations in the JPH3 (junctophilin 3) gene on chromosome 16
- ☐ It is a CTG/CAG repeat expansion disease
- ☐ The transmission is autosomal dominant
- ☐ It occurs in South African Blacks
- ☐ It presents with dementia, chorea, and oculomotor abnormalities
- ☐ It has a more severe phenotype than HD
- ☐ There is more prominent dysarthria and dystonia than in HD
- ☐ Thalamic volumes are smaller than in HD

Huntington's disease-like 3 (HDL3)

- ☐ This is a recessive HD phenocopy
- ☐ It manifests with chorea, dystonia, and seizures

Huntington's disease-like 4 (HDL4, SCA17)

- ☐ This is caused by mutations in the TATA box binding protein gene

Spinocerebellar ataxia (SCA)

- ☐ This is an HD phenotype that is most often seen with SCA 17/HDL 4
- ☐ It is also seen with SCA 1, 2, 3, 7, 8, 12, and 14

Other neurodegenerative causes of chorea

- ☐ Benign hereditary chorea (BHC)
- ☐ Wilson's disease
- ☐ McLeod syndrome
- ☐ Friedreich's ataxia (FA): delayed onset phenotype
- ☐ Ataxia telangiectasia (AT)
- ☐ Ataxia with oculomotor apraxia (AO) 1 and 2
- ☐ Kufor Rakeb
- ☐ C9orf72 gene mutation

Other causes of (HD) phenotype

- ☐ Dentatorubral-pallidolyusian atrophy (DRPLA)
- ☐ Neuroferritinopathy
- ☐ Pantothenate kinase associated neurodegeneration (PKAN)
- ☐ Neuroacanthocytosis
- ☐ Chorea acanthocytosis (VPS13A gene)
- ☐ PRNP prion disease
- ☐ RNF216 and FRRS1L gene mutations
- ☐ ADCY5-related dyskinesia: childhood-onset chorea, dystonia and myoclonus
- ☐ Xeroderma pigmentosum

HUNTINGTON'S DISEASE (HD): TREATMENT

Treatments of chorea: VMAT blockers

- ☐ Tetrabenazine
- ☐ Deutetrabenazine
- ☐ Valbenazine

Treatment of chorea: Neuroleptics

- ☐ These are Risperidone and Olanzapine
- ☐ They are probably as effective as Tetrabenazine
- ☐ They are also indicated for psychosis, aggression, and irritability

Treatment of chorea: other agents

- ☐ Amantadine
- ☐ Riluzole
- ☐ Nabilone
- ☐ Ethyl-EPA
- ☐ Minocycline
- ☐ Creatine

Treatments of depression

- ☐ Selective serotonin reuptake inhibitors (SSRIs)
- ☐ Mirtazapine
- ☐ Venlafaxine

Treatments of altered sleep-wake cycle

- ☐ Hypnotics
- ☐ Zoplicone
- ☐ Zolpidem

Mood stabilisers

- ☐ Valproate
- ☐ Carbamazepine
- ☐ Lamotrigine

Physical exercise: benefits

- ☐ It stablises motor function
- ☐ It improves cardiovascular function

Investigational treatments

- ☐ Selective histone deacylase (HDAC) inhibitors
- ☐ Rilmenidine
- ☐ CYP46A1: an enzyme in cholesterol degradation
- ☐ Statins: these reportedly delay motor progression
- ☐ Gene editing

Acronym

- ☐ VMAT: vesicular monoamine transporter

PAROXYSMAL KINESIGENIC DYSKINESIA (PKD): CLINICAL FEATURES

Triggers for attacks

- ☐ Sudden movement
- ☐ Startle
- ☐ Cannabis
- ☐ Menses
- ☐ Cold weather
- ☐ Humidity
- ☐ Hunger

Aura symptoms

- ☐ Sensory
- ☐ Osmophobia
- ☐ Dysarthria
- ☐ Tongue tingling

Dyskinesia features

- ☐ The episodes are unilateral, bilateral or alternating
- ☐ They last <1 minute
- ☐ There are frequent daily attacks
- ☐ The attacks are worse in the summer months
- ☐ There is no loss of consciousness or pain
- ☐ There is occasional associated migraine
- ☐ There is a refractory period after an attack

Associated movement disorders

- ☐ Dystonia
- ☐ Chorea
- ☐ Ballism
- ☐ Convulsions in infants
- ☐ Writer's cramp
- ☐ Essential tremor (ET)
- ☐ Galloping tongue

Associated neurological disorders

- ☐ Hemiplegic migraine
- ☐ Epilepsy

Distinctive features of PRRT2 PKD

- ☐ Younger onset age
- ☐ Longer attack duration
- ☐ Complicated clinical features

Synonyms

- ☐ Episodic kinesigenic dyskinesia 1 (EKD1)
- ☐ DYT10

DENTATORUBRAL PALLIDOLYUSIAN ATROPHY (DRPLA)

Genetics

- ☐ This is caused by mutations in the atrophin 1 gene on chromosome 12p13
- ☐ It is a CAG repeat expansion disease
- ☐ The transmission is autosomal dominant
- ☐ The onset age is 34–60 years

Clinical features

- ☐ Ataxia: this may be the only feature
- ☐ Chorea
- ☐ Dementia
- ☐ Psychiatric features
- ☐ Huntington's disease-like phenotype: this is seen in older-onset cases
- ☐ Progressive myoclonic epilepsy (PME)

Magnetic resonance imaging (MRI)

- ☐ Atrophy: of the brainstem, superior cerebellar peduncle, and cerebellum
- ☐ Abnormal signal: in the brainstem, cerebellum, and thalamus
- ☐ Leukodystrophy: this occurs occasionally
- ☐ The eye of the tiger sign: this is occasionally present

Miscellaneous movement disorders

TIC DISORDERS: CAUSES

Neurodegenerative diseases

- [ ] Parkinsonian disorders
- [ ] Huntington's disease (HD)
- [ ] Neuroacanthocytosis
- [ ] Wilson's disease
- [ ] Neurodegeneration with brain iron accumulation (NBAI)

Other neurological diseases

- [ ] Multiple sclerosis (MS)
- [ ] Torsion dystonia
- [ ] Essential tremor
- [ ] Restless legs syndrome (RLS)
- [ ] Corpus callosum dysgenesis
- [ ] Arnold Chiari malformation
- [ ] Neurofibromatosis (NF)
- [ ] Traumatic brain injury (TBI)
- [ ] Stroke
- [ ] Hypoxic-ischaemic encephalopathy
- [ ] Haemorrhage from arteriovenous malformation (AVM)

Drug-induced

- [ ] Lamotrigine
- [ ] Carbamazepine
- [ ] Levodopa
- [ ] Clozapine
- [ ] Fluphenazine
- [ ] Buspirone
- [ ] Neuroleptics and neuroleptic withdrawal
- [ ] Cocaine
- [ ] Caffeine

Infections

- [ ] Encephalitis
- [ ] Creutzfeldt Jakob disease (CJD)
- [ ] Sydenham's chorea
- [ ] Post-encephalitic
- [ ] Lyme neuroborreliosis

Developmental syndromes

- [ ] Autism
- [ ] Pervasive developmental disorder
- [ ] Asperger's syndrome
- [ ] Savant syndrome
- [ ] Down's syndrome

Other causes

- [ ] Idiopathic
- [ ] Tourette syndrome (TS)
- [ ] Carbon monoxide (CO) poisoning
- [ ] Antiphospholipid antibody syndrome
- [ ] Klinefelter's syndrome
- [ ] Fragile X syndrome
- [ ] Peripheral injuries

TOURETTE SYNDROME: CLINICAL FEATURES

Genetics

- [ ] Mutations of the ASH1L gene may confer susceptibility

Types

- [ ] Motor
- [ ] Vocal (phonic)
- [ ] Cognitive: repetitive thoughts

Onset age

- [ ] The mean onset age is 5 years
- [ ] The worst period is 8–12 years
- [ ] About 5% have adult onset tics: these start after the age of 50 years

Clinical features

- [ ] The tics start cranially and progress caudally
- [ ] Premonitory sensory urges are frequent
- [ ] Subjects have a feeling of control over the tics (intentionality)
- [ ] Subjects show enhanced habit formation
- [ ] There is social disinhibition
- [ ] The course is waxing and waning
- [ ] The tics may be relieved by concentration and sleep
- [ ] Relaxation and excitement may aggravate the tics

Diagnostic criteria

- [ ] 2 or more motor tics
- [ ] 1 phonic tic occurring most days for more than a year
- [ ] Starting before age 18 years
- [ ] Not caused by any medical condition or substance abuse

Co-morbidities

- [ ] Attention deficit hyperactivity disorder (ADHD): this is present in most cases
- [ ] Obsessive compulsive disorder (OCD)
- [ ] Autistic spectrum disorders
- [ ] Sleep disorders
- [ ] Anger control problems
- [ ] Pathological laughter

Features of adult Tourette syndrome

- [ ] Facial and trunkal tics are more frequent
- [ ] There may be a history of substance abuse
- [ ] Mood disorders are more frequent
- [ ] Phonic tics are less frequent
- [ ] Attention-deficit hyperactivity disorder is less frequent

Pathological features

- [ ] Reduced brain cortical thickness
- [ ] Positive oligoclonal bands (OCB) in 38% of patients: this may indicate an immune basis

DOI: 10.1201/9781003221258-29

TARDIVE DYSKINESIA: CLINICAL FEATURES

Defining features

- ☐ The disorder develops during treatment or within 6 months of stopping the treatment
- ☐ It requires ≥ 3 months of drug use (usually 1–2 years)
  - ○ 1 month if >60 years age
- ☐ The movements persist for ≥1 month after stopping the treatment
- ☐ Remission occurs in about 13–25% of cases: it is spontaneous in 2%
- ☐ The onset is insidious
- ☐ There is progression followed by stabilisation

Stereotypic movements

- ☐ Foot tapping
- ☐ Piano-playing finger and toe movements
- ☐ Hand rubbing
- ☐ Trunk rocking and swaying

Akathisia (inner restlessness): manifestations

- ☐ Rocking or pacing on a spot
- ☐ Crossing and uncrossing of legs
- ☐ Shifting weight from one foot to another
- ☐ Touching the face or the scalp

Other movement disorders

- ☐ Orofacial dyskinesias
- ☐ Myoclonus
- ☐ Parkinsonism
- ☐ Tremor
- ☐ Dystonia
- ☐ Chorea: trunkal or generalised
- ☐ Tics: tardive tourettism
- ☐ Tardive diaphragmatic tremor

Respiratory dyskinesia

- ☐ Gasping
- ☐ Stridor
- ☐ Irregular breathing
- ☐ Speech interruption
- ☐ Paradoxical breathing
- ☐ Dyspnoea on exertion
- ☐ Respiratory noises: humming, moaning

Other movements

- ☐ Neuroleptic malignant syndrome (NMS)
- ☐ Tardive pain

SEROTONIN SYNDROME: CAUSES

Antidepressants

- ☐ Selective serotonin reuptake inhibitors (SSRIs)
- ☐ Serotonin norepinephrine reuptake inhibitors (SNRIs)
- ☐ Tricyclic antidepressants
- ☐ Trazodone
- ☐ Buspirone
- ☐ Lithium

Monoamine oxidase inhibitors (MAOI)

- ☐ Phenelzine
- ☐ Moclobemide
- ☐ Clorgiline
- ☐ Isocarboxazid
- ☐ Selegiline

Anti-emetics and antihistamines

- ☐ Metoclopramide
- ☐ Ondansteron
- ☐ Chlorpheniramine

Abuse drugs

- ☐ Cocaine
- ☐ Ecstasy (MDMA)
- ☐ Lysergic acid diethylamine (LSD)
- ☐ Foxy methoxy
- ☐ Syrian rue

Opiates

- ☐ Tramadol
- ☐ Pethidine

Other drugs

- ☐ Triptans
- ☐ Amphetamines
- ☐ Dextromethorphan
- ☐ Ginseng
- ☐ Levodopa
- ☐ Ritonovir
- ☐ Sibutramine
- ☐ St John's wort (hypericum perforatum)
- ☐ Tryptophan
- ☐ Valproate

SEROTONIN SYNDROME: CLINICAL FEATURES

Onset features

- ☐ Rapid onset: this is within minutes
- ☐ Agitation
- ☐ Hypervigilance

Features of autonomic hyperactivity

- ☐ Tachycardia
- ☐ Hypertension
- ☐ Shivering
- ☐ Sweating
- ☐ Hyperthermia >38°C
- ☐ Mydriasis

Neuromuscular features

- ☐ Tremor
- ☐ Myoclonus
- ☐ Rigidity
- ☐ Easy startle
- ☐ Head turning behaviour
- ☐ Seizures
- ☐ Hyperreflexia
- ☐ Clonus

Hunter diagnostic criteria: core features

- ☐ There is use of a serotonergic agent within the preceding 5 weeks
- ☐ Other causes of the symptoms have been excluded
- ☐ With any one of the following:
- ☐ Myoclonus
- ☐ Agitation
- ☐ Diaphoresis
- ☐ Tremor and hyperreflexia
- ☐ Hypertonia
- ☐ Temperature >38°C

Alternative diagnostic criteria

- ☐ Radomski criteria
- ☐ Sternbach criteria

Severity

- ☐ Related to combination of medications
- ☐ Worse with monoamine oxidase inhibitors (MAOIs)
- ☐ SSRIs alone, even in overdose, do not cause severe features

RESTLESS LEGS SYNDROME (RLS): RISK FACTORS AND CAUSES

Demographic risk factors

- ☐ Women
- ☐ Pregnancy
- ☐ North Europeans
- ☐ North Americans
- ☐ Obesity

Peripheral neurological causes

- ☐ Peripheral neuropathy (PN)
- ☐ Charcot–Marie–Tooth disease (CMT)
- ☐ Lumbosacral radiculopathy
- ☐ Myasthenia gravis (MG)
- ☐ Guillain–Barre syndrome (GBS)
- ☐ Post-polio syndrome (PPS)

Central neurological causes

- ☐ Migraine
- ☐ Parkinson's disease (PD)
- ☐ Multiple sclerosis (MS)
- ☐ Myelopathy
- ☐ Vespers curse
- ☐ Ischaemic stroke

Systemic causes

- ☐ Iron deficiency
- ☐ Caffeine
- ☐ Sedative/narcotic withdrawal
- ☐ Hypothyroidism
- ☐ Peripheral vascular disease (PVD)
- ☐ Uraemia
- ☐ Cardiovascular disease
- ☐ Diabetes
- ☐ Rheumatologic disorders
- ☐ Depression
- ☐ Poor mental health
- ☐ High cholesterol
- ☐ Inflammatory bowel disease (IBD)

Exacerbating drugs

- ☐ Tricyclic antidepressants
- ☐ Selective serotonin reuptake inhibitors (SSRIs)
- ☐ Calcium channel blockers
- ☐ Anticonvulsants
- ☐ Neuroleptics
- ☐ Lithium
- ☐ Beta blockers
- ☐ Antihistamines
- ☐ Withdrawal of sedatives
- ☐ Withdrawal of vasodilators
- ☐ Metoclopramide
- ☐ Interferon alpha
- ☐ Zonisamide

RESTLESS LEGS SYNDROME (RLS): DRUG TREATMENTS

Level A evidenced drug treatment

- [ ] Pramipexole 0.125 mg daily; maximum 0.75 mg daily
- [ ] Gabapentin enacarbil 600–1200 mg daily
  - ○ Start with 300 mg if age is >65 years
- [ ] Rotigotine patch 1 mg daily; maximum is 3 mg daily
- [ ] Cabergoline: this has significant cardiac side effects

Level B evidenced drug treatment

- [ ] Ropinirole 0.25 mg daily; maximum 4 mg daily
- [ ] Pregabalin 75–450 mg daily
  - ○ Start with 75 mg if age is <65 years
  - ○ Start with 50 mg if age is >65 years
- [ ] Ferric carboxymaltose 500 mg given twice 5 days apart
- [ ] Pneumatic compression

Level C evidenced drug treatment

- [ ] Levodopa
- [ ] Oxycodone prolonged release 10–40 mg daily: start with 5–10 mg
- [ ] Near-infrared spectroscopy
- [ ] Transcranial magnetic stimulation (TMS)
- [ ] Vibrating pads: to improve subjective sleep

Optional drug treatments: Gabapentin

- [ ] Gabapentin 900–1200 mg daily
- [ ] Start with 300 mg if <65 years, and 100 mg if >65 years

Optional drug treatments: others

- [ ] Methadone 5–30 mg daily: start with 2.5 mg
- [ ] Vitamins C and E in haemodialysed patients
- [ ] Clonidine
- [ ] Carbamazepine

Guidelines for iron therapy

- [ ] Check baseline iron, ferritin, TIBC, and %TSAT
- [ ] Administer iron only if %TSAT is >45
- [ ] Give elemental oral iron 65 mg if ferritin is ≤75 µg/L
- [ ] Give intravenous (IV) iron if oral is inappropriate and ferritin is ≤100 µg/L
  - ○ Renal function must be normal

Insufficient evidenced treatment

- [ ] Clonazepam
- [ ] Lisuride
- [ ] Amantadine
- [ ] Valerian
- [ ] Zolpidem
- [ ] Topiramate
- [ ] Dihydroergocriptine
- [ ] Tramadol

Acronyms

- [ ] TSAT: transferrin saturation
- [ ] TIBC: total iron binding capacity

NEUROLEPTIC MALIGNANT SYNDROME (NMS): CAUSES AND RISK FACTORS

Causes

- [ ] Use or withdrawal of both classical and atypical neuroleptics
- [ ] Use of dopamine-depleting drugs
- [ ] Withdrawal of dopaminergic drugs

Neuroleptic-related risk factors

- [ ] Previous NMS
- [ ] Parenteral administration
- [ ] Higher doses
- [ ] Abrupt dose reduction
- [ ] Depot formulation
- [ ] Concomitant use of Lithium and SSRIs

Other risk factors

- [ ] Agitation
- [ ] Dehydration
- [ ] Restraint
- [ ] Iron deficiency
- [ ] Physical exertion
- [ ] High environmental temperature
- [ ] Hyponatraemia
- [ ] High ambient temperature
- [ ] Exhaustion
- [ ] Mental retardation

Acronym

- [ ] SSRIs: selective serotonin reuptake inhibitors

NEUROLEPTIC MALIGNANT SYNDROME (NMS): CLINICAL FEATURES

Onset features

- ☐ Symptoms start about 10–30 days after discontinuation of neuroleptic drugs
- ☐ The interval is longer with depo preparations
- ☐ Symptoms progress over 24–72 hours

Main neurological features

- ☐ Rigidity
- ☐ Trismus
- ☐ Opisthotonus

Autonomic features

- ☐ Autonomic features
- ☐ Hyperthermia
- ☐ Altered consciousness
- ☐ Dysautonomia
- ☐ Tachycardia
- ☐ Tachypnoea
- ☐ Hypertension
- ☐ Sweating

Other neurological features

- ☐ Tremor
- ☐ Dystonia
- ☐ Chorea
- ☐ Myoclonus
- ☐ Seizures
- ☐ Ataxia
- ☐ Cerebellar degeneration: this is possibly due to the high temperature

Differential diagnosis

- ☐ Serotonin syndrome
- ☐ Malignant hyperthermia (MH)
- ☐ Malignant catatonia
- ☐ Withdrawal of intrathecal Baclofen
- ☐ Effect of dopamine antagonists
- ☐ Dopaminergic withdrawal syndrome

NEUROLEPTIC MALIGNANT SYNDROME (NMS): MANAGEMENT

Investigations

- ☐ Raised creatinine kinase (CK)
- ☐ Leucocytosis
- ☐ Rhabdomyolysis
- ☐ Renal impairment
- ☐ Abnormal liver function
- ☐ Abnormal coagulation

Treatment of rigidity

- ☐ Anticholinergics in mild cases
- ☐ Lorazepam in moderate cases
- ☐ Dantrolene in severe cases

Treatment of excessive dopaminergic block

- ☐ Bromocriptine
- ☐ Amantadine
- ☐ Levodopa/Carbidopa

Non-drug treatments

- ☐ Electroconvulsive therapy (ECT)
- ☐ Cooling
- ☐ Correction of fluid and electrolyte deficits

PAINFUL LEGS MOVING TOES (PLMT)

Causes

- ☐ Idiopathic
- ☐ Peripheral neuropathy (PN)
- ☐ Radiculopathies, e.g. herpes zoster
- ☐ Myelitis
- ☐ Cauda equina lesions
- ☐ Nerve root lesions
- ☐ Neuroleptics
- ☐ Chemotherapy
- ☐ Wilson's disease
- ☐ Systemic diseases, e.g. HIV

Types

- ☐ Central: complex electromyogram (EMG) pattern
- ☐ Peripheral (lumbar roots or tibial nerve): simple EMG pattern

Clinical features

- ☐ The movements are flexion-extension or abduction-adduction
- ☐ They usually involve the lower limbs
- ☐ They are preceded by severe pain in one limb
  - ○ But they may be painless
- ☐ Bilateral symptoms may arise from unilateral lesions
- ☐ Involuntary movements occur in affected digits
- ☐ The movements are absent in sleep

Variants

- ☐ Painful limbs moving extremities (PLME)
  - ○ When the upper limbs are also affected
- ☐ Painful shoulder-moving deltoid syndrome

Drug treatments

- ☐ Gabapentin
- ☐ Pregabalin
- ☐ Benzodiazepines

Non-drug treatments

- ☐ Nerve root sympathetic block
- ☐ Epidural blocks
- ☐ Sympathectomy
- ☐ Sympathetic block
- ☐ Neurectomy
- ☐ Botulinum toxin
- ☐ Transcutaneous electrical nerve stimulation (TENS)
- ☐ Vibratory simulation
- ☐ Epidural spinal cord stimulation

CHAPTER 5

Neuroinflammatory and autoimmune disorders

Multiple sclerosis

MULTIPLE SCLEROSIS (MS): NON-MODIFIABLE RISK FACTORS

Genetic mutations

- ☐ TYK2
- ☐ CYP27B1
- ☐ NLRP1
- ☐ IL-7Ra: interleukin 7 receptor α chain
- ☐ TNFAIP3
- ☐ TNFRSF1A
- ☐ STK11: serine therorine kinase 11
- ☐ IL18: interleukin 18

Ethnicity

- ☐ Caucasians have a higher risk
- ☐ Blacks, Asians, and Hispanics have a lower risk

Age-related risk factors

- ☐ Migration to high MS incidence areas before adolescence increases the risk
- ☐ Women with earlier age of menarche have a higher risk

Month of birth

- ☐ May is a high-risk birth month in the Northern hemisphere
- ☐ November is a high-risk birth month in the Southern hemisphere

Chronic cerebrospinal venous insufficiency (CCVI)

- ☐ There is insufficient evidence for this as an MS risk factor
- ☐ It is not present at the onset of MS

MULTIPLE SCLEROSIS (MS): MODIFIABLE RISK FACTORS

Dietary

- ☐ Low vitamin D: individual, maternal, and neonatal
- ☐ Low polyunsaturated fatty acids
- ☐ Low fish consumption

Cigarette smoking

- ☐ Smoking is a risk factor for developing MS
- ☐ Secondary smoke also increases the risk of paediatric MS
- ☐ Smoking may also hasten the progression of MS
- ☐ Smoking may act synergistically with Epstein Barr virus (EBV) to increase the risk

Lifestyle

- ☐ Childhood obesity
- ☐ Stressful life events
- ☐ Traumatic head injury (TBI): especially concussion in adolescence
- ☐ Gender identity disorders in males

Infections

- ☐ Epstein Barr virus (EBV)
- ☐ Fungi
- ☐ Enterobius vermicularis

Environmental

- ☐ Poor sun exposure
- ☐ Low lifetime UV-B sunlight exposure
- ☐ Higher latitudes: also associated with earlier onset age
- ☐ Organic solvents: probably linked to HLA-DRB1*15 allele

Other risk factors

- ☐ Low testosterone
- ☐ Endometriosis
- ☐ High leptin levels

Non-risk factors

- ☐ Vaccinations

DOI: 10.1201/9781003221258-31

MULTIPLE SCLEROSIS (MS): CLASSIFICATION

Relapsing remitting MS (RRMS)

- [ ] There are repeated demyelinating attacks affecting different areas lasting >24 hours
- [ ] RRMS is also diagnosed with one attack and MRI or CSF features of dissemination in time and place

Primary progressive MS (PPMS)

- [ ] The disease is progressive from onset without relapses

Secondary progressive MS (SPMS)

- [ ] The disease is progressive after an initial phase of RRMS
- [ ] Cervical spine atrophy may be a marker of the onset of SPMS

Benign (non-progressive) MS

- [ ] This occurs in about 5% of cases
- [ ] It is predicted by a low initial relapse frequency
- [ ] The expanded disability status scale (EDSS) score is 3.0 for $\geq$ 10 years
- [ ] The initial event usually completely resolves
- [ ] Cognitive decline however progresses at the same rate as non-benign MS

Spinal onset MS

- [ ] This occurs in 33% of cases
- [ ] Affected patients are usually older at onset
- [ ] There is a high risk of progression and disability

Pure spinal MS

- [ ] This manifests as relapsing short segment spinal myelitis
- [ ] There are no cranial lesions for up to 2 years

Myelocortical MS

- [ ] There is spinal cord and cerebral cortex demyelination
- [ ] There is no involvement of the cerebral white matter

Cortically dominant MS

- [ ] There are predominantly cortical lesions
- [ ] These are best detected with phase-sensitive inversion-recovery MRI
- [ ] It is associated with cortical atrophy
- [ ] It predicts cognitive deficits

Oligoclonal band (OCB) negative MS

- [ ] This is associated with a more benign course
- [ ] It is associated with less markers of CSF inflammation: white cells and IgG concentration
- [ ] 50% convert to OCB-positive MS

Marburg variant

- [ ] There is severe axonal and myelin damage in this variant
- [ ] It follows an aggressively fulminant course associated with oedema and mass effect

Other forms and variants of MS

- [ ] Progressive relapsing MS: there is progression from onset with episodic relapses
- [ ] Silent progression MS: there is progressive brain atrophy with no relapsing activity
- [ ] Single-attack (solitary) progressive MS
- [ ] Transitional MS: this is the stage between RRMS and SPMS
- [ ] Balo's concentric sclerosis
- [ ] Tumefactive MS (TMS)

MULTIPLE SCLEROSIS (MS): TYPICAL NEUROLOGICAL FEATURES

Cerebellar and brainstem features

- ☐ Ataxia
- ☐ Tremor
- ☐ Dysphagia
- ☐ Dysarthria
- ☐ Vertigo
- ☐ Dizziness
- ☐ Diplopia

Trigeminal neuralgia

- ☐ Trigeminal neuralgia may be 15 times more frequent in MS than in the general population
- ☐ It is usually due to brainstem lesions
- ☐ It may be caused by supratentorial lesions
- ☐ It is more intractable than in people without MS

Autonomic features

- ☐ Constipation
- ☐ Incontinence
- ☐ Erectile dysfunction: with reduced libido and premature ejaculation
- ☐ Bladder dysfunction

Cognitive features

- ☐ These usually manifest as impaired memory and executive dysfunction
- ☐ They may occur pre-clinically
- ☐ They may present as isolated cognitive relapses
- ☐ These are not associated with mood impairment or fatigue
- ☐ There may be associated pseudobulbar affect (PBA): pathological laughter and crying

Psychiatric features

- ☐ Anxiety
- ☐ Depression
- ☐ Psychosis

Pyramidal features

- ☐ Transverse myelitis
- ☐ Lhermitte's phenomenon
- ☐ Tonic spasms
- ☐ Spasticity
- ☐ Positive McArdle's sign: neck flexion induces rapid reversible weakness

Ophthalmic features

- ☐ Optic neuritis
- ☐ Nystagmus
- ☐ Internuclear ophthalmoplegia (INO)
- ☐ Uhthoff's phenomenon: heat or exercise induced visual impairment
- ☐ Pulfrich effect: moving objects appear to follow a curved course

Fatigue: types

- ☐ Mental or physical
- ☐ Subjective or objective
- ☐ Primary or secondary

MULTIPLE SCLEROSIS (MS): OTHER NEUROLOGICAL FEATURES

Cranial nerve dysfunction

- ☐ Olfactory dysfunction
- ☐ Taste dysfunction
- ☐ Hyperacusis

Movement disorders

- ☐ Restless legs syndrome (RLS): this is possibly related to cervical cord damage
- ☐ Paroxysmal kinesigenic dyskinesia (PKD)

Sleep-related disorders

- ☐ Insomnia
- ☐ Sleep-related breathing disorders (SRBD)
- ☐ Periodic limb movement disorders (PLMD)
- ☐ Secondary narcolepsy
- ☐ REM sleep behaviour disorder (RBD)
- ☐ Propriospinal myoclonus

Headache disorders

- ☐ MS-related headache may present as status migrainosus
- ☐ High cervical cord lesions may manifest as occipital neuralgia

Neuromuscular features

- ☐ Focal amyotrophy: this results from cervical cord lesions involving the anterior horn cells
  - ○ It may also result from the involvement of the intraspinal nerve roots
- ☐ Acute radicular symptoms
- ☐ Peripheral nerve involvement: this is seen on magnetic resonance neurography

Other MS neurological presentations

- ☐ Foreign accent syndrome (FAS)
- ☐ Word finding difficulty
- ☐ Pain
- ☐ Heat sensitivity
- ☐ Sensory disturbance
- ☐ Paroxysmal attacks
- ☐ Impulsivity
- ☐ Seizures

Prodromal MS symptoms

- ☐ Pain
- ☐ Headache
- ☐ Gastrointestinal impairment
- ☐ Urinary symptoms
- ☐ Anorectal symptoms
- ☐ Anxiety and depression
- ☐ Insomnia
- ☐ Fatigue
- ☐ Cognitive impairment
- ☐ Frequent health care use

Disorders reported to be associated with MS

- ☐ Charcot–Marie–Tooth disease X (CMTX)
- ☐ Neurofibromatosis type 1 (NF1)
- ☐ Horner's syndrome

MULTIPLE SCLEROSIS (MS): SYSTEMIC FEATURES

Respiratory dysfunction

- ☐ Excessive daytime sleepiness (EDS)
- ☐ Respiratory impairment: this is frequent in wheelchair-bound patients
- ☐ Neurogenic pulmonary oedema (NPE): this includes flash pulmonary oedema

Cardiac dysfunction

- ☐ Takotsubo cardiomyopathy: this is due to demyelination in the medulla
  - ○ It presents with acute heart failure
- ☐ Neurogenic stunned myocardium (NSM)
- ☐ Myocardial infarction

Episodic hypothermia

- ☐ This occurs especially in advanced secondary progressive MS (SPMS)
- ☐ It is usually associated with impaired consciousness
- ☐ There are no associated hypothalamic disorders

Systemic lupus erythematosus (SLE)

- ☐ Familial clusters of SLE with MS have been reported
- ☐ Association of SLE with MS is however generally rare

Hormonal disorders

- ☐ Panhypopituitarism
- ☐ Male infertility

Gastrointestinal disorders

- ☐ Inflammatory bowel disease (IBD)
- ☐ Low vitamin K2 levels

Possible cancer risk

- ☐ The evidence for an increased cancer risk with MS is conflicting
- ☐ Some reports suggest a reduced or an absent risk of cancer
- ☐ Others report a small risk of melanoma, breast, brain, and urinary system cancer

Systemic MS associations

- ☐ Gender identity disorders
- ☐ Low intraocular pressure
- ☐ Osteoporosis

MULTIPLE SCLEROSIS (MS): DIFFERENTIAL DIAGNOSIS

Inflammatory

- ☐ Neuromyelitis optica (NMO)
- ☐ Acute disseminated encephalomyelitis (ADEM)
- ☐ Behcet's disease
- ☐ Progressive multifocal leukoencephalopathy (PML)
- ☐ Neurosarcoidosis: this has higher CSF protein, white cell count, and serum ACE than in MS
- ☐ Central nervous system (CNS) vasculitis
- ☐ Leukoencephalopathy
- ☐ Schilder's disease

Autoimmune

- ☐ Systemic lupus erythematosus (SLE)
- ☐ Antiphospholipid antibody syndrome (APS)
- ☐ Sjogren's syndrome
- ☐ Polyarteritis nodosa (PAN)
- ☐ Stiff person syndrome (SPS)

Infective

- ☐ Lyme neuroborreliosis
- ☐ Brucellosis
- ☐ Meningovascular syphilis
- ☐ HTLV associated myelopathy (HAM)

Myelopathic

- ☐ Hereditary spastic paraparesis (HSP)
- ☐ Cervical cord compression
- ☐ Subacute combined degeneration (SCD)

Ischaemic and vascular

- ☐ Small vessel disease
- ☐ Leukoaraiosis
- ☐ Binswanger's disease
- ☐ Cavernoma
- ☐ Brainstem arteriovenous malformations (AVMs)
- ☐ Dural arteriovenous fistula (dAVF)

Neoplastic

- ☐ Pontine glioma
- ☐ Lymphoma
- ☐ Intravascular lymphoma

Miscellaneous differentials

- ☐ Atopic myelitis
- ☐ Motor neurone disease (MND)
- ☐ Susac's syndrome
- ☐ Coarctation of the aorta
- ☐ Thalassaemia
- ☐ CADASIL
- ☐ Platybasia/basilar invagination
- ☐ Virchow Robin spaces
- ☐ TPP2 gene mutation

Acronym

- ☐ CADASIL: cerebral autosomal dominant arteriopathy with subcortical infarcts and leukoencephalopathy

CLINICALLY ISOLATED SYNDROMES (CIS): PREDICTORS OF CONVERSION TO MS

Clinical predictors

- ☐ Non-white ethnicity
- ☐ Female gender
- ☐ Younger age
- ☐ Smoking at the time of CIS
- ☐ Fatigue at the time of CIS
- ☐ Cognitive impairment
- ☐ Severity of disability at onset
- ☐ Non-treatment with disease modifying drugs (DMDs)
- ☐ Non-optic neuritis presentation

Radiological predictors

- ☐ Abnormal magnetic resonance imaging (MRI) scan
- ☐ Multiple lesions on MRI scan
  - ○ ≥10 lesions are highly predictive
- ☐ Progressive ventricular enlargement
- ☐ Infratentorial lesions: especially brainstem
- ☐ Grey matter brain atrophy

Cerebrospinal (CSF) potential predictors

- ☐ Soluble CD27
- ☐ Oligoclonal bands (OCBs)
- ☐ Neurofilament light chain (NFL)
- ☐ Chitinase 3 like 1 (CHI3L1)
- ☐ Immunoglobulin M (IgM)

Serum predictors

- ☐ High IgG3 level
- ☐ Neurofilaments (NfL)

Predictors of conversion of spinal cord CIS to MS

- ☐ Inflammatory cerebrospinal fluid (CSF)
- ☐ 3 or more periventricular lesions
- ☐ Age ≤40 years

Predictors of conversion of optic neuritis (ON) to MS

- ☐ Spinal lesions
- ☐ Infratentorial lesions
- ☐ Enhancing lesions
- ☐ Pericalcarine cortical atrophy

CIS conversion rate to MS

- ☐ Risk of conversion with normal MRI is 11% after 10 years
- ☐ Risk of conversion with abnormal MRI is 83%
- ☐ 20% convert to relapsing remitting (RRMS)
- ☐ 24% convert to secondary progressive (SPMS)
- ☐ 39% convert to benign MS

RADIOLOGICALLY ISOLATED SYNDROME (RIS): PREDICTORS OF CONVERSION TO MS

Clinical

- ☐ Younger age
- ☐ Pregnancy
- ☐ Abnormal visual evoked potentials (VEPs)

Radiological

- ☐ Cervical cord lesions
- ☐ Infratentorial lesions
- ☐ Cortical lesions: especially frontotemporal
- ☐ Lesion load: >9 T2 MRI lesions
- ☐ Contrast enhancing lesions

Cerebrospinal fluid (CSF)

- ☐ Positive CSF oligoclonal bands (OCBs)
- ☐ Positive CSF neurofilament light chain (NFL)

Predictors of progression to primary progressive MS (PPMS)

- ☐ Males
- ☐ Older age
- ☐ Spinal cord lesions

RIS conversion and progression rate to MS

- ☐ 30–50% convert to clinical syndrome over 5–10 years respectively
- ☐ 66% develop radiological progression over 5 years
- ☐ 84% of cervical RIS lesions progress to CIS or PPMS over a median of 1.6 years
- ☐ 5% of asymptomatic multiple sclerosis (MS) relatives have incidental RIS
  - ○ About 50% were scanned for headaches

Acronyms

- ☐ CIS: clinically isolated syndrome
- ☐ PPMS: primary progressive multiple sclerosis

MULTIPLE SCLEROSIS (MS): SYMPTOMATIC TREATMENTS

Fatigue: drug treatments

- ☐ Amantadine
- ☐ Modafinil
- ☐ Methylphenidate
- ☐ A recent systematic review however suggested that these are all no better than placebo

Fatigue: non-drug treatments

- ☐ Mindfulness-based training
- ☐ Cognitive behaviour therapy (CBT)
- ☐ Flavinoid-rich cocoa

Urinary symptoms

- ☐ Oxybutynin
- ☐ Tolterodine
- ☐ Self-catheterisation
- ☐ Suprapubic bladder neck vibration
- ☐ Urinary diversion
- ☐ Intravesical capsaicin
- ☐ Intermittent vasopressin
- ☐ Botulinum toxin

Spasticity

- ☐ Baclofen
- ☐ Gabapentin
- ☐ Tizanidine
- ☐ Dantrolene
- ☐ Diazepam
- ☐ Botulinum toxin
- ☐ Intrathecal (IT) Baclofen
- ☐ Cannabinoid (Sativex)
- ☐ Nabiximols as add-on
- ☐ Intrathecal phenol
- ☐ Surgical tenotomy

Tremors

- ☐ Mechanical damping, e.g. with weights
- ☐ Isoniazid (INH)
- ☐ Clonazepam
- ☐ Betablockers
- ☐ Stereotactic radiosurgery: gamma knife thalamotomy
- ☐ Deep brain stimulation (DBS)

Tonic spasms

- ☐ Carbamazepine
- ☐ Phenytoin

Emotional lability

- ☐ Amitriptyline
- ☐ Citalopram

Oscillopsia

- ☐ Gabapentin
- ☐ Memantine

DISEASE MODIFYING TREATMENTS (DMTS): TYPES

Interferons

- ☐ Interferon β 1a
- ☐ Interferon β 1b
- ☐ Pegylated interferon (PEG interferon) β-1a

Monoclonal antibodies

- ☐ Natalizumab
- ☐ Alemtuzumab
- ☐ Daclizumab (now withdrawn)
- ☐ Ocrelizumab

Oral agents

- ☐ Dimethyl fumarate
- ☐ Teriflunomide
- ☐ Fingolimod

Other agents

- ☐ Glatiramer acetate
- ☐ Mitoxantrone
- ☐ Cladribine
- ☐ Cyclophosphamide

Conventional first line DMTs for MS

- ☐ Interferons
- ☐ Pegylated interferon beta 1a
- ☐ Glatiramer acetate
- ☐ Teriflunomide
- ☐ Dimethyl fumarate

First line DMTs for aggressive disease

- ☐ Natalizumab
- ☐ Fingolimod
- ☐ Alemtuzumab

Second line DMTs for aggressive disease

- ☐ Cladribine
- ☐ Rituximab
- ☐ Cyclophosphamide
- ☐ Autologous stem cell transplant (ASCT)

Newer DMTs

- ☐ Siponimod
- ☐ Ozanimod
- ☐ Ofatumumab
- ☐ Diroximel fumarate

Neuromyelitis optica (NMO)

NEUROMYELITIS OPTICA (NMO): CENTRAL NEUROLOGICAL FEATURES

Demographic features

- [ ] The mean onset age is 30 years
  - ○ It is 20 years in multiple sclerosis (MS)
- [ ] It predominantly affects females in the fertile ages
- [ ] Females are more likely than men to be antibody positive
- [ ] The course is relapsing in 80% of cases and monophasic in 20%
- [ ] One case has been reported following Zika virus infection

Cranial nerve features

- [ ] Visual impairment: from optic neuritis (ON)
- [ ] Foveal thinning without optic neuritis
- [ ] Olfactory dysfunction
- [ ] Lower cranial nerve dysfunction

Cerebral features

- [ ] Depression
- [ ] Cognitive impairment
- [ ] Rapidly progressive leukoencephalopathy: case report
- [ ] Fatigue
- [ ] Short acting neuralgiform headache attacks with cranial autonomic symptoms (SUNA)

Brainstem features

- [ ] Intractable hiccup and nausea (IHN): with medullary extension or relapse
- [ ] Respiratory failure
- [ ] Paroxysmal sneezing
- [ ] Eye movement disorders: especially abnormal saccades
- [ ] Pathological yawning

Spinal cord features

- [ ] Gait difficulty
- [ ] Paroxysmal tonic spasms of the limbs and trunk: these occur more frequently than in MS
- [ ] Prominent radicular and dysaesthetic symptoms
- [ ] Pruritus
- [ ] Occipital neuralgia: with high spinal cord lesions

Spinal movement disorders (SMDs)

- [ ] Tonic spasms
- [ ] Focal dystonia
- [ ] Spinal myoclonus
- [ ] Spontaneous clonus
- [ ] Tremors

NMO relapses

- [ ] These may occur in clusters
- [ ] They are associated with new or enhancing radiological lesion: unlike in pseudo-relapse
- [ ] Visual loss predicts a true relapse from pseudo-relapse

Late onset NMO

- [ ] This is defined as onset after the age of 50 years: it may present as late as >75 years
- [ ] It presents less frequently with cervical cord and optic nerve presentations
- [ ] It is associated with fewer lesions around the fourth ventricle
- [ ] There are more hemispheric lesions with more motor and sensory disability
- [ ] It is associated with higher serum C3 and C4 levels

DOI: 10.1201/9781003221258-32

NEUROMYELITIS OPTICA (NMO): SYSTEMIC FEATURES

Endocrine

- ☐ Morbid obesity
- ☐ Hyperinsulinaemia
- ☐ Hyperandrogenism
- ☐ Amenorrhoea
- ☐ Galactorrhoea
- ☐ Hyponatraemia
- ☐ Panhypopituitarism

Paraneoplastic

- ☐ Paraneoplastic NMO usually occurs in older people and in males
- ☐ It is less likely in patients with anti-AQP4 antibodies
- ☐ It is more likely to present with nausea and vomiting
- ☐ The typical primary cancers are lung, breast, and oesophageal

NMO and pregnancy

- ☐ There is a high risk of NMO relapse in pregnancy and post-partum
- ☐ There is an increased risk of premature births
- ☐ Pregnancy is associated with a poor prognosis

Autoimmune associations

- ☐ Systemic lupus erythematosus (SLE)
- ☐ Systemic sclerosis (SS)
- ☐ Myasthenia gravis (MG)
- ☐ Autoimmune thyroid dysfunction: low T3 levels and positive anti-thyroid antibodies

Other systemic NMO associations

- ☐ Clostridium perfringens infection
- ☐ Low vitamin D level
- ☐ Nivolumab treatment
- ☐ Coeliac disease

NEUROMYELITIS OPTICA (NMO): CLINICAL DIFFERENTIALS AND PROGNOSIS

Inflammatory

- ☐ Multiple sclerosis (MS)
  - ○ Free light chain kappa (FLC-k) may differentiate MS from NMO
- ☐ Anti MOG antibody syndrome
  - ○ C4 complement levels are higher than in Aquaporin 4 NMO
- ☐ Acute disseminated encephalomyelitis (ADEM)
- ☐ Idiopathic acute transverse myelitis
- ☐ Idiopathic optic neuritis
- ☐ Neuro Behcet's disease
- ☐ Sarcoidosis
- ☐ Sjogren's syndrome
- ☐ Systemic lupus erythematosus (SLE)

Viral

- ☐ Human T-lymphotrophic virus 1 (HTLV-1)
- ☐ Herpes simplex
- ☐ Epstein–Barr virus (EBV)
- ☐ Cytomegalovirus
- ☐ Dengue virus

Other infections

- ☐ Syphilis
- ☐ Lyme neuroborreliosis
- ☐ Tuberculosis
- ☐ Mycoplasma pneumoniae
- ☐ Streptococcus pneumoniae
- ☐ Cladophialophora bantiana

Other clinical differentials

- ☐ Leber hereditary optic neuropathy (LHON)
- ☐ Central nervous system (CNS) lymphoma
- ☐ Spinal dural arteriovenous fistula (SDAVF)
- ☐ Hypertrophic olivary degeneration: disrupted Mollaret's triangle (dentato-rubro-olivary circuit)
  - ○ This may mimic an NMO relapse

Poor prognostic features

- ☐ African ancestry
- ☐ Younger onset age
- ☐ Older age
- ☐ Women >40 years
  - ○ They are less treatment-responsive and they achieve less complete remission
- ☐ Aquaporin4 (AQP4) antibody: this carries a higher risk of relapses
  - ○ AQP4 status however does not affect treatment response

NEUROMYELITIS OPTICA (NMO): DIFFERENTIALS OF LETM

Muscle sclerosis (MS)

- [ ] LETM may result from coalescence of smaller MS lesions
- [ ] There is more grey matter atrophy in MS than in NMO
- [ ] Plasma complement biomarker levels are higher in NMO

Other inflammatory differentials

- [ ] Acute disseminated encephalomyelitis (ADEM)
  - ○ Putamen lesions occur more often than in NMO
- [ ] Neuromyelitis optica (NMO)
  - ○ This shows dorsal subpial enhancement
- [ ] Neurosarcoidosis
  - ○ This shows ring enhancement and the trident sign
- [ ] Systemic lupus erythematosus (SLE)
- [ ] Sjögren's syndrome
- [ ] Anti-MOG antibody syndrome
- [ ] Chronic lymphocytic inflammation with pontine perivascular enhancement responsive to steroids (CLIPPERS)
- [ ] Behçet's disease
- [ ] Anti GFAP meningoencephalomyelitis

Infections

- [ ] Tuberculosis (TB)
- [ ] Spirochetes: Syphilis, Lyme neuroborreliosis
- [ ] Retroviruses: HIV, HTLV-1
- [ ] Other viruses: Herpesvirus, Dengue fever
- [ ] Campylobacter jejuni
- [ ] Parasites: Schistosomiasis, Toxocara myelitis
- [ ] Creutzfeldt Jakob disease (CJD)

Neoplastic

- [ ] Astrocytoma
- [ ] Ependymoma
- [ ] B-cell lymphoma
- [ ] Paraneoplastic

Metabolic

- [ ] Vitamin B12 deficiency: subacute combined degeneration (SCD)
- [ ] Copper deficiency
- [ ] Biotidinase deficiency
- [ ] Nitric oxide (NO) myelopathy: causing subacute combined degeneration
- [ ] Mitochondrial encephalopathy, lactic acidosis and stroke-like episodes (MELAS)
- [ ] Cerebrotendinous xanthomatosis (CTX)

Other radiological differentials

- [ ] Spinal cord infarction
- [ ] Spinal cord arteriovenous malformation (AVM)
- [ ] Dural arteriovenous fistula (dAVF)
- [ ] Fibrocartilaginous embolism
- [ ] Spinal cord contusion
- [ ] Common variable immunodeficiency
- [ ] Erdheim Chester disease (ECD)

Acronym

- [ ] LETM: longitudinally extensive transverse myelitis

NEUROMYELITIS OPTICA (NMO): LONG-TERM IMMUNOSUPPRESSION TREATMENT

Indications

- [ ] Antibody positive
- [ ] Optic neuritis (ON) with LETM
- [ ] Severe relapsing ON or LETM
- [ ] Absence of MS features on MRI brain
- [ ] No alternative diagnoses

Rituximab: use

- [ ] Rituximab has the best evidence for effectiveness in NMO
- [ ] It is better than Azathioprine
- [ ] The risk of long-term adverse events is very low
- [ ] It is given on Day 1 and 14: then repeated 6-monthly
- [ ] FCGR3A polymorphism predicts relapses

Rituximab: side effects

- [ ] Infection
- [ ] Leukopenia
- [ ] Posterior reversible encephalopathy syndrome (PRES)
- [ ] Interstitial lung disease
- [ ] Secondary hypogammaglobulinaemia

Azathioprine

- [ ] Azathioprine is given with oral steroids
- [ ] It may be the first choice in low income situations

Alternative agents

- [ ] Mycophenolate: it may be better tolerated than Azathioprine
- [ ] Mitoxantrone
- [ ] Methotrexate
- [ ] Cyclophosphamide
- [ ] Intravenous immunoglobulins (IVIg)
- [ ] Satralizumab: this is an IL-6 receptor monoclonal recycling antibody
- [ ] Inebilizumab: this is anti-CD19 B cell-depleting antibody

Emerging agents

- [ ] Eculizumab
- [ ] Tocilizumab
- [ ] Aquaporumab
- [ ] Ruxolitinib
- [ ] Bortezomib
- [ ] Tacrolimus
- [ ] Ofatumumab: for refractory paediatric cases
- [ ] Haematopoietic stem cell transplantation (HSCT)

Other neuroinflammatory disorders

ANTI-MOG ANTIBODY DISORDERS: PHENOTYPES

Acute disseminated encephalomyelitis (ADEM)

- ☐ This is associated with large bilateral lesions
- ☐ It is more likely to manifest with longitudinally extensive transverse myelitis (LETM)
- ☐ It has a better outcome than ADEM without anti MOG antibodies

Optic neuritis (ON)

- ☐ About 80% of anti-MOG antibody disorders have ON
- ☐ It is frequently bilateral and recurrent
- ☐ There is prominent optic disc swelling
- ☐ There are fewer periventricular lesions than in multiple sclerosis (MS)
- ☐ There are no ovoid or perpendicular lesions
- ☐ It is frequently relapsing remitting
- ☐ It is often steroid responsive and dependent

Neuromyelitis optica spectrum disorders (NMOSD)

- ☐ Anti-MOG antibody is present in a third of aquaporin 4 antibody-negative NMO
- ☐ NMOSD may be the most frequent phenotype of anti-MOG disorders
- ☐ It is more frequent in males
- ☐ It presents with coincident optic neuritis and transverse myelitis
- ☐ It more frequently follows a benign monophasic than a relapsing course

Multiple sclerosis (MS)

- ☐ Anti-MOG MS is usually associated with brainstem and spinal cord lesions
- ☐ It follows a severe course with frequent relapses

Multiphasic disseminated encephalomyelitis (MDEM)

- ☐ This usually occurs in children
- ☐ It may also present in adults

Leukodystrophy-like phenotype

- ☐ This manifests with large confluent symmetrical lesions
- ☐ It only occurs in children under the age of 7 years
- ☐ It has a poor response to immunosuppression

Other anti-MOG antibody disorder phenotypes

- ☐ Isolated transverse myelitis (TM)
  - ○ This may show patchy gadolinium enhancement
- ☐ Cerebral cortical encephalitis: unilateral or bilateral
- ☐ Combined central and demyelinating syndrome (CCPD)
  - ○ This is usually spinal cord and optic nerve involvement
- ☐ Acute flaccid myelitis
- ☐ Brainstem encephalitis mimicking CLIPPERS
  - ○ This is associated with punctate and curvilinear enhancement
- ☐ Synchronised steroid-responsive epilepsy with relapsing optic neuritis (SERON)
  - ○ Paroxysms of seizures and relapsing optic neuritis

Acronym

- ☐ CLIPPERS: chronic lymphocytic inflammation with pontine perivascular enhancement responsive to steroids

DOI: 10.1201/9781003221258-33

NEUROSARCOIDOSIS: CRANIAL FEATURES

Demographic features

- [ ] Neurosarcoidosis occurs in about 5–10% of sarcoidosis
- [ ] It is isolated in 1% of cases
- [ ] The mean onset age is 33–41 years
- [ ] It is commoner in Blacks
- [ ] It is more frequent in females

Ophthalmological features

- [ ] Optic neuritis (ON): this is subacute or slowly progressive
  - ○ It is painful in only a third of cases
- [ ] Optic atrophy
- [ ] Rapid papilloedema: especially in young women
- [ ] Uveitis
- [ ] Ocular pain
- [ ] Diplopia
- [ ] Horner's syndrome
- [ ] Adie's pupil
- [ ] Argyll Robertson pupils

Cranial nerve features

- [ ] Facial nerve palsy
  - ○ This may present as Heerfordt's syndrome with uveitis, parotitis, and fever
- [ ] Anosmia: this may be the initial presentation of neurosarcoidosis
- [ ] Vocal cord palsy
- [ ] Other cranial neuropathies

Cerebral features

- [ ] Hemiparesis
- [ ] Hemianopia
- [ ] Seizures: often steroid resistant
- [ ] Movement disorders
- [ ] Mass lesions: especially in the hypothalamus and pituitary
- [ ] Hydrocephalus
  - ○ This may be the presenting feature of sarcoidosis and neurosarcoidosis
- [ ] Ataxia
- [ ] Somnolence and confusion
- [ ] Depression
- [ ] Headache

NEUROSARCOIDOSIS ASSOCIATED MYELOPATHY

Clinical features

- [ ] This is a chronically evolving myelopathy
- [ ] It may be the only feature of neurosarcoidosis
- [ ] It may present with a 'corset-like' lower chest pressure sensation
- [ ] It may present at the site of compressive cervical myelopathy
- [ ] It may mimic non-inflammatory myelopathy
  - ○ Positron emission tomography (PET) scan may help differentiate
- [ ] It is often steroid-resistant

Magnetic resonance imaging (MRI): patterns

- [ ] Longitudinally extensive transverse myelitis (LETM)
  - ○ This has a propensity for the dorsal surface of the spinal cord
  - ○ It is most often cervical followed by thoracic
- [ ] Short tumefactive myelitis
- [ ] Spinal meningitis/meningoradiculitis
- [ ] Anterior myelitis associated with areas of disc degeneration

Magnetic resonance imaging (MRI): other features

- [ ] Spinal cord atrophy
- [ ] Arachnoiditis
- [ ] Intra/extradural lesions
- [ ] Cauda equina syndrome (CES)
- [ ] Lumbosacral plexopathy
- [ ] Bony involvement

Magnetic resonance imaging (MRI): enhancement patterns

- [ ] Dorsal subpial enhancement
- [ ] Meningeal/radicular enhancement
- [ ] Ventral subpial enhancement
- [ ] Enhancement at sites of coexisting structural abnormalities, e.g. spondylosis
- [ ] Intramedullary (central canal): with a positive trident sign

Cerebrospinal fluid (CSF) features

- [ ] Raised protein
- [ ] Raised white cell count (pleocytosis)
- [ ] Low glucose

NEUROSARCOIDOSIS: MRI FEATURES

Typical brain MRI features

- ☐ Hydrocephalus
- ☐ Non-specific white matter lesions
- ☐ Mass lesions (granulomas)
- ☐ Meningeal enhancement
- ☐ Cerebral atrophy
- ☐ Cerebellar high signal changes
- ☐ Optic nerve enhancement
- ☐ Granulomatous angiitis
- ☐ Cockscrew medullary veins: dilated veins
- ☐ Cranial base lesions

Spinal MRI features

- ☐ Longitudinally extensive transverse myelitis (LETM)
- ☐ Short tumefactive myelitis
- ☐ Spinal meningitis/meningoradiculitis
- ☐ Anterior myelitis associated with areas of disc degeneration
- ☐ Trident sign: this is due to associated central canal involvement
  - ○ This helps to exclude neuromyelitis optica (NMO)
- ☐ Contrast enhancement: this is characteristically dorsal subpial
  - ○ Ventral subpial enhancement shows as the Braid-like sign

Venous sinus features

- ☐ This shows as venous sinus obstruction
- ☐ It is possibly secondary to meningeal disease
- ☐ There may be associated features of raised intracranial pressure (ICP)

Ischaemic lesions

- ☐ These usually appear as small infarcts
- ☐ They are secondary to vasculitis or embolism
- ☐ They present clinically as stroke or transient ischaemic attacks (TIAs)

Haemorrhagic lesions

- ☐ These are usually parenchymal and small-sized
- ☐ They are probably secondary to vasculitis

Other lesions

- ☐ Enhancing cavernous sinus masses
- ☐ Moyamoya-like vasculopathy
- ☐ Skull base lesions

NEUROSARCOIDOSIS: TREATMENT

Steroids alone

- ☐ Oral Prednisolone
- ☐ Intravenous Methlyprednisolone

Steroids with other immunosuppression

- ☐ Azathioprine
- ☐ Methotrexate
- ☐ Mycophenolate: this is less effective than Methotrexate
- ☐ Ciclosporin
- ☐ Cyclophosphamide

Immunomodulators in refractory cases

- ☐ Infliximab
- ☐ Hydroxychloroquine
- ☐ Pentoxifylline
- ☐ Thalidomide
- ☐ Adalimumab
- ☐ Etanercept

Other treatments

- ☐ Cranial irradiation: low dose whole brain radiation
- ☐ Neurosurgery: for hydrocephalus and sarcoid pseudotumours

PROGRESSIVE MULTIFOCAL LEUKOENCEPHALOPATHY (PML): RISK FACTORS

JC virus infection

- ☐ JC (John Cunningham) virus is responsible for PML
- ☐ It belongs to the BK viruses
- ☐ It infects oligodendrocytes
- ☐ JC virus DNA is also found in urine and lymphocytes
- ☐ 80–90% of adults are JC virus antibody positive
- ☐ It may jointly co-infect with herpes viruses
  - ○ Varicella zoster (VZV) and Epstein Barr virus (EBV)
- ☐ JC virus also causes encephalitis and meningitis

Immunosuppressive disorders

- ☐ AIDS
- ☐ Cancer
- ☐ Autoimmune diseases
- ☐ Immunosuppressive treatment
- ☐ Lymphoproliferative diseases
- ☐ Myeloproliferative diseases
- ☐ Sarcoidosis
- ☐ Tuberculosis (TB)
- ☐ Whipple's disease
- ☐ Transplantation
- ☐ Coeliac disease

Natalizumab: high risk features for PML

- ☐ Duration of treatment ≥25 months
- ☐ Prior immunosuppression
- ☐ Positive JC virus antibody
- ☐ Anti JC virus antibody index ≥1.5

Other drugs

- ☐ Rituximab
- ☐ Fingolimod
- ☐ Alemtuzumab
- ☐ Mycophenolate mofetil
- ☐ Fumarate

PROGRESSIVE MULTIFOCAL LEUKOENCEPHALOPATHY (PML): CLINICAL FEATURES

Demographic features

- ☐ PML develops after a mean interval of about 2 years after Natalizumab treatment
- ☐ It evolves over weeks
- ☐ The mortality is 29%
- ☐ The one-year survival is 38–62%

Neurological features

- ☐ Cognitive impairment
- ☐ Language dysfunction
- ☐ Visual impairment
- ☐ Personality change
- ☐ Ataxia
- ☐ Seizures
- ☐ Fever
- ☐ Immune reconstitution inflammatory response (IRIS)
- ☐ There is no optic nerve or spinal cord involvement

Poor prognostic features

- ☐ Older age
- ☐ Late diagnosis
- ☐ Generalised disease on MRI
- ☐ Lack of enhancing lesions at diagnosis
- ☐ Presence of disability before diagnosis

Factors that do not affect prognosis

- ☐ Gender
- ☐ Disease duration
- ☐ Prior immunosuppression
- ☐ Cerebrospinal fluid (CSF) JC viral load

Causes of death

- ☐ Immune reconstitution inflammatory syndrome (IRIS)
- ☐ Aspiration pneumonia
- ☐ Hypoventilation syndrome/respiratory failure
- ☐ Status seizures

PROGRESSIVE MULTIFOCAL LEUKOENCEPHALOPATHY (PML): INVESTIGATIONS

Magnetic resonance imaging (MRI)

- ☐ This shows multifocal, asymmetric, and subcortical white matter lesions
- ☐ They are hypointense on T1 sequences
- ☐ They show as high signal on T2 and FLAIR sequences
- ☐ They are relatively non-enhancing
- ☐ A punctate pattern of lesions is sensitive for Natalizumab PML
- ☐ There is a thin and linear gyriform hypointense rim in paralesional U-fibers
  - ○ This is seen on susceptibility weighted imaging

Cerebrospinal fluid (CSF)

- ☐ JC virus polymerase chain reaction (PCR)
  - ○ This may be negative with small PML lesions
- ☐ JC virus DNA level: this is low in 50% of cases
  - ○ Low copy numbers may not indicate PML

Diagnostic criteria for PML

- ☐ Magnetic resonance imaging (MRI) which is consistent with PML
- ☐ Positive JC virus DNA in the cerebrospinal fluid (CSF)
- ☐ PML demonstrated on histopathology
- ☐ JC virus identified on electron microscopy, immunohistochemistry, or PCR

Differential diagnosis from PML-IRIS on MRI

- ☐ PML-IRIS enhances on contrast MRI: unlike PML
- ☐ Patchy or punctate enhancement is the earliest sign of PML-IRIS

Acronyms

- ☐ PCR: Polymerase chain reaction
- ☐ PML-IRIS: PML immune reconstitution inflammatory syndrome

PROGRESSIVE MULTIFOCAL LEUKOENCEPHALOPATHY (PML): MANAGEMENT

Pre-Natalizumab assessments: JC virus antibody

- ☐ Serum anti JC virus antibody is checked within 6 months before starting treatment
- ☐ Consider alternative treatments to Natalizumab if JC virus is positive
- ☐ Alternative treatments can be instituted at the outset or during the first 12 months of Natalizumab
- ☐ This is because PML is unlikely to develop within 12 months of treatment

Pre-Natalizumab assessments: others

- ☐ Magnetic resonance imaging (MRI): this is done within 3 months of starting treatment
- ☐ Urine JC virus DNA polymerase chain reaction (PCR)

PML monitoring on Natalizumab therapy

- ☐ Anti-JC virus antibody
  - ○ Six-monthly in seronegative cases or if the antibody index is ≤1.5
  - ○ There is no need to routinely re-check it within the first year of treatment
- ☐ Magnetic resonance imaging (MRI)
  - ○ This is done 6–12 monthly depending on risk stratification and treatment duration

Treatment guidelines in suspected PML

- ☐ Stop Natalizumab treatment
- ☐ Check magnetic resonance imaging (MRI)
- ☐ Check cerebrospinal fluid (CSF)
- ☐ Monitor for IRIS with contrast MRI 12–14 weeks after stopping Natalizumab
  - ○ IRIS occurs in almost all cases after stopping treatment
- ☐ Treat PML

Treatment of PML

- ☐ Plasma exchange (PE) or immune-absorption to remove Natalizumab
- ☐ Antiviral agents: Mirtazapine or Mefloquine
- ☐ Intravenous steroids to prevent IRIS
  - ○ Especially with brainstem or large hemispheric lesions
- ☐ Maraviroc: this may be effective in Natalizumab-induced PML-IRIS

Re-starting treatment in suspected PML

- ☐ This is indicated if the patient is well and there is no PML after 2 years
- ☐ Patient should be re-consented at a higher risk
- ☐ Monitoring is with annual MRI scans

Investigational treatments: immune checkpoint inhibitors

- ☐ Pembrolizumab
- ☐ Nivolumab

Acronym

- ☐ IRIS: immune reconstitution inflammatory syndrome

Autoimmune encephalitis

ANTI-LGI1 VGKC AUTOIMMUNE ENCEPHALITIS: CLINICAL FEATURES

Epidemiology

- ☐ Anti-LG1 accounts for most cases of anti-VGKC encephalitis
- ☐ It may co-exist with anti-CASPR2 antibodies (double positive)
- ☐ Seropositivity may be delayed
- ☐ The onset age is about 65 years
- ☐ Males are affected more frequently by a ratio of 2:1

Possible associated HLA haplotypes

- ☐ DRB1*07:01-DQB1*02:02
- ☐ B*44:03
- ☐ C*07:06
- ☐ DR7
- ☐ DRB4

Clinical triad

- ☐ Memory loss
- ☐ Confusion
- ☐ Seizures

Psychiatric features

- ☐ Anxiety
- ☐ Depression
- ☐ Agitation

Cognitive features

- ☐ Amnesia: this is due to damage to the hippocampus
- ☐ Encephalitis

Other features

- ☐ Seizures
- ☐ Neuromyotonia
- ☐ Morvan's syndrome
- ☐ Hemianaesthesia: this may be a frequent initial symptom
- ☐ Hypothermic attacks
- ☐ Neuropathic pain
- ☐ Hyponatraemia
- ☐ Demyelinating polyneuropathy: case report
- ☐ Tumours: these are uncommon unlike in anti-CASPR2 encephalitis
- ☐ Sleep disturbance
- ☐ Sudden cardiac death: this is due to seizure-related cardiac ischaemia
- ☐ Rapidly progressive global cerebral atrophy

Outcome

- ☐ Amnesia and spatial disorientation often persist
- ☐ 35% of cases relapse: some relapses are delayed by >8 years
- ☐ New onset psychosis has been reported after recovery

Differential diagnosis: anti-CASPR2

- ☐ There are no faciobrachial dystonic seizures or paroxysmal dizziness

ANTI-LG1 VGKC AUTOIMMUNE ENCEPHALITIS: FACIOBRACHIAL DYSTONIC SEIZURES

Presentation

- ☐ They start before the onset of encephalitis
- ☐ They may present as isolated epilepsy

Clinical features

- ☐ They manifest as brief unilateral posturing of the face and limbs
- ☐ They may present as subtle jerks or dropping of objects
- ☐ There may be a sensory aura
- ☐ Episodes are very frequent: up to 100/day
- ☐ Seizures may alternate sides

Triggers

- ☐ Rapid movements
- ☐ Emotion
- ☐ Stress
- ☐ Noise

Implications

- ☐ Seizures predict cognitive decline
- ☐ Only 10% response to antiepileptic drugs alone
- ☐ About 90% respond to the addition of immunotherapy

DOI: 10.1201/9781003221258-34

ANTI-CASPR2 VGKC AUTOIMMUNE ENCEPHALITIS: CLINICAL FEATURES

Causes of anti CASPR2 positivity

- ☐ Hashimoto thyroiditis
- ☐ Thymoma
- ☐ Systemic lupus erythematosus (SLE)
- ☐ Pembrolizumab
- ☐ Association with HLA-DRB1*11:01 haplotype

Clinical presentations

- ☐ Limbic encephalitis
- ☐ Neuromyotonia
- ☐ Morvan's syndrome
- ☐ Cerebellar ataxia
- ☐ Progressive encephalomyelitis, rigidity and myoclonus (PERM)
- ☐ Stiff person syndrome (SPS)

Central features

- ☐ Encephalopathy
- ☐ Insomnia
- ☐ Transient epileptic amnesia (TEA)
- ☐ Episodic ataxia
- ☐ Cerebellar ataxia
- ☐ Myoclonic status epilepticus
- ☐ Spinal myoclonus
- ☐ Parkinsonism

Peripheral features

- ☐ Peripheral nerve hyperexcitability (PNH)
- ☐ Dysautonomia
- ☐ Neuropathic pain
- ☐ Weight loss
- ☐ Thymoma: in about 20% of cases

Clinical outcome

- ☐ It is treatment-responsive in >90% of cases
- ☐ Clinical relapses occur in 25% of cases

ANTI-CASPR2 VGKC AUTOIMMUNE ENCEPHALITIS: MANAGEMENT

Anti-VGKC antibody testing

- ☐ Positive VGKC antibody test is not pathogenic unless either CASPR2 or LGI1 is positive
  - ○ Low levels may however indicate malignancy
- ☐ Anti-CASPR2 may co-exist with anti-LGI1: this is double seropositivity

Initial treatment

- ☐ Steroids: oral or intravenous
- ☐ Intravenous immunoglobulins (IVIg)
  - ○ Combination with steroids may be better
- ☐ Plasma exchange

Secondary treatment for refractory cases

- ☐ Azathioprine
- ☐ Mycophenolate
- ☐ Tacrolimus
- ☐ Rituximab

ANTI-NMDAR AUTOIMMUNE ENCEPHALITIS: CLINICAL FEATURES

Epidemiology

- ☐ The median onset age is about 22 years: the age range is 5–76 years
- ☐ Females account for 70–90% of cases

Triggers

- ☐ Herpes simplex virus (HSV): encephalitic and non-encephalitic
- ☐ Japanese B encephalitis
- ☐ Methamphetamine abuse: case report

Encephalitic features

- ☐ Prodrome of fever and headache for 1–3 weeks
- ☐ Seizures
- ☐ Short term memory deficits
- ☐ Reduced consciousness
- ☐ Mutism

Movement disorders

- ☐ Chorea
- ☐ Athetosis
- ☐ Dystonia: including hemidystonia
- ☐ Opisthotonus
- ☐ Ballismus
- ☐ Blepharospasm
- ☐ Oculogyric crisis
- ☐ Dyskinesias: grimacing, masticatory, and jaw opening/closure
- ☐ Paroxysmal exercise-induced foot weakness
- ☐ Myorhythmia-like dyskinesias of the face and ears
- ☐ Isolated nocturnal orofacial dyskinesia
- ☐ Dystonic posturing

Sleep disorders

- ☐ Insomnia
- ☐ Hypersomnia
- ☐ Nightmares
- ☐ Sleep-related hyperphagia and hypersexuality

Psychiatric features

- ☐ Hallucinations: visual or auditory
- ☐ Acute schizoaffective episodes
- ☐ Depression and mania
- ☐ Addictive and eating disorders
- ☐ Catatonia
- ☐ Post-partum psychosis
- ☐ Suicidality

Systemic features

- ☐ Neuroleptic intolerance in 50% of cases
  - ○ This presents with hyperthermia, rigidity, rhabdomyolysis, or coma
- ☐ Hypoventilation
- ☐ Cardiac dysrhythmias
- ☐ Lymphocytosis
- ☐ Dysautonomia
- ☐ Low uric acid levels

ANTI-NMDAR AUTOIMMUNE ENCEPHALITIS: INVESTIGATIONS

HLA associations

- ☐ HLA-DRB1*16:02 in Han Chinese
- ☐ HLA-B*07:02 in Germans

Genetics

- ☐ It may be associated with GRIN1 mutations
- ☐ GRIN1 encodes an NMDA receptor subunit

Associated glial and neuronal surface antibodies

- ☐ Myelin oligodendrocyte glycoprotein (MOG)
- ☐ Glial fibrillary acidic protein (GFAP)
- ☐ Aquaporin 4 (AQP4)
- ☐ AMPA receptor (AMPAR)
- ☐ GABAA receptor (GABAAR)
- ☐ GABAB receptor (GABABR)

Serum antibody titers

- ☐ Serum antibodies are negative in 15% of cases
- ☐ Negative serum titres occur especially in the elderly and with mild disease
- ☐ Negative serum titres also occur in cases without tumours

Cerebrospinal fluid (CSF): antibody titers

- ☐ CSF is more sensitive than serum
- ☐ CSF titres are higher than in serum
- ☐ Higher titres are seen with teratoma
- ☐ Higher titres correlate with relapse and poorer outcome

Cerebrospinal fluid (CSF): other features

- ☐ Pleocytosis
- ☐ Oligoclonal bands: in the late stages

Magnetic resonance imaging (MRI) brain

- ☐ The MRI is abnormal in about half of cases
- ☐ Hippocampal lesions are the most frequent abnormalities
- ☐ Hippocampal lesions predict a poor prognosis
- ☐ Superficial white matter damage may also be seen

Positron emission tomography (PET)

- ☐ PET is more sensitive than MRI
- ☐ It shows occipital hypometabolism
- ☐ This is probably a biomarker of anti-NMDA encephalitis

Electroencephalography (EEG) features

- ☐ Focal or diffuse slowing
- ☐ Disorganised activity
- ☐ Seizure activity
- ☐ Extreme delta brush (EDB): this resembles the waveforms in premature infants

ANTI-NMDAR AUTOIMMUNE ENCEPHALITIS: TREATMENT

First line immunotherapy

- ☐ Methylprednisolone
- ☐ Intravenous immunoglobulins (IVIg)
- ☐ Plasma exchange

Second line immunotherapy

- ☐ Azathioprine
- ☐ Methotrexate
- ☐ Mycophenolate
- ☐ Cyclophosphamide
- ☐ Rituximab
- ☐ Alemtuzumab

Emerging treatments

- ☐ Electroconvulsive therapy (ECT)
- ☐ Bortezomib
- ☐ Tocilizumab

Surgery

- ☐ This is indicated for associated tumours

Possible markers of treatment response

- ☐ Serum cystatin C
- ☐ Serum uric acid

ANTI-AMPAR AUTOIMMUNE ENCEPHALITIS

Pathology

- ☐ The antibodies target AMPAR receptors
- ☐ They are made up of tetramers of the glutamate receptors (GluR) types 1, 2, 3 or 4

Epidemiology

- ☐ It typically affects middle aged women
- ☐ The median onset age is about 60 years

Clinical features

- ☐ Subacute onset
- ☐ Prominent psychosis
- ☐ Confusion
- ☐ Memory impairment (amnesia)
- ☐ Seizures
- ☐ Frequent relapses

Associated tumours

- ☐ Lung
- ☐ Breast
- ☐ Thymus
- ☐ Ovarian
- ☐ Melanoma

Investigations

- ☐ The brain magnetic resonance imaging (MRI) shows bilateral medio-temporal abnormalities
- ☐ The cerebrospinal fluid (CSF) is lymphocytic
- ☐ The electroencephalogram (EEG) is normal

Treatment

- ☐ Prednisolone
- ☐ Intravenous immunoglobulin (IVIg)
- ☐ Plasma exchange
- ☐ Azathioprine
- ☐ Mycophenolate
- ☐ Rituximab

Acronym

- ☐ AMPAR: α-amino-3-hydroxy-5-methyl-4-isoxazolepropionic acid receptors

Peripheral autoimmune disorders

NEUROMYOTONIA: CLINICAL FEATURES

Peripheral features

- [ ] Cramps: these are triggered by muscle contractions and cold exposure
- [ ] Myokymia
- [ ] Pseudomyotonia: this is impaired muscle relaxation worse with exertion
- [ ] Excessive sweating
- [ ] Paraesthesias
- [ ] Mild weakness
- [ ] Muscle hypertrophy
- [ ] Painless involuntary flexion of ring and middle fingers
- [ ] Armadillo syndrome (laborious gait)
- [ ] Finger flexion

Central features

- [ ] Insomnia
- [ ] Delusions, hallucinations
- [ ] Prolonged paralysis after general anaesthesia

Synonym

- [ ] Isaacs syndrome

MORVAN'S SYNDROME

Aetiology

- [ ] This is usually associated with CASPR2 antibody
- [ ] It may be antibody-negative

Neurological features

- [ ] Neuromyotonia
- [ ] Subacute insomnia
- [ ] Psychiatric features
- [ ] Confusion
- [ ] Memory problems
- [ ] Circadian dysregulation
- [ ] Hallucinations
- [ ] Frontotemporal dysfunction

Systemic features

- [ ] Pain
- [ ] Weight loss
- [ ] Hyperhidrosis
- [ ] Excessive salivation
- [ ] Excessive lacrimation
- [ ] Impotence
- [ ] Cardiac arrhythmia
- [ ] Associated thymoma

DOI: 10.1201/9781003221258-35

ANTI-GAD SYNDROMES: PHENOTYPES

Classic anti-GAD syndromes

- ☐ Stiff person syndrome (SPS)
- ☐ Progressive encephalomyelitis with rigidity and myoclonus (PERM)
- ☐ Autoimmune encephalitis

Temporal lobe epilepsy

- ☐ This may present as musicogenic seizures
- ☐ It is often drug- and immunotherapy-resistant
- ☐ It may respond best to steroids
- ☐ It often does not respond to temporal lobe surgery

Cerebellar ataxia

- ☐ The onset is subacute
- ☐ It usually affects females with late onset diabetes
- ☐ It presents with persistent vertigo and vertical diplopia
- ☐ There may be recurrent cerebellar events
- ☐ It is often associated with other endocrinopathies
- ☐ It is responsive to early immunotherapy

Eye movement disorders

- ☐ Opsoclonus myoclonus
- ☐ Downbeat nystagmus (DBN)
- ☐ Periodic alternating nystagmus (PAN)
- ☐ Ocular flutter

Other anti-GAD associated neurological disorders

- ☐ Myasthenia gravis (MG)
- ☐ Paraneoplastic encephalomyelitis
- ☐ Batten's disease: juvenile neuronal ceroid lipofuscinosis (NCL)
- ☐ Neuromyotonia
- ☐ Miller Fisher syndrome (MFS)
- ☐ Inflammatory myopathy: presenting with dropped head syndrome

Other anti-GAD associated medical disorders

- ☐ Diabetes mellitus
- ☐ Possibly gluten sensitivity

STIFF PERSON SYNDROME (SPS): CLINICAL FEATURES

Epidemiology

- ☐ The onset is typically in the 4th to 6th decade
- ☐ Females predominate 2:1
- ☐ Symptoms improve in pregnancy

Features of rigidity

- ☐ Spine and leg rigidity: this is often asymmetric
- ☐ Both hands and feet are involved in 25% of cases
- ☐ It may result in lumbar hyperlordosis

Features of spasms

- ☐ These are painful
- ☐ They may be triggered by noise, stress, contact, and emotional stress
- ☐ They cause gait difficulty because of hyperextended legs
- ☐ Status spasticus may develop
  - ○ This results from respiratory and thoracic paraspinal muscle involvement
- ☐ Serotonin-norepinephrine reuptake inhibitors may exacerbate symptoms

Other features

- ☐ Psychological features: these may predominate
- ☐ Epilepsy
- ☐ Ataxia
- ☐ About two-thirds are unable to function independently

Associated autoimmune disorders

- ☐ Diabetes mellitus
- ☐ Autoimmune thyroiditis
- ☐ Pernicious anaemia
- ☐ Coeliac disease
- ☐ Systemic lupus erythematosus (SLE) rarely

Associated cancers

- ☐ Breast
- ☐ Small cell lung cancer (SCLC)
- ☐ Thymoma
- ☐ Colon
- ☐ Hodgkin's lymphoma

Differential diagnoses

- ☐ Parkinson's disease (PD)
- ☐ Primary lateral sclerosis (PLS)
- ☐ Multiple sclerosis (MS)
- ☐ Psychiatric phobia/anxiety
- ☐ Status dystonicus

STIFF PERSON SYNDROME (SPS): VARIANTS

Stiff limb syndrome

- ☐ The sphincters are affected in half of cases
- ☐ The brainstem is involved in a third of cases
- ☐ Most cases are anti-GAD antibody negative

Stiff person syndrome (SPS) plus: types

- ☐ Cerebellar ataxia without atrophy
- ☐ Epilepsy
- ☐ Abnormal eye movements
- ☐ Phobic/anxious personality

Stiff person syndrome (SPS) with encephalomyelitis

- ☐ Anti-amphiphysin antibody is frequently positive
- ☐ It is possibly paraneoplastic: breast, lung, colon, and Hodgkin's lymphoma
- ☐ It presents with myoclonus and cognitive decline
- ☐ There may be associated brainstem signs
- ☐ The course is progressive
- ☐ The prognosis is poor

Other SPS variants

- ☐ Progressive encephalomyelitis with rigidity and myoclonus (PERM)
- ☐ Persistent focal stiff man/leg
- ☐ Cerebellar subtype
- ☐ Jerking stiffman syndrome

STIFF PERSON SYNDROME (SPS): TREATMENT

Spasticity treatment: benzodiazepines

- ☐ Diazepam primarily
- ☐ Clonazepam
- ☐ Alprazolam
- ☐ Lorazepam

Spasticity treatment: others

- ☐ Baclofen
- ☐ Dantrolene
- ☐ Tizanidine
- ☐ Gabapentin
- ☐ Valproate
- ☐ Carbamazepine
- ☐ Tiagabine
- ☐ Levetiracetam
- ☐ Propofol
- ☐ Intramuscular (IM) botulinum toxin

Treatment of respiratory crisis

- ☐ Midazolam: intravenous or intranasal

Immunosuppression

- ☐ Corticosteroids
- ☐ Intravenous immunoglobulins (IVIg)
- ☐ Plasma exchange
- ☐ Azathioprine
- ☐ Methotrexate
- ☐ Mycophenolate
- ☐ Chemotherapy for paraneoplastic cases
- ☐ Autologous haematopoietic stem cell transplantation (HSCT)
  - ○ For patients who are refractory to other treatments
- ☐ Rituximab: this is probably not better than placebo

CHAPTER 6

Infections

Viral infections

VIRAL ENCEPHALITIS: AETIOLOGICAL INDICATORS

Recent travel

- ☐ Dengue
- ☐ Japanese B
- ☐ Vaccinations

Skin rash

- ☐ Measles
- ☐ Chickenpox
- ☐ Parvovirus
- ☐ HHV6

Contact with animals

- ☐ Rabies, e.g. dogs
- ☐ West Nile (sick birds)

Tremors (basal ganglia involvement)

- ☐ West Nile
- ☐ Japanese B

Acute flaccid paralysis

- ☐ Polio
- ☐ Enterovirus 71

Immunocompromised state

- ☐ Herpes simplex (HSV) 1 and 2
- ☐ Varicella zoster (VZV)
- ☐ Enteroviruses
- ☐ Epstein Barr virus (EBV)
- ☐ Cytomegalovirus (CMV)
- ☐ Human herpes virus 6 (HHV6)
- ☐ Human herpes virus 7 (HHV7)
- ☐ JC/BK virus

Other indicative features of aetiology

- ☐ Mumps: parotitis and testicular pain
- ☐ Norovirus: gastroenteritis
- ☐ Influenza: seasonal epidemics
- ☐ HIV: risky sexual behaviour
- ☐ Herpes simplex virus (HSV): olfactory hallucinations
- ☐ Varicella zoster (VZV): acute cerebellar ataxia

VIRAL ENCEPHALITIS: MANAGEMENT

Investigations

- ☐ Cerebrospinal fluid (CSF) polymerase chain reaction (PCR)
  - ○ For herpes simplex (HSV)
  - ○ Consider repeating in 3–7 days if it is initially negative
- ☐ HIV screening is indicated in all cases
- ☐ Throat and rectal swabs: for enterovirus

Treatment of infection

- ☐ Treat all suspected cases with intravenous Acyclovir
- ☐ Administer high dose oral Valaciclovir (HDVA) if IV Acyclovir is not possible or available
- ☐ Treat all patients for 14–21 days
- ☐ Treat the immunocompromised for at least 21 days
  - ○ Then continue with oral treatment until CD4 count is >200

Treatment of raised intracranial pressure

- ☐ 30° head-up position
- ☐ Craniectomy if severe
- ☐ Consider steroids

Indications for steroids in viral encephalitis

- ☐ Brain swelling with herpes simplex virus (HSV)
  - ○ Consider steroids even if there is no brain swelling
- ☐ Varicella zoster virus (VZV): it has a strong vasculitic component
- ☐ Acute demyelinating encephalomyelitis (ADEM)
- ☐ Acute haemorrhagic leukoencephalitis
- ☐ Diffuse encephalopathy with systemic viral infections

DOI: 10.1201/9781003221258-37

HIV ASSOCIATED NEUROLOGICAL SYNDROMES: CLASSIFICATION

HIV associated central neurological syndromes

- ☐ HIV associated neurocognitive disorder (HAND)
- ☐ HIV leukoencephalopathy
- ☐ HIV associated myelopathies
- ☐ HIV associated drug-induced syndromes
- ☐ HIV associated neurological opportunistic infections
- ☐ HIV associated tumours
- ☐ HIV associated cerebral vasculopathy: presents with multiple aneurysms
- ☐ Immune reconstitution inflammatory syndrome (IRIS)
- ☐ HIV related movement disorders: opsoclonus-myoclonus-ataxia syndrome
- ☐ HIV associated pure cerebellar degeneration and ataxia

HIV associated myopathies

- ☐ Polymyositis (PM-HIV)
- ☐ Inclusion body myositis (IBM)
- ☐ Immune mediated necrotising myopathy (IMNM)
- ☐ Non-specific myositis (NSM)
- ☐ Sporadic late onset nemaline myopathy (SLONM)

HIV associated neuropathy (HAN)

- ☐ HIV associated sensory neuropathy
- ☐ HIV associated vasculitic neuropathy
- ☐ Opportunistic vasculitic neuropathy
- ☐ Diffuse infiltrative lymphocytosis syndrome (DILS)
- ☐ Acute inflammatory demyelinating polyradiculoneuropathy (AIDP)
- ☐ Chronic inflammatory demyelinating polyradiculoneuropathy (CIDP)

Other HIV associated neurological disorders

- ☐ HIV associated neurological opportunistic infections
- ☐ HIV associated motor neurone disease: this may be associated with HERV-K
- ☐ Bibrachial amyotrophic diplegia (BAD)

HIV ASSOCIATED NEUROCOGNITIVE DISORDERS (HAND): CLINICAL FEATURES

Classification

- ☐ Asymptomatic neurocognitive impairment (ANI)
  - ○ There is no impairment of activities of daily living
- ☐ Mild neurocognitive disorder (MND)
- ☐ HIV associated dementia (HAD): this is a subcortical dementia
  - ○ It is less prevalent than ANI and MND because of the use of combined antiretrovirals (cARTs)

HIV-associated dementia (HAD)

- ☐ Impaired concentration and attention
- ☐ Memory deficits
- ☐ Psychomotor slowing
- ☐ Behavioural symptoms
- ☐ Apathy
- ☐ Gait disturbance
- ☐ Impaired manual dexterity
- ☐ Tremor
- ☐ Seizures in advanced cases

Infective differential diagnoses

- ☐ Cytomegalovirus (CMV) encephalitis
- ☐ Progressive multifocal leukoencephalopathy (PML)
- ☐ Cryptococcal meningitis
- ☐ Tuberculous meningitis (TBM)
- ☐ Neurosyphilis
- ☐ Varicella zoster encephalitis
- ☐ Hepatitis C virus (HCV) infection
- ☐ Creutzfeldt-Jakob disease (CJD)

Other differential diagnoses

- ☐ Neurodegenerative dementias
- ☐ Pseudodementia
- ☐ Metabolic encephalopathy
- ☐ Primary CNS lymphoma
- ☐ Immune reconstitution inflammatory syndrome (IRIS)

Neurocognitive screening tools

- ☐ Revised HIV dementia scale
- ☐ International HIV dementia scale
- ☐ MoCA test
- ☐ NEU screen
- ☐ CogState

Neurocognitive testing

- ☐ Trail-making
- ☐ Grooved peg board
- ☐ Digit-symbol test
- ☐ Reaction time
- ☐ Reye figure copying
- ☐ Mosaic test
- ☐ Rey-Auditory-Verbal Learning test

HIV ASSOCIATED NEUROPATHY (HAN)

Sensory neuropathy

- ☐ This is a painful distal neuropathy
- ☐ Pain is worse at night or after walking
- ☐ Weakness is rare

Acute and chronic inflammatory demyelinating polyradiculoneuropathy

- ☐ This is possibly autoimmune
- ☐ The cerebrospinal fluid (CSF) is typically lymphocytic

Opportunistic vasculitic neuropathy: causes

- ☐ Cytomegalovirus (CMV)
- ☐ Varicella zoster virus (VZV)
- ☐ Hepatitis B virus (HBV)
- ☐ Hepatitis C virus (HCV)

Herpes zoster associated neuropathy: types

- ☐ Radiculopathy
- ☐ Myeloradiculopathy

Diffuse infiltrative lymphocytosis syndrome (DILS)

- ☐ This is a Sjogren-like disorder
- ☐ It presents with painful distal sensory peripheral neuropathy (DSPN)
- ☐ There may be multiple mononeuropathies

Other HIV associated neuropathies

- ☐ HIV associated vasculitic neuropathy
- ☐ CMV polyradiculopathy
- ☐ Optic neuropathy as a presenting feature of HIV infection

Treatment

- ☐ Lamotrigine: Level B evidence
- ☐ Cannabis: Level A evidence
- ☐ Capsaicin patches: Level A evidence

RABIES ENCEPHALITIS: CLINICAL FEATURES

Types of rabies infection

- ☐ Encephalitic (furious rabies): this accounts for 80% of cases
- ☐ Paralytic (dumb rabies): this is seen in 20% of cases

General features

- ☐ Altered sensorium
- ☐ Fever
- ☐ Myalgia
- ☐ Headache
- ☐ Irritability
- ☐ Depression

Hydrophobia

- ☐ This is a phobia of swallowing water
- ☐ It manifests with inspiratory spasms
- ☐ There may be painful laryngospasms
- ☐ It may progress to aerophobia
- ☐ It may be absent in paralytic rabies

Peripheral neurological features

- ☐ Paraesthesias at site of the bite
- ☐ Fasciculations
- ☐ Radiculopathy

Autonomic features

- ☐ Excessive sweating
- ☐ Hypersalivation
- ☐ Blood pressure changes

Sexual features

- ☐ Excessive libido and hypersexuality
- ☐ Priapism
- ☐ Penile hyperexcitability and recurrent ejaculation
- ☐ Penile pain

Differential diagnosis

- ☐ Schizophrenia
- ☐ Delirium tremens
- ☐ Acute psychosis
- ☐ Hypomania
- ☐ Hysteria
- ☐ Tetanus
- ☐ Paralytic poliomyelitis
- ☐ Guillain–Barre syndrome (GBS)
- ☐ Botulism
- ☐ Diphtheria

Course and outcome

- ☐ The mean incubation period is 2 months: the range is 7 days to 4 years
- ☐ The mean duration of illness is 2 weeks: the range is 4–24 days
- ☐ It is almost uniformly fatal but survival up to a year has been reported

RABIES ENCEPHALITIS: VIROLOGY AND MANAGEMENT

Virology

- ☐ Rabies is a Lyssavirus: a rhabdovirus zoonosis
- ☐ Transmission is by direct animal bites or saliva contamination of wounds

Transmitting animals

- ☐ Dogs
- ☐ Cats
- ☐ Foxes
- ☐ Jackals
- ☐ Wolves
- ☐ Mongooses
- ☐ Racoons
- ☐ Skunks
- ☐ Bats
- ☐ Human-to-human transmission is possible

Investigations

- ☐ Immunology
- ☐ Cerebrospinal fluid (CSF): for cells and viral titres
- ☐ Neuropathology: this shows Negri bodies

Post-exposure management

- ☐ Post-exposure human rabies immunoglobulin (HRIG)
- ☐ Barrier nursing
- ☐ Wound care

Pre-exposure management

- ☐ Human diploid cell or chick cell vaccination
- ☐ This is indicated for relatives, staff, animal handlers, laboratory workers, and travellers

VARICELLA ZOSTER VIRUS (VZV) INFECTION: CENTRAL FEATURES

Virology

- ☐ This is a human neurotrophic alphavirus
- ☐ It is latent in ganglionic neurons

Risk factors for reactivation

- ☐ Age
- ☐ Immunosuppression
- ☐ Diabetes
- ☐ Extracorporeal shock wave lithotripsy (case report)

Cerebral presentations

- ☐ Aseptic meningitis: especially with craniocervical zoster
- ☐ Meningoencephalitis
- ☐ Meningo-encephalo-radiculo-neuropathy: cranial and peripheral nerve involvement
- ☐ Focal encephalitis
- ☐ Brainstem encephalitis
- ☐ Cerebellitis
- ☐ Encephalomyelitis
- ☐ SUNCT

Spinal cord presentations

- ☐ Acute ascending and necrotising myelitis: vanishing spinal cord
- ☐ Haemorrhagic myelitis
- ☐ Longitudinally extensive transverse myelitis (LETM) with positive aquaporin 4 antibody

Herpes zoster ophthalmicus

- ☐ This is zoster of the ophthalmic division of the trigeminal nerve
- ☐ It may present as herpes zoster optic neuropathy (HZON)

Cranial nerve palsies

- ☐ Optic neuritis
- ☐ Ischaemic optic neuropathy
- ☐ Ophthalmoplegia: diplopia may be the only feature of zoster
- ☐ Ramsay Hunt syndrome: facial nerve
- ☐ Laryngeal paralysis: vagus nerve
- ☐ Polyneuritis cranialis: lower cranial nerves

Ocular features

- ☐ Acute retinal necrosis
- ☐ Progressive outer retinal necrosis (PORN)

Acronym

- ☐ SUNCT: Short-lasting unilateral neuralgiform headache attacks with conjunctival injection and tearing

VARICELLA ZOSTER VIRUS (VZV) INFECTION: PERIPHERAL FEATURES

Dermatological features

- ☐ Chicken pox
- ☐ Herpes zoster
- ☐ Bilateral herpes zoster

Herpes zoster plexopathy

- ☐ This may cause segmental zoster-associated limb paresis (ZALP)
- ☐ MRI shows T2 signal hyperintensity, nerve enlargement, and enhancement

Zoster mononeuropathies

- ☐ Ulnar
- ☐ Median
- ☐ Sciatic
- ☐ Femoral

Zoster paresis

- ☐ Limb weakness
- ☐ Diaphragmatic weakness
- ☐ Urinary retention
- ☐ Abdominal hernia

Other peripheral neurological features

- ☐ Preherpetic neuralgia
- ☐ Post herpetic neuralgia
- ☐ Subclinical reactivation of herpes zoster
- ☐ Zoster sine herpete: chronic radicular pain without rash

VARICELLA ZOSTER (VZV) VASCULOPATHY

Risk factors

- ☐ Immune compromise
- ☐ HIV infection
- ☐ Systemic lupus erythematosus (SLE)
- ☐ Rheumatoid arthritis
- ☐ Steroid therapy
- ☐ Natalizumab

Possible pathogenetic mechanisms

- ☐ Inflammation
- ☐ Dysregulation of programmed death ligand-1 (PD-1)
- ☐ Downregulation of major histocompatibility complex class 1 (MHC1)

Onset features

- ☐ Skin rash: this occurs in about 60% of cases
- ☐ Vasculopathy: this starts 6 weeks to 4 months after the rash
- ☐ Headache
- ☐ Ophthalmic zoster: this is more frequent in the elderly

Vascular features

- ☐ Transient ischaemic attack (TIA)
- ☐ Stroke
- ☐ Aneurysm formation
- ☐ Intracerebral haemorrhage (ICH)
- ☐ Subarachnoid haemorrhage (SAH)
- ☐ Carotid dissection
- ☐ Peripheral artery disease
- ☐ Cerebral vein thrombosis (CVT)
- ☐ Giant cell arteritis (GCA)
- ☐ Granulomatous aortitis

Non-vascular features

- ☐ Radiculitis
- ☐ Myelitis
- ☐ Meningitis

VARICELLA ZOSTER (VZV) VASCULOPATHY: MANAGEMENT

Cerebrospinal fluid (CSF) analysis: features

- ☐ Pleocytosis: this occurs in a third of cases
- ☐ VZV DNA: this is detected in 30% of cases
- ☐ Anti-VZV IgG: this is present in 90% of cases

Magnetic resonance imaging (MRI): infarcts

- ☐ These are single or multifocal ovoid infarcts
- ☐ They are more often deep than cortical
- ☐ They are especially at gray-white matter junctions

Magnetic resonance imaging (MRI): vasculitis

- ☐ This appears as diffusely irregular blood vessels
- ☐ There is stenosis and post-stenotic dilatation
- ☐ Vascular enhancement is present
- ☐ A moyamoya pattern is possible
- ☐ It may be multifocal: especially in the immunocompromised
- ☐ Angiography is abnormal in 70% of cases

Treatment

- ☐ Intravenous Aciclovir
- ☐ Oral steroids for 5 days

DENGUE VIRUS INFECTION (DENV): NEUROLOGICAL FEATURES

Encephalopathy

- ☐ Altered sensorium
- ☐ Behavioural symptoms
- ☐ Headache
- ☐ Dizziness
- ☐ Confusion
- ☐ Seizures
- ☐ Non-convulsive status epilepticus
- ☐ Epilepsia partialis continua (EPC)
- ☐ Myoclonus

Meningoencephalitis

- ☐ Viral encephalitis
- ☐ Haemorrhagic encephalitis
- ☐ Mild encephalitis/encephalopathy with reversible splenial lesions (MERS)
- ☐ Meningitis

Neuroinflammatory syndromes

- ☐ Acute disseminated encephalomyelitis (ADEM)
- ☐ Neuromyelitis optica (NMO)

Cerebellitis

- ☐ Nystagmus
- ☐ Dysarthria
- ☐ Ataxia

Vascular features

- ☐ Intracranial haemorrhage
- ☐ Subdural haematoma (SDH)
- ☐ Subdural effusion
- ☐ Stroke
- ☐ Cerebral vein thrombosis (CVT)
- ☐ Cerebral vasculitis

Cranial nerve palsies

- ☐ Abducens
- ☐ Facial
- ☐ Oculomotor

Spinal cord features

- ☐ Acute transverse myelitis (ATM)
- ☐ Longitudinally extensive transverse myelitis (LETM)
- ☐ Compressive myelopathy: by haematoma

Other central features

- ☐ Post encephalitic Parkinsonism
- ☐ Mania
- ☐ Hydrocephalus
- ☐ Opsoclonus myoclonus syndrome (OMS)
- ☐ Dementia

DENGUE VIRUS INFECTION (DENV): OPHTHALMOLOGICAL FEATURES

Optic nerve features

- ☐ Optic neuritis
- ☐ Blurred vision
- ☐ Papilloedema
- ☐ Reduced visual acuity
- ☐ Metamorphorpsia
- ☐ Micropsia

Retinal features

- ☐ Vasculitis
- ☐ Haemorrhage
- ☐ Detachment
- ☐ Cotton wool spots
- ☐ Retinal pigment epithelial detachment
- ☐ Maculopathy
- ☐ Visual field defects
- ☐ Subconjunctival haemorrhages

Vitreal features

- ☐ Anterior uveitis
- ☐ Vitreous haemorrhage
- ☐ Floaters

DENGUE VIRUS INFECTION (DENV): SYSTEMIC FEATURES

Dengue haemorrhagic fever

- ☐ This is especially frequent in travellers
- ☐ Haemorrhage results from increased vascular permeability and plasma leakage
- ☐ It causes ecchymosis and petechial haemorrhages
- ☐ It is associated with thrombocytopenia
- ☐ The frequent bleeding sites are the gums, vagina, and gastrointestinal tract
- ☐ The fever is biphasic

Dengue shock syndrome: features

- ☐ Haemorrhagic fever
- ☐ Circulatory failure

Hepatic features

- ☐ Hepatitis
- ☐ Portal hypertension
- ☐ Acalculous cholecystitis

Gastrointestinal features

- ☐ Nausea
- ☐ Appendicitis
- ☐ Febrile diarrhoea
- ☐ Splenomegaly
- ☐ Pancreatitis

Cardiac features

- ☐ Cardiac conduction defects
- ☐ Myocarditis
- ☐ Pericardial effusion

Haematological features

- ☐ Lymphadenopathy
- ☐ Thrombocytopaenia
- ☐ Leukopaenia

Metabolic features

- ☐ Hyponatraemia
- ☐ Hypokalaemia

Other systemic features

- ☐ Arthralgia
- ☐ Transient skin rash
- ☐ Vasculitis
- ☐ Renal failure
- ☐ Acute respiratory distress syndrome (ARDS)
- ☐ Disseminated intravascular coagulopathy (DIC)
- ☐ Most infections are asymptomatic

WEST NILE VIRUS (WNV) INFECTION: CENTRAL FEATURES

Meningitis

- ☐ Headache
- ☐ Neck stiffness
- ☐ Altered mental status
- ☐ Vasculitis with intracerebral haemorrhage (ICH)

Movement disorders

- ☐ Myoclonus
- ☐ Opsoclonus-myoclonus
- ☐ Tremor: postural and kinetic
- ☐ Parkinsonism
- ☐ Ataxia
- ☐ Chorea

Ophthalmic features

- ☐ Vitritis
- ☐ West Nile virus retinopathy (WNVR)
- ☐ Optic neuritis

Psychiatric features

- ☐ Anxiety
- ☐ Depression
- ☐ Apathy

Other central features

- ☐ Deafness

WEST NILE VIRUS (WNV) INFECTION: PERIPHERAL AND SYSTEMIC FEATURES

Muscle weakness: types

- ☐ Poliomyelitis
- ☐ Asymmetrical flaccid paralysis

Peripheral neuropathy (PN): types

- ☐ Pure motor neuropathy: this is the usual type
- ☐ Sensory neuropathy
- ☐ Autonomic neuropathy
- ☐ Guillain–Barre syndrome (GBS)

Neuromuscular disorders

- ☐ Diaphragmatic paralysis
- ☐ Isolated hypercapnic respiratory failure
- ☐ Brachial plexopathy
- ☐ Unilateral faciobrachial weakness
- ☐ Radiculopathy
- ☐ Vocal cord paralysis: from recurrent laryngeal nerve involvement
- ☐ Myasthenia gravis (MG)
- ☐ Rhabdomyolysis

Dermatological features

- ☐ Erythematous macular, papular, or morbilliform rash: this spares the palms and soles
- ☐ Purpura fulminans

Systemic features

- ☐ Influenza-like illness
- ☐ West Nile fever
- ☐ Nausea
- ☐ Vomiting
- ☐ Isolated respiratory failure: due to phrenic nerve involvement

Risk factors for mortality

- ☐ Older age
- ☐ Diabetes mellitus
- ☐ Encephalitis: this has a worse prognosis than meningitis

CORONAVIRUS (SARS-COV-2) INFECTION: SYSTEMIC FEATURES

Cardiorespiratory features

- ☐ Cough
- ☐ Dyspnoea
- ☐ Haemoptysis
- ☐ Chest pain
- ☐ Acute respiratory distress syndrome (ARDS)
- ☐ Sore throat
- ☐ Rhinorrhoea
- ☐ Sputum production
- ☐ Wheezing
- ☐ Pneumothorax
- ☐ Acute myocardial infarction
- ☐ Myocarditis
- ☐ Heart failure

Ophthalmic features

- ☐ Conjunctivitis: viral, immune, and follicular
- ☐ Oculomotor palsies
- ☐ Retinopathy

Dermatological features

- ☐ Exanthematous rash
- ☐ Urticaria
- ☐ Chickenpox like vesicles
- ☐ Petechiae
- ☐ Acute haemorrhagic oedema of infancy
- ☐ Pityriasis rosea
- ☐ Chilblains
- ☐ Diffuse or disseminated erythema
- ☐ Livedo racemose
- ☐ Blue toe syndrome
- ☐ Retiform purpura
- ☐ Purpuric exanthema

Multisystem inflammatory syndrome in children (MIS-C)

- ☐ Paediatric multisystem inflammatory syndrome temporally associated with SARS-Cov-2 infection
  - ○ PIMS-TS
- ☐ It is similar to Kawasaki disease
- ☐ It mainly affects children of African ancestry
- ☐ There may be associated bilateral thalamic and corpus callosum splenium lesions

Other systemic features

- ☐ Acute kidney injury
- ☐ Liver dysfunction
- ☐ Coagulopathy with antiphospholipid antibodies
- ☐ Acute symptomatic hyponatremia
- ☐ Syndrome of inappropriate ADH secretion (SIADH)
- ☐ Autoimmune haemolytic anaemia (AIHA)
- ☐ Systemic vasculitis
- ☐ Nausea, vomiting, and diarrhoea: rarely

Synonym

- ☐ COVID-19

CORONAVIRUS (SARS-COV-2) INFECTION: CENTRAL VASCULAR FEATURES

Ischaemic stroke: pathology

- ☐ This is caused by large vessel occlusion
- ☐ It is frequent in the vertebrobasilar territory
- ☐ There may be acute thrombus in the common carotid artery bifurcation
- ☐ Pathology shows thrombotic microangiopathy with secondary endotheliopathy
- ☐ It has a haemorrhagic predisposition

Ischaemic stroke: presentation

- ☐ Stroke may occur early or late in the course of the infection
- ☐ The incidence is 1.4%
- ☐ Multiple territories are affected in half of cases
- ☐ There may be concurrent cerebral vein thrombosis (CVT)
- ☐ There is associated elevated D-dimer of ≥1000 µg/L

Ischaemic stroke: management

- ☐ Consider prophylactic and early therapeutic low molecular weight heparin (LMWH)
- ☐ Thrombolysis appears to be safe and effective

Haemorrhagic features

- ☐ Intracerebral haemorrhage (ICH)
- ☐ Subarachnoid haemorrhage (SAH)
- ☐ Microbleeds
- ☐ Subdural haematomas (SDH)
- ☐ Intraventricular haemorrhage (IVH)
- ☐ Haemorrhagic posterior reversible encephalopathy syndrome (PRES)
- ☐ Haemorrhagic venous infarction
  - ○ This is secondary to cerebral vein thrombosis (CVT)
- ☐ Anticoagulation related haemorrhage

Other vascular features

- ☐ Central nervous system vasculitis
- ☐ Posterior reversible encephalopathy syndrome (PRES)
- ☐ Cerebral vein thrombosis (CVT)

Synonym

- ☐ COVID-19

CORONAVIRUS (SARS-COV-2) INFECTION: CENTRAL NON-VASCULAR FEATURES

COVID encephalopathy

- ☐ This is associated with elevated CSF IL-1β, IL-6, and ACE
- ☐ It may mimic a glial tumour
- ☐ MRI may show cytotoxic corpus callosum lesions

Other forms of encephalopathy

- ☐ Acute necrotising encephalopathy
- ☐ Acute haemorrhagic necrotising encephalopathy
- ☐ Hypoxic encephalopathy

SARS-Cov-2 related encephalitis

- ☐ This is a cytokine release syndrome
- ☐ The MRI shows olfactory tract hyperintensity
- ☐ It may respond to steroids and plasma exchange (PE)

Other forms of encephalitis

- ☐ Post-infectious brainstem encephalitis
- ☐ Anti-NMDAR autoimmune encephalitis

Inflammatory and demyelinating features

- ☐ Demyelination: it may present as enhancing tumefactive demyelination
- ☐ Acute disseminated encephalomyelitis (ADEM)
- ☐ Cytotoxic corpus callosum lesions: secondary to systemic inflammation
- ☐ Coronavirus disease-related disseminated leukoencephalopathy (CRDL)
- ☐ Acute transverse myelitis (ATM)

Headache

- ☐ Headache is the presenting feature in 6–26% of COVID19 cases
- ☐ It is moderate to severe
- ☐ It may be throbbing or pressing
- ☐ It may be holocranial, hemicranial, frontal or occipital
- ☐ It may be worsened by physical exertion and head movements
- ☐ There may be associated hypersensitivity to stimuli
- ☐ It may be associated with isolated intracranial hypertension
- ☐ It responds poorly to analgesics
- ☐ Headache may also be associated with PPE use

Other central presentations

- ☐ Dysexecutive syndrome
- ☐ Generalised myoclonus
- ☐ Dizziness
- ☐ Ataxia
- ☐ Transient global amnesia (TGA): case report
- ☐ Prolonged unconsciousness

Unconfirmed associations

- ☐ Seizures: there are many case reports of an association with COVID19
  - ○ But a multi-centre trial found no association
- ☐ Parkinsonism: a causal association with COVID19 has not been established

Synonym

- ☐ COVID-19

CORONAVIRUS (SARS-COV-2) INFECTION: CRANIAL NERVE DISORDERS

Olfactory and gustatory features: epidemiology

- ☐ Both smell and taste impairments occur in more >50% of COVID19 cases
- ☐ Both symptoms appear simultaneously and within 4 days of infection
- ☐ Smell and taste are not affected in about 40% of cases
- ☐ Smell impairment alone occurs in 3.8% of cases
- ☐ Taste impairment alone occurs in 1.5% of cases

Olfactory and gustatory features: presentation

- ☐ Taste impairment may be complete loss of taste or loss of sweet flavour
- ☐ Taste may also be metallic, bitter, or salty flavour
- ☐ MRI may show oedema and signal abnormality of the olfactory bulb with anosmia

Olfactory and gustatory features: prognosis

- ☐ Taste recovers totally in 45–50% of cases and partially in about 40% of cases
- ☐ Anosmia recovers in 40–50% of cases
- ☐ Smoking history predicts poor recovery of olfactory function

Other cranial neuropathies

- ☐ Trigeminal neuropathy: secondary to reactivation of latent herpes zoster
- ☐ Hearing impairment and tinnitus
- ☐ Facial nerve palsy

Synonym

- ☐ COVID-19

CORONAVIRUS (SARS-COV-2) INFECTION: PERIPHERAL FEATURES

Guillain–Barre syndrome (GBS)

- ☐ The mean onset age is 55–59 years: the range is 11–94 years
- ☐ The mean onset time is 11 days after COVID
- ☐ Males account for about 65–68% of cases
- ☐ The features are usually typical of classic GBS
- ☐ It is demyelinating in about 50% of cases
- ☐ Cerebrospinal fluid (CSF) was negative for SARS-CoV-2 RNA in all cases
- ☐ Most cases respond to a single course of intravenous immunoglobulin (IVIg)
- ☐ Causality is uncertain as the incidence is not considered higher than expected
- ☐ There are also many case reports of Miller Fisher syndrome (MFS)

Neuromuscular junction (NMJ) features

- ☐ Myasthenia gravis (MG)

Muscle features

- ☐ Skeletal muscle injury
- ☐ Necrotising autoimmune myositis (NAM): with myalgia, high CK, and rhabdomyolysis
- ☐ Myositis
- ☐ Critical illness myopathy

Peripheral nerve features

- ☐ Motor peripheral neuropathy (PN)
- ☐ Critical illness neuropathy
- ☐ Neuralgic amyotrophy

Synonym

- ☐ COVID-19

Bacterial infections

BACTERIAL MENINGITIS: CLINICAL FEATURES

Commonest causative organisms

- [ ] *Neisseria meningitidis*
- [ ] *Streptococcus pneumoniae*
- [ ] *Listeria monocytogenes*
- [ ] *Haemophilus influenza*

Risk factors

- [ ] Otitis media
- [ ] Sinusitis
- [ ] Pneumonia
- [ ] Endocarditis
- [ ] Head injury
- [ ] Neurosurgery
- [ ] Immune compromise
- [ ] Diabetes mellitus
- [ ] Alcoholism
- [ ] Cerebrospinal fluid (CSF) leak
- [ ] Fossa navicularis: this is persistent dehiscence of the base of the occiput

Clinical features

- [ ] Fever
- [ ] Neck stiffness
- [ ] Altered consciousness
- [ ] Positive Kernig's and Brudzinski's signs
- [ ] Jolt accentuation sign
- [ ] Seizures
- [ ] Skin rash
- [ ] Papilloedema
- [ ] Cranial nerve palsies
- [ ] Gaze palsy
- [ ] Visual field defects
- [ ] Focal limb weakness

Complications

- [ ] Cerebral vein thrombosis (CVT)
- [ ] Arterial vasospasm
- [ ] Brain abscess
- [ ] Subdural empyema
- [ ] Hydrocephalus
- [ ] Brain infarction
- [ ] Recurrence: this occurs in 9% of cases

Predictor of poor outcome: the FOUR score

- [ ] Full Outline of UnResponsiveness score: range is 0 to 16
- [ ] Factors: eye response, motor response, brainstem reflexes, and respiratory pattern

Differential diagnosis: crowned dens syndrome

- [ ] This is pseudogout of the atlantoaxial joint
- [ ] This appears as a crown-like calcification of the dens
- [ ] It presents with fever, neck pain and stiffness, and headache
- [ ] CT shows linear calcification along the transverse ligament of the atlas (TLA)
- [ ] FDG PET shows increased uptake
- [ ] Treatment is with non-steroidal anti-inflammatory drugs (NSAIDs)

DOI: 10.1201/9781003221258-38

BACTERIAL MENINGITIS: MANAGEMENT

Management guidelines

- ☐ Take blood cultures
- ☐ Perform lumbar puncture (LP)
  - ○ Delay for 30 minutes following brief seizures
  - ○ Consider withholding LP if there are prolonged seizures
- ☐ Administer antibiotics within 60 minutes
- ☐ Administer dexamethasone with or shortly before the 1st dose of antibiotic
  - ○ With Streptococcus pneumonia or Haemophilus influenza
- ☐ Report all suspected meningococcal or Haemophilus influenza meningitis

Indications for head CT before lumbar puncture (LP)

- ☐ Immunocompromised states
- ☐ Central nervous system (CNS) disease: mass lesion, stroke, focal infection
- ☐ New onset seizure within 1 week of presentation
- ☐ Features of raised intracranial pressure (ICP)
- ☐ Impaired consciousness
- ☐ Focal neurologic deficits

Antibiotic choice

- ☐ 3rd generation cephalosporins are the first choice
  - ○ Ceftriaxone 2g 12–24 hourly
  - ○ Cefotaxime 2g 6–8 hourly
- ☐ Amoxicillin 2g 4 hourly: for Listeria
- ☐ Vancomycin: for Penicillin-resistant pneumococcal meningitis
- ☐ Benzylpenicillin: for rapidly evolving Neisseria meningitidis

Duration of antibiotic treatment

- ☐ Neisseria meningitidis: 7 days
- ☐ Haemophilus influenza: 7–14 days
- ☐ Streptococcus pneumonia: 10–14 days
- ☐ Listeria monocytogenes: 21 days
- ☐ Gram negative bacilli: 21–28 days
- ☐ Pseudomonas aeruginosa: 21–28 days
- ☐ Unspecified aetiology: 10–14 days

Contact prophylaxis: for meningococcal meningitis

- ☐ Rifampicin 600 mg 12 hourly for 48 hours
- ☐ Ciprofloxacin 500 mg stat
- ☐ Ceftriaxone 1g IV/IM stat
- ☐ Amoxicillin or Phenoxymethyl Penicillin for 7 days if <15 years age

Vaccination

- ☐ Infant 4CMenB meningococcal vaccination is effective

TUBERCULOUS MENINGITIS (TBM): CLINICAL FEATURES

Risk factors

- ☐ Recent contact
- ☐ HIV infection
- ☐ Alcoholism
- ☐ Malnutrition
- ☐ Diabetes mellitus
- ☐ Malignancy
- ☐ Steroid use
- ☐ Possibly genetic and racial factors

Prodrome

- ☐ Low-grade fever
- ☐ Malaise
- ☐ Headache
- ☐ Dizziness
- ☐ Vomiting
- ☐ Personality change

Meningeal features

- ☐ Headache
- ☐ Fever
- ☐ Neck stiffness
- ☐ Limb weakness
- ☐ Seizures in children

Cranial nerve palsies

- ☐ Optic
- ☐ Oculomotor
- ☐ Trochlear
- ☐ Abducens
- ☐ Facial
- ☐ Vestibulocochlear

Neuroimaging features

- ☐ Hydrocephalus
- ☐ Infarcts: from vasculitis
- ☐ Tuberculomas
- ☐ Basilar meningeal thickening (exudates) and enhancement
- ☐ Cerebral oedema

Indicators of TBM v Cryptococcal meningitis

- ☐ Significant neck stiffness
- ☐ Higher body temperature
- ☐ Impaired consciousness
- ☐ Lower cerebrospinal fluid (CSF) opening pressures
- ☐ Higher CSF leucocyte count
- ☐ CD4 cell count <200/μL
- ☐ CSF to plasma glucose of ≤0.2
- ☐ CSF lymphocytes >200/μL
- ☐ Negative CSF cryptococcal antigen test

TUBERCULOUS MENINGITIS (TBM): CSF ANALYSIS

Cell count

☐ Lymphocytic pleocytosis: usually 100–1000 cells/cubic mm
☐ Polymorphs may predominate in the first 10 days

Protein

☐ Elevated protein: usually 100–500 mg/dL

Glucose

☐ Low: usually <45 mg/dL
☐ CSF to plasma ratio is <0.5

Microscopy

☐ Ziehl Neelsen (ZN) staining for acid-fast bacilli (AFB)
☐ Gram staining for bacteria
☐ India ink for fungi

Culture

☐ The is the gold standard CSF test
☐ The yield is higher with multiple, large volume (10ml) samples

Other CSF tests

☐ CSF adenosine deaminase level of ≥10 U/L: this has >90% sensitivity and specificity
☐ Antigen testing for Cryptococcus neoformans
☐ Polymerase chain reaction (PCR)
☐ Nucleic acid amplification techniques (NAATs)
☐ Interferon-gamma release assay
☐ The Xpert MTB/RIF assay

TUBERCULOUS MENINGITIS (TBM): TREATMENT

Anti TB drug treatment

☐ Isoniazid, Rifampicin, Pyrazinamide, and Ethambutol: for 2 months
☐ Isoniazid and Rifampicin: for 10 months

Adjunctive treatments

☐ Dexamethasone: this improves survival in HIV-negative cases but not disability
☐ Fluid restriction: for syndrome of inappropriate ADH secretion (SIADH)

Treatment of hydrocephalus

☐ Repeated lumbar puncture
☐ External ventricular drainage
☐ Ventriculoperitoneal shunt placement
☐ Endoscopic third ventriculostomy

LYME NEUROBORRELIOSIS: CLINICAL FEATURES

Onset features

- ☐ Tick bite: this is remembered by 40% of patients
- ☐ Erythema migrans
- ☐ Lymphocytoma

Lymphocytic meningitis

- ☐ Opsoclonus myoclonus
- ☐ Parkinsonism
- ☐ Amnesia

Cranial neuropathies

- ☐ Facial weakness: this is bilateral in a third of cases
- ☐ Diplopia
- ☐ Optic neuritis
- ☐ Hearing loss
- ☐ Dizziness

Peripheral nerve features

- ☐ Mononeuropathy
- ☐ Mononeuritis multiplex
- ☐ Polyneuropathy

Other features

- ☐ Stroke: secondary to vasculitis: it may be multiple and recurrent
- ☐ Encephalomyelitis
- ☐ Brainstem encephalitis
- ☐ Diaphragmatic paralysis
- ☐ Guillain–Barre syndrome (GBS) rarely
- ☐ Postganglionic Horner syndrome with Raeder syndrome
- ☐ Spinal radiculitis: it is Banwarth's syndrome if there is associated facial weakness

Late Lyme neuroborreliosis (post-Lyme syndrome): clinical features

- ☐ Encephalopathy
- ☐ Encephalomyelitis
- ☐ Radiculoneuropathy
- ☐ Insomnia
- ☐ Pain: myalgia and arthralgia
- ☐ Headache
- ☐ Paraesthesias
- ☐ Cognitive deficits
- ☐ Subcortical dementia
- ☐ Chronic fatigue
- ☐ The symptoms last more than 6 months

Late Lyme neuroborreliosis (post-Lyme syndrome): causes of persistent symptoms

- ☐ Misdiagnosis
- ☐ Slowly resolving symptoms
- ☐ Irreversible tissue damage
- ☐ Inadequate treatment: but antibiotics are ineffective in treating it

NEUROSYPHILIS: CLINICAL FEATURES

Clinical phenotypes

- ☐ Asymptomatic neurosyphilis
  - ○ There is only abnormal cerebrospinal fluid (CSF)
- ☐ Acute or subacute myelopathy
  - ○ This is frequently in the thoracolumbar region
- ☐ Tabes dorsalis
- ☐ General paresis of the insane (GPI)
- ☐ Taboparesis
- ☐ Vascular-stroke
- ☐ Meningovascular syphilis
- ☐ Optic neuritis (ON)

Tabes dorsalis: features

- ☐ Lightning pains
- ☐ Ataxia
- ☐ Argyll Robertson pupil
- ☐ Areflexia
- ☐ Charcot joints
- ☐ Paraesthesias

General paresis of the insane (GPI): features

- ☐ Delirium
- ☐ Psychosis
- ☐ Dementia
- ☐ Emotional symptoms
- ☐ Personality change
- ☐ Seizures
- ☐ Hemiparesis

Meningovascular syphilis: types

- ☐ Hydrocephalic type
- ☐ Basilar type: with facial and vestibulochochlear neuropathy

Syphilis in association with HIV

- ☐ HIV leads to a faster progression to neurosyphilis
- ☐ Do CSF analysis in HIV-positive cases if the CD4 cell count is ≤350 cells/µL
- ☐ CSF analysis in HIV-positive cases is also indicated if the VDRL/RPR titer is ≥1:32

Other presentations of neurosyphilis

- ☐ Parkinsonism
- ☐ Myoclonus
- ☐ Chorea
- ☐ Dystonia
- ☐ Progressive supranuclear palsy (PSP)
- ☐ Corticobasal degeneration (CBD)
- ☐ Orofacial dyskinesias: the candy sign

Differential diagnosis

- ☐ Creutzfeldt Jakob disease (CJD)

NEUROSYPHILIS: MANAGEMENT

Indications for syphilis screening

- ☐ Men who have sex with men
- ☐ People living with HIV
- ☐ History of incarceration
- ☐ History of commercial sex work
- ☐ All pregnant women

Cerebrospinal fluid (CSF) analysis: indications

- ☐ All cases of neurosyphilis
- ☐ Poor treatment response in early syphilis
- ☐ HIV infection: if the CD4 cell count is ≤350 cells/μL or VDRL/RPR titer is ≥1:32

Cerebrospinal fluid (CSF) analysis: features

- ☐ Cells are >5/cubic mm in most symptomatic cases
- ☐ Positive CSF VDRL/RPR is diagnostic if the sample is not contaminated by blood
- ☐ CSF TPHA index is >70
- ☐ TPHA titre is >320
- ☐ A negative treponemal CSF analysis excludes the diagnosis

Brain magnetic resonance imaging (MRI): features

- ☐ Subcutaneous lesions
- ☐ Medullary oedema: in the adjacent bone
- ☐ Dural thickening

Treatment

- ☐ Benzathine Penicillin G intramuscular (IM)
- ☐ Procaine Penicillin
- ☐ Doxycycline
- ☐ Azithromycin: if Penicillin and Doxycycline are contraindicated
  - ○ But Azithromycin does not treat maternal infection
- ☐ Amoxicillin
- ☐ Ceftriaxone

Cerebrospinal fluid (CSF) monitoring

- ☐ The CSF is monitored by cell counts
- ☐ It is repeated at 6 months if it is initially abnormal
- ☐ The CSF is usually normal by 2 years

TETANUS: CLINICAL FEATURES

Tetanus syndromes

- ☐ Generalised
- ☐ Localised
- ☐ Neonatal
- ☐ Cephalic

Painful spasms

- ☐ They are spontaneous
- ☐ They are stimulus-sensitive: to touch, visual, auditory, and emotional triggers
- ☐ They are worst in the first 2 weeks
- ☐ They may cause laryngospasm

Rigidity: manifestations

- ☐ Masseter rigidity (lockjaw, trismus)
- ☐ Risus sardonicus
- ☐ Neck stiffness
- ☐ Opisthotonus
- ☐ Camptocormia: this may be the initial symptom

Autonomic dysfunction

- ☐ Profuse sweating
- ☐ Diarrhoea
- ☐ Bronchorrhoea

Other features

- ☐ Facial weakness
- ☐ Back pain
- ☐ Headache

The spatula test

- ☐ Stimulation of the pharynx with a spatula provokes masseter spasm
- ☐ This causes the patient to bite on the spatula
- ☐ It is a very sensitive and specific test
- ☐ It carries a risk of respiratory arrest

Differential diagnosis

- ☐ Tetany
- ☐ Strychnine poisoning
- ☐ Drug induced dystonic reactions
- ☐ Rabies
- ☐ Hypocalcaemia
- ☐ Hypoglycaemia
- ☐ Seizures
- ☐ Meningitis

Magnetic resonance imaging (MRI) brain: features

- ☐ Enhancing cortical and subcortical brain lesions

Poor prognostic features

- ☐ A short period of onset: this is the interval from the first symptom to the onset of spasms

TETANUS: TREATMENT

Main antibiotics

- ☐ Metronidazole with Penicillin
- ☐ Penicillin may cause hyperexcitability and seizures in high doses

Alternative antibiotics

- ☐ Tetracycline
- ☐ Erythromycin
- ☐ Clindamycin
- ☐ Doxycycline
- ☐ Chloramphenicol

Treatment of spasms

- ☐ Benzodiazepines
  - ○ Diazepam is the treatment of choice
  - ○ Midazolam is the 2nd option
- ☐ Muscle relaxants: in severe cases
- ☐ Magnesium sulphate: for autonomic control in severe cases
- ☐ Intrathecal Baclofen: this shows varying success but it is risky

Other treatments

- ☐ Morphine: this may aid sedation and autonomic control
- ☐ Early wound debridement
- ☐ Enteral feeding: as early as possible
- ☐ Tetanus immunoglobulin or intravenous immunoglobulins (IVIg)
- ☐ Tetanus toxoid immunisation

Treatment of complications

- ☐ Fractures
- ☐ Tendon rupture
- ☐ Contractures
- ☐ Seizures
- ☐ Bed sores
- ☐ Myoclonus
- ☐ Intramuscular haemorrhage
- ☐ Sleep disturbance

Parasitic infections

PARASITIC INFECTIONS OF THE NERVOUS SYSTEM: CLASSIFICATION

Cestode infections

- ☐ Cerebral alveolar echinococcosis: caused by *Echinococcus multilocularis*
- ☐ Cerebral cystic echinococcosis (hydatid disease): caused by *Echinococcus granulosus*
- ☐ Neurocysticercosis: caused by *Taenia solium*
- ☐ Neurosparganosis: caused by *Spirometra mansoni*
- ☐ Other cestodes: caused by *Taenia multiceps*

Trematode infections

- ☐ Neuroschistosomiasis: caused by *Schistosoma mansoni*, haematobium, and japonicum
- ☐ Neuroparagonimiasis: caused by *Paragonimus westermani*
- ☐ Alaria americana
- ☐ Schistosoma mekongi
- ☐ Schistosoma intercalatum

Nematode infections

- ☐ Baylisascariosis: caused by *Baylisascaris procyonis*
- ☐ Neuroangiostrongyliasis: caused by *Angiostrongylus cantonensis* and *costaricensis*
- ☐ Gnathostomiasis: caused by *Gnathostoma spinigerum*
- ☐ Neurotoxocariasis: caused by *Toxocara canis* and *cati*
- ☐ Neurotrichinelliasis: caused by *Trichinella spiralis*
- ☐ Ascaris suum
- ☐ *Gnathostoma hispidum*
- ☐ Loa loa
- ☐ Strongyloides stercoralis

Protozoan infections

- ☐ Brain abscess: caused by *Entamoeba histolytica*
- ☐ Cerebral Chagas disease: caused by *Trypanosoma cruzi*
- ☐ Cerebral malaria: caused by *Plasmodium falciparum*
- ☐ Neurotoxoplasmosis: caused by *Toxoplasma gondii*
- ☐ Primary amoebic meningoencephalitis: caused by *Naegleria fowleri*
- ☐ Sleeping sickness: caused by *Trypanosoma brucei gambiense* and *rhodesiense*
- ☐ *Babesia* species
- ☐ *Balamuthia mandrillaris*

CEREBRAL MALARIA: PATHOLOGY AND CLINICAL FEATURES

Pathology of malaria

- ☐ Cerebral malaria is caused by *Plasmodium falciparum* (*P. falciparum*)
- ☐ It is especially prevalent in sub-Saharan Africa
- ☐ It usually affects children

Pathogenesis of cerebral malaria

- ☐ *P. falciparum* infected red blood cells (PfRBC) adhere to blood vessels
- ☐ This is mediated by *P. falciparum* erythrocyte membrane protein 1 (PfEMP1)
- ☐ This malarial vasculopathy is due to a hyperactive immune response
- ☐ There is associated disruption of the blood-brain barrier
- ☐ There is also associated neuroinflammation
- ☐ Severe haemolysis also contributes to the pathology

Brainstem features

- ☐ Pupillary abnormalities
- ☐ Absent corneal reflexes
- ☐ Breathing abnormalities
- ☐ Decorticate and decerebrate rigidity

Other neurological features

- ☐ Subarachnoid haemorrhage (SAH)
- ☐ Subconjunctival haemorrhage
- ☐ Ataxia
- ☐ Extra pyramidal rigidity
- ☐ Psychosis
- ☐ Neck stiffness
- ☐ Hemiparesis
- ☐ Epilepsy
- ☐ Coma

Malarial retinopathy

- ☐ This manifests as retinal whitening and haemorrhages
- ☐ It is caused by sequestration of infected red blood cells
- ☐ Its presence differentiates malarial from non-malarial causes of coma
- ☐ It predicts a poor prognosis

Systemic features

- ☐ Hypoglycaemia
- ☐ Metabolic acidosis
- ☐ Hyponatraemia
- ☐ Hyperpyrexia
- ☐ Anaemia
- ☐ Disseminated intravascular coagulopathy (DIC)
- ☐ Pulmonary oedema
- ☐ Adult respiratory distress syndrome (ARDS)

Long-term neurocognitive features

- ☐ Speech and hearing impairments
- ☐ Behavioural abnormalities

DOI: 10.1201/9781003221258-39

CEREBRAL MALARIA: INVESTIGATIONS AND TREATMENT

Blood investigations

- [ ] Blood glucose
- [ ] Acidosis
- [ ] Blood film: thick and thin
- [ ] Microscopy
- [ ] Polymerase chain reaction (PCR): this is more sensitive than microscopy

Emerging biomarkers

- [ ] Plasma angiopoietin levels
- [ ] sTNF-R2
- [ ] IL-8
- [ ] IL-1ra
- [ ] RANTES

Computed tomography (CT) head: features

- [ ] Cerebral oedema
- [ ] Obstructive hydrocephalus
- [ ] Focal atrophy

Magnetic resonance imaging (MRI) brain: features

- [ ] Brain swelling
- [ ] Increased brain volume
- [ ] Abnormal T2 signal changes
- [ ] Diffusion weighted imaging (DWI) abnormalities
- [ ] Bilateral hippocampal sclerosis

Other investigations

- [ ] Cerebrospinal fluid (CSF) analysis: to exclude meningitis
  - ○ Biomarkers include CXCL10 and VEGF
- [ ] Electroencephalogram (EEG): this shows diffuse slowing

Emerging ophthalmologic investigations

- [ ] Optical coherence tomography (OCT): this may demonstrate retinopathy
- [ ] Fluorescence angiography

Main treatments

- [ ] Artemisinin derivatives: Artesunate, Artemethar, or Arteether
  - ○ Artesunate is the first line treatment
- [ ] Cinchona alkaloids: Quinine, Quinidine, or Cinchonine
  - ○ Monitor for hypoglycaemia on Quinine

Follow up treatment: for seven days

- [ ] Oral sulfadoxine/pyrimethamine or Tetracycline/doxycycline
- [ ] Clindamycin in pregnant women and children

Ancillary treatments

- [ ] Blood transfusion: this is indicated if the packed cell volume is <20%
- [ ] Exchange blood transfusion: this is indicated if parasitaemia is >10% of peripheral erythrocytes
- [ ] Phenobarbitone for seizures

POST MALARIA NEUROLOGICAL SYNDROME (PMNS)

Pathology

- [ ] This is an autoimmune encephalitis
- [ ] It is associated with neurexin-3α antibodies
- [ ] It is also associated with voltage-gated potassium channel (VGKC) antibodies
- [ ] It usually follows falciparum malaria infection
- [ ] There is an increased risk in Mefloquine-treated patients

Systemic features

- [ ] Fever
- [ ] Headache

Cognitive features

- [ ] Somnolence
- [ ] Apathy
- [ ] Disorientation
- [ ] Confusion
- [ ] Impaired memory
- [ ] Disrupted sleep-awake cycle

Psychiatric features

- [ ] Abnormal behaviour
- [ ] Emotional lability
- [ ] Confabulation
- [ ] Catatonia with waxy flexibility
- [ ] Hallucinations

Other features

- [ ] Cerebellar ataxia
- [ ] Ophthalmoparesis
- [ ] Tremors
- [ ] Seizures

Other post malaria neurological syndromes

- [ ] Delayed cerebellar ataxia
- [ ] Guillain–Barre syndrome (GBS)

Course

- [ ] The onset is 2–60 days after recovery from malaria
- [ ] It is usually self-limiting: the median duration is 6 hours

Magnetic resonance imaging (MRI) brain: features

- [ ] There are FLAIR signals in the caudate-capsule-lenticulate regions
- [ ] There is no contrast enhancement

Other investigations

- [ ] Electroencephalogram (EEG): this shows subcortical encephalopathy
- [ ] Cerebrospinal fluid (CSF) analysis: this shows no infective features

Treatment

- [ ] IV Methylprednisolone

NEUROCYSTICERCOSIS: PARENCHYMAL TYPE

Biology

- ☐ This is caused by infection with the larval stage of *Taenia solium*
- ☐ It is known as pork tapeworm

Pathology

- ☐ There is pathological evidence of parenchymal cysts
- ☐ The cysts are usually in different stages of maturation
- ☐ The cysts are usually in the cerebral hemispheres
- ☐ They are usually at the grey-white matter junction
- ☐ They are rare in the cerebellar hemispheres
- ☐ There is initial surrounding cerebral oedema followed by calcification

Diagnostic criteria

- ☐ Seizures and at least one cyst with scolex visible on imaging
- ☐ Multiple cysts and a positive immunological test in the absence of a visible scolex on imaging

Clinical features

- ☐ Seizures: including epilepsia partialis continua (EPC)
- ☐ Focal neurological deficits
- ☐ Raised intracranial pressure (ICP)
- ☐ Hydrocephalus
- ☐ Cognitive deficits
- ☐ Headache
- ☐ Stroke: this may be due to cysticercal arteritis
- ☐ Movement disorders
- ☐ Acute psychosis
- ☐ Subdural effusion
- ☐ Bilateral ptosis

NEUROCYSTICERCOSIS: EXTRAPARENCHYMAL (RACEMOSE) TYPE

Diagnostic criteria

- ☐ Diagnosis requires at least one cyst with scolex visible on imaging
- ☐ If without visible scolex it requires ≥2 of hydrocephalus, inflammatory CSF, positive immunological test, and calcifications or parenchymal cysts

Intracranial features

- ☐ Meningitis
- ☐ Ependymitis
- ☐ Raised intracranial pressure
- ☐ Hydrocephalus
- ☐ Cranial neuropathies: extraocular and optic nerves
- ☐ Vasculitis causing TIA and stroke
- ☐ Intracerebral haemorrhage (ICH)
- ☐ Dementia

Fourth ventricle features (Brun's syndrome)

- ☐ Episodic headache
- ☐ Vomiting
- ☐ Papilloedema
- ☐ Neck stiffness
- ☐ Sudden positional vertigo: induced by rotatory head movements
- ☐ Drop attacks
- ☐ Transient loss of consciousness

Isolated brainstem features

- ☐ Oculomotor nerve palsy
- ☐ Trochlear nerve palsy
- ☐ Internuclear ophthalmoplegia (INO)
- ☐ Isolated one-and-a-half syndrome
- ☐ Vertical one-and-a-half syndrome
- ☐ Claude syndrome: oculomotor nerve palsy with contralateral ataxia

Orbital features

- ☐ Periocular swelling
- ☐ Proptosis
- ☐ Ptosis
- ☐ Papilloedema
- ☐ Restricted ocular movements
- ☐ Atypical optic neuritis
- ☐ Subretinal parasites on fundoscopy

Spinal cord involvement

- ☐ This presents as a subacute or chronic transverse myelopathy
- ☐ Intramedullary forms usually involve the thoracic spinal cord
- ☐ Extramedullary (leptomeningeal) forms may occur in any part of the spinal cord
- ☐ The lesions are usually single
- ☐ Spinal cord involvement may rarely present with hydrocephalus

Other extraparenchymal sites

- [ ] Intrasellar: this presents with impaired visual acuity, visual field defects, and hypopituitarism
- [ ] Intraventricular: this may show a 'full moon' sign on endoscopy
- [ ] Cisternal: this presents with hydrocephalus

NEUROCYTICERCOSIS: MANAGEMENT

Serology

- [ ] Enzyme-linked immunosorbent assay (ELISA)
- [ ] Enzyme-linked immunoelectrotransfer blot (EITB)

Magnetic resonance imaging (MRI): cyst types

- [ ] Vesicular
- [ ] Colloidal
- [ ] Granular-nodular
- [ ] Calcified

Magnetic resonance imaging (MRI): other features

- [ ] Single enhancing nodules
- [ ] Neurocysticercosis-associated inflammation

Magnetic resonance imaging (MRI): differentials

- [ ] Cerebral microbleeds
- [ ] Cystic brain tumours

Computed tomography (CT)

- [ ] Cysts
- [ ] Calcifications

Cerebrospinal fluid (CSF)

- [ ] CSF constituents are usually normal
- [ ] ELISA and EITB may be positive

Other tests

- [ ] Plain X-ray: this shows cigar shaped calcifications
- [ ] Histology: of muscle and subcutaneous tissues
- [ ] Polymerase chain reaction (PCR)

Treatment

- [ ] Albendazole: 15–30 mg/kg/day for 10 days
- [ ] Prednisolone 1 mg/kg/day: it is administered with Albendazole
- [ ] Praziquantel
- [ ] Surgery for symptomatic cysts
- [ ] Shunt for hydrocephalus

TOXOPLASMOSIS: CLINICAL FEATURES

Biology

- ☐ Toxoplasma gondii is the causative parasite
- ☐ Transmission of *T. gondii* cysts is food borne via raw meat, and water-borne via cat faeces
- ☐ Transmission may also be congenital

Maturation forms

- ☐ Sporozoites: these are released from oocysts
- ☐ Bradyzoites: these are released from the tissue cysts
- ☐ Tachyzoites: these are the fast-replicating forms

Risk factors for infection and reactivation

- ☐ HIV infection
- ☐ Malignancies
- ☐ Organ transplantation

Encephalitic features

- ☐ Headache
- ☐ Fever
- ☐ Lethargy
- ☐ Weakness
- ☐ Altered mentation
- ☐ Speech disturbance
- ☐ Visual impairment
- ☐ Seizures
- ☐ Cranial nerve dysfunction
- ☐ Dementia
- ☐ Ataxia

Other neurological features

- ☐ Brain mass lesions
- ☐ Polymyositis

Ocular toxoplasmosis

- ☐ Retinochoiroditis
- ☐ Primary retinal lesions
- ☐ Retinochoroidal scars

Congenital toxoplasmosis: features

- ☐ Chorioretinitis
- ☐ Intracranial calcifications
- ☐ Hydrocephalus
- ☐ Epilepsy
- ☐ Deafness

Congenital toxoplasmosis: differentials (TORCH complex)

- ☐ Rubella
- ☐ Cytomegalovirus
- ☐ Herpes simplex virus (HSV)

Other features

- ☐ Cervical lymphadenopathy

TOXOPLASMOSIS: MANAGEMENT

Parasite identification

- ☐ Serology
- ☐ Culture
- ☐ Polymerase chain reaction (PCR)

Computed tomography (CT) scan

- ☐ This usually shows multiple abscesses
- ☐ They are hypoattenuating or isoattenuating
- ☐ They demonstrate smooth or nodular enhancement
- ☐ There is surrounding vasogenic oedema and mass effect
- ☐ There are calcifications in congenital forms

Magnetic resonance imaging (MRI): features

- ☐ Multiple T1 hypointense mass lesions
- ☐ Rim-like enhancement
- ☐ Peripheral hyperintensity due to haemorrhages
- ☐ Surrounding vasogenic oedema
- ☐ Eccentric target sign
- ☐ Concentric target sign

Radiological differentials: cerebral lymphoma

- ☐ Lymphoma lesions are larger and more periventricular than toxoplasma abscesses
- ☐ They also show a more butterfly pattern of spread
- ☐ They are more enhancing than toxoplasma abscesses
- ☐ They take up more thallium on SPECT

Radiological differentials: others

- ☐ Pyogenic abscesses: central restricted diffusion unlike in toxoplasma abscesses
- ☐ Tuberculoma
- ☐ Aspergillosis
- ☐ Progressive multifocal leukoencephalopathy (PML)
- ☐ Cryptococcosis

Prevention

- ☐ Washing fruits and vegetables
- ☐ Avoiding raw and undercooked meat
- ☐ Hand-washing after gardening or handling cats

Drug treatments

- ☐ Pyrimethamine
- ☐ Sulphadiazine
- ☐ Folinic acid
- ☐ Clindamycin if allergic to sulphadiazine

Drug prophylaxis in immunosuppressed people

- ☐ Trimethoprim-sulfamethoxazole

Fungal infections

FUNGAL INFECTIONS OF THE NERVOUS SYSTEM: CLASSIFICATION

Major nervous system fungal infections

- ☐ Aspergillus species: especially *Aspergillus fumigatus*
- ☐ Cryptococcus species: *Cryptococcus neoformans* and *gattis*
- ☐ Candida species: *Candida albicans*

Dimorphic fungi

- ☐ Histoplasma capsulatum
- ☐ Coccidioides immitis

Non-aspergillus moulds

- ☐ Mucormycetes
- ☐ Hyalohyphomycetes
- ☐ Phaeohyphomycetes

Other nervous system fungal infections

- ☐ Non-candida non-cryptococcus species
- ☐ Zygomycetes
- ☐ *Cladophialophora bantiana*
- ☐ *Exophiala dermatitidis*
- ☐ *Ramichloridium Mackenzie*
- ☐ *Ochroconis gallopava*
- ☐ Melanised fungi
- ☐ *Scedosporium apiospermum*

CRYPTOCOCCAL MENINGITIS: CLINICAL FEATURES

Pathology

- ☐ This is caused by *Cryptococcus neoformans* and *gatti*
- ☐ It is acquired by inhalation
- ☐ It resides in lymph nodes
- ☐ It disseminates after a latent period
- ☐ It has a predilection for the nervous system
- ☐ It causes a subacute meningoencephalitis

Risk factors: cell-mediated immunodeficiency syndromes

- ☐ Idiopathic CD4+ lymphopaenia
- ☐ Pulmonary alveolar proteinosis
- ☐ X linked CD40L deficiency (Hyper-IgM syndrome)
- ☐ Hyper-IgE recurrent infection syndrome (Job syndrome)

Risk factors: others

- ☐ HIV infection
- ☐ Organ transplant recipients: except stem cell transplantation
- ☐ Malignancies: especially hematopoietic

Neurological features

- ☐ Headache
- ☐ Seizures
- ☐ Confusion
- ☐ Coma
- ☐ Hearing impairment: from auditory neuropathy
- ☐ Stroke: especially basal ganglia

Ophthalmic features

- ☐ Visual impairment
- ☐ Diplopia
- ☐ Intermittent oculomotor nerve palsy
- ☐ Blindness

Systemic features

- ☐ Fever
- ☐ Nausea
- ☐ Vomiting

Cryptococcal immune reconstitution inflammatory syndrome (IRIS)

- ☐ This follows treatment of HIV infection
- ☐ It is associated with lymphadenitis and lung cavities
- ☐ It is classified into paradoxical and unmasking types

DOI: 10.1201/9781003221258-40

Cryptococcal meningitis associated disorders

- [ ] HIV infection
- [ ] Tuberculosis (TB)
- [ ] Sarcoidosis
- [ ] Autoimmune disorders

Outcome

- [ ] Mortality is the same or lower in cases associated with HIV infection

CRYPTOCOCCAL MENINGITIS: MANAGEMENT

Magnetic resonance imaging (MRI) brain: features

- [ ] Intraparenchymal nodules
- [ ] Leptomeningeal enhancement:
  - This is prominent in the basal ganglia
  - It may show a micronodular pattern
- [ ] Dilated Virchow-Robin spaces (VRS)
- [ ] Ventriculomegaly
- [ ] Brain abscess
- [ ] Posterior fossa cysts
- [ ] Choroid plexitis
- [ ] Multiple lacunar infarcts
- [ ] Soap bubble appearance: due to gelatinous periventricular pseudocysts

Cerebrospinal fluid (CSF) analysis: routine tests

- [ ] High opening pressure
- [ ] Lymphocytic pleocytosis: it may be eosinophilic
- [ ] High protein
- [ ] Low glucose

Cerebrospinal fluid (CSF) analysis: fungal tests

- [ ] Latex agglutination cryptococcal antigen test
- [ ] Lateral flow dipstick cryptococcal antigen test
- [ ] India ink stain
- [ ] Fungal culture

Antifungal treatment

- [ ] Amphotericin B and Flucytosine combination for 2 weeks
- [ ] Monitor Flucytosine for bone marrow suppression
- [ ] Monitor Amphotericin for renal impairment

Management of raised intracranial pressure

- [ ] Daily therapeutic lumbar puncture: this improves survival
- [ ] Lumbar drainage
- [ ] Ommaya reservoir
- [ ] Ventriculo-peritoneal shunting
- [ ] Some authors recommend Mannitol
- [ ] Avoid Dexamethasone: it is associated with poorer outcomes

Preventative treatment

- [ ] Primary antifungal prophylaxis in HIV infection: Itraconazole or Fluconazole

Aseptic, recurrent, and chronic meningitis

ASEPTIC MENINGITIS: CAUSES

Infectious

- ☐ Viruses are the commonest infections: especially Enteroviruses
- ☐ Bacteria: including syphilis
- ☐ Tuberculosis
- ☐ Fungal
- ☐ Parasitic

Drug-induced

- ☐ Non-steroidal anti-inflammatory drugs (NSAIDs): especially Ibuprofen
- ☐ Antimicrobials
- ☐ Intravenous immunoglobulin (IVIg)
- ☐ Intrathecal drugs
- ☐ Vaccines
- ☐ Monoclonal antibodies
- ☐ Carbamazepine
- ☐ Lamotrigine

Autoimmune

- ☐ Systemic lupus erythematosus (SLE)
- ☐ Sjogren's syndrome
- ☐ Rheumatoid arthritis (RA)
- ☐ Kawasaki disease
- ☐ Behcet's syndrome
- ☐ Vogt-Koyanagi-Harada disease

Other causes

- ☐ Neurosarcoidosis
- ☐ Neurosurgery
- ☐ Neoplasms
- ☐ Cerebral aneurysms
- ☐ Relapsing polychondritis: this may cause recurrent and purulent meningitis

RECURRENT MENINGITIS: CAUSES

Tumours

- ☐ Cranial
- ☐ Spinal

Chemical

- ☐ Cysts
- ☐ Craniopharyngioma

Other causes

- ☐ Drugs
- ☐ Biologic products
- ☐ Chronic inflammation
- ☐ Mollaret's meningitis
- ☐ Immunodeficiency
- ☐ Congenital lesions
- ☐ Connective tissue diseases
- ☐ Fossa navicularis: persistent base of skull dehiscence
- ☐ Surgery
- ☐ Trauma

DOI: 10.1201/9781003221258-41

CHRONIC MENINGITIS: CAUSES

Infective

- [ ] Tuberculosis (TB)
- [ ] Lyme disease
- [ ] Listeria
- [ ] Syphilis
- [ ] HIV
- [ ] Cytomegalovirus (CMV)
- [ ] Cryptococcus
- [ ] Candida
- [ ] Aspergillus
- [ ] Parasitic

Drug-induced

- [ ] Non-steroidal anti-inflammatory drugs (NSAIDS)
- [ ] Intravenous immunoglobulins (IVIg)
- [ ] Immunosuppressants
- [ ] Antibiotics
- [ ] Chemotherapy

Chemical

- [ ] Contrast media
- [ ] Local anaesthetics
- [ ] Microvascular collagen (Ativene)

Neoplastic

- [ ] Cancer
- [ ] Lymphoma
- [ ] Leukaemia

Neuroinflammatory

- [ ] Neurosarcoidosis
- [ ] Central nervous system (CNS) vasculitis
- [ ] Systemic lupus erythematosus (SLE)

Uveomeningitis

- [ ] Behcet's disease
- [ ] Vogt-Koyanagi-Harada disease

Other causes

- [ ] Hypertrophic pachymeningitis
- [ ] Idiopathic: this accounts for 15–30% of cases

CHAPTER 7

Headache

Migraine

MIGRAINE: NON-MODIFIABLE RISK FACTORS

Individual risk factors

- ☐ Caucasian ethnicity
- ☐ Male sex: this is a risk factor for migraine starting before puberty
- ☐ Female sex: this is a risk factor for migraine starting after puberty
- ☐ Early puberty
- ☐ Excessive female hormones in males
- ☐ Family history of migraine

Familial hemiplegic migraine (FMH) gene mutations

- ☐ CACNAA1
- ☐ ATP1A2
- ☐ SCN1A

High homocysteine gene mutations

- ☐ MTHFR C677T gene mutation
- ☐ NNMT rs694539 gene mutation

Other genetic risk factors

- ☐ CADASIL
- ☐ 3243A>G mitochondrial DNA mutation
- ☐ Diamine oxidase rs10156191 and rs2052129 variants
- ☐ Glutamate receptor (GRIA1 rs2195450) gene variant
- ☐ Endothelin receptor type A (EDNRA): vascular gene polymorphism
- ☐ ROSAH syndrome: autosomal dominant ALPK1 gene mutations

Hypercoagulable risk factors

- ☐ von Willebrand factor (vWF) antigen
- ☐ Fibrinogen
- ☐ Tissue plasminogen activator (tPA) antigen
- ☐ Endothelial microparticles
- ☐ Thrombocytosis
- ☐ Erythrocytosis
- ☐ Antiphospholipid syndrome (APS)

Protective factors

- ☐ Diabetes may be protective against migraine

Acronyms

- ☐ CADASIL: Cerebral autosomal dominant arteriopathy, subcortical infarcts, and leukoencephalopathy
- ☐ MTHFR: Methyl-tetrahydrofolate reductase
- ☐ NNMT: Nicotinamide-N-Methyltransferase
- ☐ ROSAH: retinal dystrophy, optic nerve oedema, splenomegaly, anhidrosis, migraine headache

MIGRAINE: MODIFIABLE RISK FACTORS

Individual risk factors

- ☐ Lower socioeconomic status
- ☐ Obesity
- ☐ Underweight

Patent foramen ovale (PFO)

- ☐ PFO with atrial septal aneurysm (ASA)
- ☐ Isolated PFO is probably not associated with migraine

Environmental risk factors

- ☐ Hot climate
- ☐ High altitude
- ☐ Playing on the computer
- ☐ Loud noises
- ☐ Domestic violence

Dietary and endocrine risk factors

- ☐ Low dietary sodium
- ☐ High serum calcium
- ☐ Low vitamin D
- ☐ Subclinical hypothyroidism

DOI: 10.1201/9781003221258-43

MIGRAINE: TRIGGERS

Physiological

- [ ] Menstruation
- [ ] Hormones

Stress

- [ ] Insufficient sleep
- [ ] Sleeping late
- [ ] Hunger

Dietary

- [ ] Chocolate
- [ ] Sugar
- [ ] Seasoning
- [ ] Cheese
- [ ] Red wine
- [ ] Alcohol

Environmental

- [ ] Reflected sunlight
- [ ] Perfumes
- [ ] Odours
- [ ] Smoke
- [ ] Passive smoking
- [ ] Heat
- [ ] Weather changes

Physical exertion

- [ ] Exercise
- [ ] Sexual activity
- [ ] Overwork

Radiotherapy

- [ ] Stroke-like migraine attacks after radiation therapy (SMART) syndrome

MIGRAINE AURAS

General aura features

- [ ] Auras occur in about a third of people with migraine
- [ ] They may also occur with or after the headache
- [ ] They may be associated with sensory, motor, and speech symptoms
- [ ] Visual auras are visible even with the eyes shut
  - ○ They gradually expand and are fully reversible
- [ ] The mean attack frequency is 12 per year

Classification of auras by duration

- [ ] Typical auras: the duration is 5–60 minutes
- [ ] Prolonged auras: the duration is >60 minutes
- [ ] Migraine aura status: when three auras occur within 3 days

Scintillating scotomas

- [ ] These are the commonest types of migraine aura
- [ ] They present as fortification spectra (teichopsias)
- [ ] Their edges are flickering, coloured, and jagged
- [ ] They expand in a C-shape towards the peripheral visual field
- [ ] They are associated with small blind spots

Other visual aura types

- [ ] Blind spot without jagged edges or colours
- [ ] Black and white lines with a central onset
- [ ] Flashes (photopsias)
- [ ] Distortion (metamorphopsia)
- [ ] Transient visual snow
- [ ] Orgasmic aura: usually acephalgic (without headache)
- [ ] Prolonged stuttering

Associated visual phenomena

- [ ] Alice in Wonderland syndrome (AIWS)
- [ ] Visual splitting
- [ ] Visual blurring or fogginess
- [ ] Seeing heat waves
- [ ] Diplopia

Differential diagnoses

- [ ] Seizures
- [ ] Stroke
- [ ] Amyloid spells

Prophylactic treatment

- [ ] Beta-blockers
- [ ] Candesartan
- [ ] Topiramate
- [ ] Valproate
- [ ] Amitriptyline
- [ ] Nortriptyline
- [ ] Lamotrigine

Treatment of migraine aura status

- [ ] Acetazolamide
- [ ] Valproate

MIGRAINE: HEADACHE FEATURES

Typical headache features

- ☐ Disabling
- ☐ Pulsating
- ☐ Unilateral
- ☐ Duration is 4–72 hours

Defining accompanying features

- ☐ Photophobia (light sensitivity): this may precede the headache
- ☐ Phonophobia (noise sensitivity)
- ☐ Nausea
- ☐ Vomiting
- ☐ Neck pain: this is more frequent than nausea
- ☐ Cutaneous allodynia: this occurs in about 80% of cases

Cranial autonomic features

- ☐ Cranial autonomic features occur in >50% of cases
- ☐ They usually accompany severe attacks
- ☐ They are mild to moderate in intensity
- ☐ They are usually bilateral except facial sweating
- ☐ Unilateral symptoms may occur: usually with intense peripheral trigeminal nerve activation
- ☐ They vary between headache attacks

Unusual migraine features

- ☐ Auditory hallucinosis (paracusis): usually of human voices
- ☐ Hemifacial spasm
- ☐ Hypothermia
- ☐ Palinopsia
- ☐ Hiccups
- ☐ Yawning
- ☐ Laughter: gelastic migraine
- ☐ The red forehead dot syndrome
- ☐ Migraine-tic syndrome: migraine with concomitant trigeminal neuralgia
- ☐ Crash migraine (old terminology): sudden onset severe headache
  - ○ It is probably the same as idiopathic thunderclap headache (TCH)

Migraine postdrome

- ☐ Tiredness
- ☐ Difficulty concentrating
- ☐ Head pain
- ☐ Neck stiffness
- ☐ Hangover feeling
- ☐ Mood changes
- ☐ Weakness
- ☐ Gastrointestinal symptoms

Significant differential diagnoses

- ☐ Colloid cyst of the third ventricle
- ☐ Subarachnoid haemorrhage (SAH)
- ☐ Seizures: a differential of migraine with aura
- ☐ Stroke: a differential of migraine with aura

OPHTHALMOPLEGIC MIGRAINE

Clinical features

- ☐ This is recurrent severe migraine with ophthalmoplegia
- ☐ It begins in childhood to early adult years
- ☐ The oculomotor nerve is the most affected nerve
- ☐ Ophthalmoplegia usually develops within a week of headache onset
- ☐ It may also involve the trigeminal nerve
- ☐ It is associated with ptosis and mydriasis
- ☐ The deficits may become persistent in a third of cases
- ☐ The headache is not migrainous in a third of cases
- ☐ It takes a median of 3 weeks to resolve

Pathogenesis

- ☐ It is possibly a recurrent cranial neuralgia: an ophthalmoplegic cranial neuropathy
- ☐ It may be caused by recurrent demyelination
- ☐ There is focal oculomotor nerve thickening and enhancement in ¾ of cases

Differential diagnosis

- ☐ Tolosa Hunt syndrome

Treatment

- ☐ Steroids may be effective

Synonym

- ☐ Recurrent painful ophthalmoplegic neuropathy (RPON)

RETINAL MIGRAINE

Pathogenesis and epidemiology

- ☐ Most cases are probably caused by retinal vasospasm
- ☐ It usually affects women in the 2nd or 3rd decade
- ☐ Subjects usually have a history of migraine with aura

Clinical features

- ☐ Recurrent and stereotyped unilateral visual loss
  - ○ Unlike typical migraine visual aura which is bilateral
- ☐ Episodes last 5–20 minutes
- ☐ Headache develops during the episode or afterwards
- ☐ The headache is usually on the same side
- ☐ Headaches may be absent
- ☐ Permanent visual loss occurs in about 40% of cases

Associated visual phenomena

- ☐ Scintillations
- ☐ Scotomas
- ☐ Blindness

Differential diagnosis

- ☐ Transient monocular blindness (TMB)
- ☐ Optic neuropathies
- ☐ Giant cell arteritis (GCA)
- ☐ Glaucoma
- ☐ Raised intracranial pressure (ICP)
- ☐ Steal phenomenon
- ☐ Optic nerve compression
- ☐ Isolated orbital vasculitis

Red flags against migraine

- ☐ Absence of headache
- ☐ Onset age >50 years
- ☐ Incomplete resolution
- ☐ Presence of risk factors of transient monocular blindness (TMB)
- ☐ Atypical symptoms and signs

Acute treatment

- ☐ Aspirin
- ☐ Pre-exercise Aspirin or Nifedipine: in exercise-induced cases

Prophylaxis

- ☐ Topiramate
- ☐ Valproate
- ☐ Tricyclics

Contraindicated drugs

- ☐ Triptans
- ☐ Ergots
- ☐ Oral contraceptive pills (OCPs)

Synonyms

- ☐ Ocular migraine
- ☐ Ophthalmic migraine

VESTIBULAR MIGRAINE

Diagnostic criteria

- ☐ History of migraine
- ☐ ≥2 attacks of vestibular vertigo
- ☐ Concomitant migraine in at least 2 vertigo attacks

Genetic risk factor

- ☐ Vestibular migraine may be familial
- ☐ The first locus is mapped to chromosome 5q35
- ☐ The transmission is autosomal dominant

Features of vertigo

- ☐ The triggers are the same as for typical migraine
- ☐ The attacks last minutes to days: but they may last seconds
- ☐ The vertigo attacks usually occur in clusters
- ☐ 3% of cases present as benign paroxysmal positional vertigo (BPPV)

Features of headache

- ☐ Headaches occur in 50% of patients
- ☐ The headache may precede, accompany, or follow the vertigo
- ☐ The headache may improve in attacks

Associated features

- ☐ Hearing loss
- ☐ Tinnitus
- ☐ Nystagmus: this occurs in 70–90% of patients in attacks
  - ○ It occurs in 60% of patients between attacks
- ☐ Photophobia
- ☐ Migraine aura
- ☐ Absence of dizziness between attacks

Acute treatment

- ☐ Triptans
- ☐ Aspirin
- ☐ Topiramate
- ☐ Vestibular suppressants

Prophylaxis

- ☐ Betablockers
- ☐ Calcium channel blockers
- ☐ Tricyclics
- ☐ Valproate
- ☐ Acetazolamide
- ☐ Methysergide
- ☐ Gabapentin

FAMILIAL HEMIPLEGIC MIGRAINE (FHM)

Genetic types and mutations

- [ ] FHM1: CACNA1 gene
- [ ] FHM2: ATP1A2 gene
- [ ] FHM3: SCN1 gene

Triggers

- [ ] Stress
- [ ] Bright light
- [ ] Intense emotion
- [ ] Excess or inadequate sleep
- [ ] Physical exertion
- [ ] Menstruation
- [ ] Smoke, fumes, and strong scents
- [ ] Alcohol
- [ ] Change in weather
- [ ] Foods and seasonings
- [ ] Medications
- [ ] Massage
- [ ] High altitude flying

Clinical features

- [ ] Migraine
- [ ] Ataxia
- [ ] Nystagmus
- [ ] Cerebellar degeneration
- [ ] Learning difficulty
- [ ] Transient encephalopathy
- [ ] Confusion: this occurs in 20% of cases
- [ ] Recurrent coma and fever
- [ ] The digiti quinti sign (DQS)
  - ○ Impaired abduction of little finger with the arms extended forward
- [ ] Elicited repetitive daily blindness (ERDB): these are unilateral or bilateral episodes of blindness
  - ○ They are caused by retinal spreading depression and last about 10 seconds
  - ○ They are triggered by eye rubbing, direct light, dark to light transition, and standing

Complications

- [ ] Seizures
- [ ] Brain atrophy: this results from prolonged, repeated, or severe attacks

Differential diagnosis: sporadic hemiplegic migraine (SHM)

- [ ] Most cases of SHM have a family history of migraine
- [ ] About a fifth of cases convert to familial hemiplegic migraine (FHM) on follow up
- [ ] Consider FHM genetic testing in cases of SHM

Treatment

- [ ] Lamotrigine
- [ ] Acetazolamide
- [ ] Verapamil

STATUS MIGRAINOSUS

Clinical features

- [ ] These are prolonged migraine attacks
- [ ] The attacks last >72 hours
- [ ] They may be episodic
- [ ] They usually affect people with low frequency of migraine attacks

Pathology

- [ ] They may be caused by cerebral vasogenic oedema
- [ ] This is supported by brain imaging studies

Secondary causes

- [ ] Withdrawal of oral contraceptive pills
- [ ] CADASIL
- [ ] Multiple sclerosis (MS)
- [ ] Cluster headaches

Drug treatments

- [ ] Dopamine receptor antagonists: they have the best evidence
- [ ] Serotonergic agents: dihydroergotamine and triptans
- [ ] Nonsteroidal anti-inflammatory drugs (NSAIDs)
- [ ] Valproate
- [ ] Corticosteroids
- [ ] Magnesium sulphate
- [ ] Mannitol
- [ ] Droperidol

Non-drug treatments

- [ ] Intravenous fluids
- [ ] High flow oxygen
- [ ] Sphenopalatine ganglion block
- [ ] General anaesthesia

MIGRAINE ACUTE DRUGS: ANALGESICS AND ANTI-EMETICS

Non-steroidal anti-inflammatory drugs (NSAIDs)

- ☐ Ibuprofen 400–600 mg PO
- ☐ Naproxen 750–825 mg PO
- ☐ Diclofenac Potassium 50–100 mg PO
- ☐ Diclofenac 100 mg suppository
- ☐ Combination with triptans, e.g. Sumatriptan and Naproxen

Analgesics

- ☐ Aspirin 600–900 mg PO
- ☐ Paracetamol 1000 mg PO

Anti-emetics: Prochlorperazine

- ☐ 5–10 mg PO
- ☐ 5–10 mg IV
- ☐ 25 mg suppository
- ☐ 3–6 mg bid buccal

Anti-emetics: others

- ☐ Metoclopramide 5–20 mg PO or IV
- ☐ Domperidone 10–20 mg PO
- ☐ Domperidone 30–60 mg bid suppository
- ☐ Chlorpromazine 25–100 mg PO
- ☐ Chlorpromazine 6.35–37.5 mg IV

Acronyms

- ☐ IV: intravenously
- ☐ PO: orally
- ☐ PR: per rectum

TRIPTANS: TYPES AND CLINICAL USE

Mode of action and indications

- ☐ These are selective serotonin 5-HT1B/1D agonists
- ☐ They cause intracranial vasoconstriction
- ☐ They inhibit the release of vasoactive neuropeptides
- ☐ They block the transmission of pain signals
- ☐ They do not interact with adrenergic and dopaminergic receptors: unlike ergots
- ☐ They are metabolised by the CYP 450 and monoamine oxidase A (MAO-A) systems
  - ○ But Naratriptan and Almotriptan depend on renal elimination
- ☐ They are indicated for severe or disabling migraine
- ☐ They are also indicated when analgesics fail to control mild migraines

Triptan types and doses

- ☐ Sumatriptan: 6 mg SC, 50–100 mg PO, 20 mg IN, 25 mg PR
- ☐ Rizatriptan: 5 mg and 10 mg PO
- ☐ Zolmitriptan: 2.5 mg and 5 mg PO
- ☐ Naratriptan: 2.5 mg PO
- ☐ Eletriptan: 80 mg PO
- ☐ Almotriptan: 12.5 mg PO
- ☐ Frovatriptan: 2.5 mg PO

Specific indications

- ☐ Frequent migraine recurrences: Naratriptan, Eletriptan or Frovatriptan
- ☐ Menstrual migraine: Frovatriptan or Rizatriptan with Dexamethasone 4 mg
- ☐ Migraine in pregnancy: Sumatriptan
- ☐ Severe nausea: use SC or IN Triptans with anti-emetic, e.g. Metoclopramide
- ☐ For greater efficacy: combine Triptans with Naproxen

Drug interactions: anti-depressants

- ☐ SSRIs: but risk of serious serotonin syndrome is low
- ☐ Tricyclics
- ☐ Nefazodone
- ☐ Trazodone
- ☐ Venlafaxine
- ☐ Bupropion
- ☐ Monoamine oxidase inhibitors (MAOI): these increase the bioavailability of some triptans
- ☐ Lithium
- ☐ Buspirone

Drug interactions: others

- ☐ Propranolol: interaction increases the bioavailability of Rizatriptan
- ☐ Cimetidine: this interacts with Zolmitriptan
- ☐ CYP3A4 metabolised drugs: these interact with Eletriptan
- ☐ P-glycoprotein pump inhibitors: these interact with Eletriptan
- ☐ Dextromethorphan
- ☐ Amantadine
- ☐ Cocaine
- ☐ Ergot drugs

Acronyms

- ☐ IN: intra-nasally

- ☐ NSAIDs: non-steroidal anti-inflammatory drugs
- ☐ PO: orally
- ☐ PR: per rectum
- ☐ SSRI: selective serotonin reuptake inhibitors

CGRP RECEPTOR ANTAGONISTS (CGRP-RAS): GENERAL ASPECTS

CGRP gene family members

- ☐ α- CGRP: this is the conventional CGRP
- ☐ β-CGRP
- ☐ Adrenomedullin
- ☐ Adrenomedullin 2
- ☐ Amylin
- ☐ Calcitonin

CGRP receptor subunits

- ☐ Calcitonin-like receptor (CLR)
- ☐ Receptor activity-modifying protein 1 (RAMP1)
- ☐ Receptor component protein (RCP)

CGRP role in migraine pathogenesis

- ☐ The level of CGRP is elevated during and between migraine attacks
- ☐ Triptans reduce CGRP levels
- ☐ People with migraine are sensitive to injections of CGRP
- ☐ CGRP-induced migraines are reversible with triptans
- ☐ Selective CGRP receptor antagonists effectively treat migraine

Indications for CGRP-RAs

- ☐ Migraine in subjects unable to take triptans

Types

- ☐ Ubrogepant
- ☐ Rimegepant
- ☐ Atogepant

Emerging CGRP-RAs

- ☐ Vazegepant: intranasal

Discontinued CGRP-RAs

- ☐ Olcegepant: because it is not orally available
- ☐ Telcagepant: because it causes liver toxicity

Synonym

- ☐ Gepants

LASMIDITAN

Pharmacology

- [ ] Lasmiditan is a serotonin 1F receptor agonist
- [ ] It belongs to the Ditan drug family
- [ ] It is suitable for patients with cardiovascular risks: it does not cause vasoconstriction

Dosing

- [ ] The dose is 50 mg, 100 mg, or 200 mg orally as required
- [ ] Only one dose is indicated in 24 hours
- [ ] A second dose is ineffective for the same headache episode

Contraindications and precautions

- [ ] Driving and operating heavy machinery within 8 hours of a dose
- [ ] Concomitant alcohol
- [ ] Concomitant use of drugs that slow the heart rate
- [ ] Severe liver impairment

Side effects

- [ ] Dizziness
- [ ] Paraesthesias
- [ ] Fatigue
- [ ] Somnolence
- [ ] Nausea
- [ ] Weakness
- [ ] Hypoaesthesia
- [ ] Bradycardia
- [ ] Hypersensitivity reaction
- [ ] Serotonin syndrome: especially when co-administered with serotonergic drugs

MIGRAINE NON-DRUG TREATMENTS

Lifestyle modification

- [ ] Diet
- [ ] Avoiding trigger factors
- [ ] Relaxation
- [ ] Exercise

Psychological treatments

- [ ] Biofeedback
- [ ] Cognitive behaviour therapy (CBT)

Complementary treatments

- [ ] Acupuncture
- [ ] Petasites (butterbur)
- [ ] MIG-99 (feverfew)
- [ ] Ginger
- [ ] Ginger and feverfew combination

Other interventional treatments

- [ ] Occipital nerve block
- [ ] Occipital nerve stimulation (ONS)
- [ ] Transcranial magnetic stimulation (TMS)

Emerging treatments

- [ ] Hyperbaric oxygen therapy (HBOT)
- [ ] High flow oxygen
- [ ] Normoxic hypercapnia: using a partial rebreathing device
- [ ] External trigeminal neurostimulation (ACME)

MIGRAINE PROPHYLACTIC DRUGS: CLASSIFICATION

Level A evidenced drugs

- ☐ Sodium valproate
- ☐ Topiramate: this is not effective in childhood migraine
- ☐ Propranolol
- ☐ Metoprolol
- ☐ Timolol eye drops: this is probably as effective as Propranolol
- ☐ Frovatriptan: for menstrual migraine

Level B evidenced drugs

- ☐ Amitriptyline: especially with co-morbid TTH, depression, or disturbed sleep
- ☐ Venlafaxine
- ☐ Atenolol 25–100 mg bid
- ☐ Nadolol

Level C evidenced drugs

- ☐ Lisinopril
- ☐ Candesartan
- ☐ Clonidine
- ☐ Guanfacine
- ☐ Nebivolol
- ☐ Pindolol
- ☐ Cyproheptadine

Insufficient evidenced drugs

- ☐ Gabapentin
- ☐ Pizotifen
- ☐ Acetazolamide
- ☐ Bisoprolol
- ☐ Verapamil
- ☐ Fluoxetine
- ☐ Nifedipine
- ☐ Nimodipine
- ☐ Olanzapine
- ☐ Quetiapine
- ☐ Petasites

Other drugs

- ☐ Methysergide 1–2 mg tid
- ☐ Betablocker with Amitriptyline combination
- ☐ Melatonin 3 mg: this is as effective as Amitriptyline 25 mg
- ☐ Flunarizine 10 mg: this is reportedly better than Topiramate
- ☐ Memantine 10–20 mg daily
- ☐ Magnesium
- ☐ Atogepant: this is the only CGRP-receptor antagonist indicated for migraine prophylaxis

Investigational prophylactic drugs

- ☐ Coenzyme Q
- ☐ Kappa opioid receptor antagonists
- ☐ Levetiracetam
- ☐ Glibenclamide: an ATP-sensitive potassium channel inhibitor

Acronym

- ☐ CGRP: calcitonin gene related peptide
- ☐ TTH: tension type headache

MIGRAINE PROPHYLAXIS: CGRP MONOCLONAL ANTIBODIES (CGRP MABS)

General aspects

- ☐ The CGRP mAbs are indicated for episodic or chronic migraine
- ☐ They are used after the failure of ≥2 other prophylactic drugs
- ☐ Other oral drugs should be stopped before starting treatment if possible
- ☐ They are used for 6–12 months if effective

Erenumab

- ☐ This is indicated for episodic and chronic migraine
- ☐ The dose is 70 or 140 mg monthly SC

Fremanezumab

- ☐ The dose for episodic migraine is 225 mg monthly or 675 mg quarterly SC
- ☐ The quarterly dose for chronic migraine is 675 mg SC
- ☐ The monthly dose for chronic migraine is 675 mg loading dose and 225 mg monthly SC

Galcanezumab

- ☐ The dose for episodic and chronic migraine is 240 mg monthly SC
- ☐ Alternatively, 240 mg loading dose and 120 mg monthly SC

Eptinezumab

- ☐ This is indicated for episodic migraine
- ☐ The dose is 1000 mg quarterly IV

Contraindications

- ☐ Pregnancy
- ☐ Lactation
- ☐ Concomitant alcohol use
- ☐ Concomitant drug abuse

Acronym

- ☐ CGRP: calcitonin gene related peptide
- ☐ IV: intravenously
- ☐ SC: subcutaneously

Trigeminal autonomic cephalalgias

CLUSTER HEADACHE (CH): CAUSES

Familial

- ☐ There is a family history in about 6 to 8% of cases
- ☐ This is more often in female patients
- ☐ The transmission pattern is mainly autosomal dominant

Vascular

- ☐ Cerebral aneurysms
- ☐ Dural arteriovenous fistula (dAVF)
- ☐ Cerebral vein thrombosis (CVT)
- ☐ Cerebral artery dissection (CAD)

Neoplastic

- ☐ Pituitary adenomas
- ☐ Meningiomas
- ☐ Paranasal carcinomas
- ☐ Metastases

Infectious

- ☐ Sphenoidal aspergillosis
- ☐ Herpes simplex virus (HSV)
- ☐ Varicella zoster virus (VZV)
- ☐ Maxillary sinusitis
- ☐ Periostitis

Drug-induced

- ☐ Chemotherapy
- ☐ Warfarin
- ☐ Cocaine

Dental

- ☐ Wisdom tooth
- ☐ Dental extraction

Developmental

- ☐ Syrinx
- ☐ Chiari malformation

Other causes

- ☐ Trauma
- ☐ Multiple sclerosis (MS)
- ☐ Idiopathic intracranial hypertension (IIH)

Lifestyle risk factors

- ☐ Smoking
- ☐ Large body mass index (BMI)
- ☐ Illicit drug use
- ☐ High alcohol consumption

CLUSTER HEADACHE (CH): CLINICAL FEATURES

Episodic CH

- ☐ This is defined as the occurrence of two or more cluster periods
- ☐ Each period lasts 7 days to 1 year
- ☐ Pain-free periods last ≥ 1 month

Chronic CH

- ☐ This is defined as cluster attacks occurring for more than one year
- ☐ There are no remissions, or the remissions last <1 month

Premonitory symptoms

- ☐ Fatigue
- ☐ Apathy
- ☐ Irritability and restlessness
- ☐ Difficulty concentrating
- ☐ Mood changes
- ☐ Panic
- ☐ Elation
- ☐ Sensitivity to light, touch, and noise
- ☐ Yawning
- ☐ Stiffness
- ☐ Paraesthesias
- ☐ Blurred vision
- ☐ Sleep disorders

Headache features

- ☐ The headaches are usually strictly unilateral
- ☐ They are usually orbito-temporal in location
- ☐ They have an abrupt onset and ending
- ☐ The episodes may alternate sides
- ☐ Attacks last 45–90 minutes: the range is 15–180 minutes
- ☐ The natural course is for improvement over time

Autonomic features: conjunctival injection

- ☐ This is often bilateral: unlike in SUNCT
- ☐ It spares the peri-corneal vessels: unlike in glaucoma and uveitis

Autonomic features: others

- ☐ Lacrimation
- ☐ Nasal congestion or rhinorrhoea
- ☐ Ptosis and miosis
- ☐ Eyelid or facial oedema
- ☐ Forehead or facial sweating

Associated attack features

- ☐ Restlessness
- ☐ Agitation
- ☐ Post ictal fatigue and impaired concentration

DOI: 10.1201/9781003221258-44

Associated migrainous symptoms

- ☐ Photophobia occurs in about 70% of cases
- ☐ There is associated nausea in 50% of cases
- ☐ The headache is bilateral in 9–16% of cases
- ☐ There may be associated visual and olfactory aura
- ☐ The headache may side-switch during an attack: but this occurs less frequently than in migraine

CLUSTER HEADACHE (CH): ACUTE TREATMENT

Level A evidence

- ☐ 100% oxygen: at least 7L/minute for 15 minutes
  - ○ It is best given with demand valve oxygen (DVO) or O$_2$ptimask
- ☐ Sumatriptan 6 mg SC
- ☐ Zolmitriptan 5–10 mg IN

Level B evidence

- ☐ Sumatriptan 20 mg IN
- ☐ Zolmitriptan 5 mg and 10 mg PO
- ☐ Sphenopalatine ganglion stimulation

Level C evidence

- ☐ Octreotide 100microgram SC
- ☐ Lidocaine 4–10% 1mL IN

Galcanezumab

- ☐ This is a calcitonin gene related peptide (CGRP) antagonist
- ☐ It is approved for episodic cluster headache
- ☐ The dose is 300 mg SC at onset: then monthly until the end of the cluster period

Insufficient-evidence

- ☐ Dihydroergotamine 1 mg nasal spray
- ☐ Somatostatin 25 microgram
- ☐ Lignocaine solution 4–6% topical IN

Vagus nerve stimulation (VNS)

- ☐ This is probably effective in episodic cluster headache
- ☐ It may not be effective for chronic cluster headache

Investigational acute treatments

- ☐ Ketamine ± magnesium: case reports

Acronyms

- ☐ IN: intranasally
- ☐ SC: subcutaneously
- ☐ PO: orally

CLUSTER HEADACHE (CH): TRANSITIONAL PROPHYLAXIS

Prednisolone

- ☐ The dose is 60 mg daily for 5 days
  - ○ It is then tapered down by 10 mg every 3 days
- ☐ Alternatively, 100 mg daily for 5 days
  - ○ It is then tapered down by 20 mg every 3 days

Suboccipital steroid injection

- ☐ This has level A evidence
- ☐ It is administered once or it may be repeated

Methysergide

- ☐ The starting dose is 1 mg daily
- ☐ The dose is increased by 1 mg every 3 days to 5 mg daily
- ☐ It is then increased every 5 days to a maximum of 12 mg daily

Ergotamine tartrate

- ☐ The dose is 1–2 mg in divided doses
- ☐ It is administered orally or rectally

Dihydroergotamine

- ☐ The dose is 1 mg bid
- ☐ It is administered subcutaneous or intramuscularly

CLUSTER HEADACHE (CH): CHRONIC DRUG PROPHYLAXIS

Verapamil

- ☐ This has level C evidence
- ☐ The initial dose is at least 240 mg daily (80 mg tid)
- ☐ The maintenance dose is usually 480 mg: up to 960 mg daily may be required
- ☐ ECG is required at baseline, before dose increments, and 10 days after dose increments
- ☐ Monitor ECG for bradycardia, arrhythmias, and heart block
- ☐ The onset of cardiac side effects may be delayed by up to 2 years

Civamide nasal spray

- ☐ This has level B evidence
- ☐ The dose is 100 µL of 0.025% to each nostril daily

Lithium

- ☐ This has level C evidence
- ☐ The dose is 600–900 mg daily
- ☐ Avoid concomitant diuretics, carbamazepine, and NSAIDS

Warfarin

- ☐ This has level C evidence
- ☐ Maintain INR at 1.5–1.9

Melatonin

- ☐ This has level C evidence
- ☐ The dose is 10 mg every night

Insufficient evidenced treatments (Level U)

- ☐ Frovatriptan 5 mg daily
- ☐ Capsaicin 0.025% cream intranasal twice daily
- ☐ Prednisolone 25 mg alternate daily

Probably ineffective treatments

- ☐ Valproate
- ☐ Cimetidine/Chlorpheniramine
- ☐ Misoprostol
- ☐ Candesartan
- ☐ Hyperbaric oxygen
- ☐ Galcanezumab 300 mg monthly subcutaneously

Other reported treatments

- ☐ Topiramate 50–200 mg daily
- ☐ Baclofen 15–30 mg daily
- ☐ Botulinum toxin
- ☐ Gabapentin 800–3600 mg daily
- ☐ Clonidine 0.2–0.3 mg daily
- ☐ Methylprednisolone 500 mg orally for 5 days then taper down
- ☐ Methysergide
- ☐ Pizotifen
- ☐ Ergotamine

Acronym

- ☐ NSAIDs: non-steroidal anti-inflammatory drugs

PAROXYSMAL HEMICRANIA (PH)

Pathology

- [ ] There may be a potential secondary cause
- [ ] This is usually a pituitary lesion

Clinical features

- [ ] It has an abrupt onset and offset
- [ ] It may be triggered by head bending or rotation
- [ ] Episodes last 2–30 minutes
- [ ] There may be up to 40 attacks daily
- [ ] There is no nocturnal preference

Associated features

- [ ] Migrainous symptoms
- [ ] Restlessness
- [ ] Agitation
- [ ] Co-morbid cluster headache: chronic paroxysmal hemicrania-tic (CPH-tic) syndrome

Main treatment

- [ ] It is Indomethacin-responsive
- [ ] The dose may go as high as 225 mg daily

Other treatments

- [ ] Topiramate
- [ ] Other non-steroidal anti-inflammatory drugs (NSAIDs)
- [ ] Greater occipital nerve injection (GONI)
- [ ] Non-invasive vagus nerve stimulation (VNS)

HEMICRANIA CONTINUA (HC)

Clinical features

- [ ] This predominantly affects females
- [ ] Its intensity is moderate to severe
- [ ] It is usually unilateral and side-locked
- [ ] It is continuous or remitting
- [ ] Visual auras may occur before or with attacks
- [ ] Exacerbations are often nocturnal
- [ ] It may occur with trigeminal neuralgia: hemicrania continua-tic (HC-tic) syndrome

Associated features

- [ ] Ipsilateral autonomic features
- [ ] Jabs and jolts
- [ ] Conjunctival injection
- [ ] Rhinorrhoea
- [ ] Nasal stuffiness
- [ ] Eyelid oedema
- [ ] Forehead sweatiness

Treatment: Indomethacin

- [ ] The dose is 25–75 mg tid orally for 3–4 days
- [ ] It may also be administered as a 50 mg dose intramuscularly
- [ ] It provides sustained relief within 2 hours

Other treatments

- [ ] Ibuprofen
- [ ] Piroxicam
- [ ] Rofecoxib

LONG LASTING AUTONOMIC SYMPTOMS WITH ASSOCIATED HEMICRANIA (LASH)

Definition
- ☐ This is a trigeminal autonomic cephalalgia (TAC)
- ☐ It is an Indomethacin-responsive headache

Triggers
- ☐ Trauma
- ☐ Menses
- ☐ Secondary cases may occur with pituitary microadenomas

Clinical features
- ☐ It is an episodic head pain
- ☐ It is usually unilateral and pulsating
- ☐ It is of moderate severity
- ☐ Episodes last up to 72 hours

Autonomic features
- ☐ Lacrimation, rhinorrhoea, and conjunctival injection
- ☐ They may precede the headache
- ☐ They predominate over the headache
- ☐ They may occur without the headache
- ☐ They mast last several days

Treatment
- ☐ Indomethacin
- ☐ Melatonin may also be effective

SUNCT: CAUSES AND TRIGGERS

Vascular causes
- ☐ Posterior fossa arteriovenous malformation (AVM)
- ☐ Brainstem cavernoma
- ☐ Vascular loops
- ☐ Brainstem infarct

Neoplastic causes
- ☐ Prolactinoma
- ☐ Astrocytoma

Other causes
- ☐ Basilar impression
- ☐ Idiopathic hypertrophic pachymeningitis
- ☐ Varicella zoster (VZV) encephalomyelitis

Triggers
- ☐ Touching the scalp or face
- ☐ Washing
- ☐ Showering
- ☐ Shaving
- ☐ Chewing
- ☐ Eating
- ☐ Talking
- ☐ Coughing
- ☐ Brushing the teeth
- ☐ Brushing the hair
- ☐ Blowing the nose
- ☐ Light
- ☐ Exercise
- ☐ Neck movements

Acronym
- ☐ SUNCT: Short lasting unilateral neuralgiform headache attacks with conjunctival injection and tearing

SUNCT: CLINICAL FEATURES

Demographic features

- ☐ The mean onset age is 50 years

Typical features

- ☐ It is an episodic or chronic headache
- ☐ It occurs as single or multiple stabs
- ☐ It may be neuralgic or throbbing
- ☐ It may be spontaneous or triggered
- ☐ It is usually unilateral and side-locked
- ☐ Episodes last 2 seconds to 20 minutes
- ☐ There may be up to 60 attacks per hour
- ☐ It has a diurnal periodicity
- ☐ There is no refractory period in most cases: unlike in trigeminal neuralgia
- ☐ There is associated ipsilateral injection and tearing

Location of headaches

- ☐ Orbital
- ☐ Supraorbital
- ☐ Temporal

Associated features

- ☐ Cutaneous trigger: this is present in about 75% of cases
- ☐ Agitation in attack: this occurs in almost 60% of cases
- ☐ Interictal background pain: this is present in about 50% of cases
- ☐ Migraine: this is more frequent than in the general population

Atypical features

- ☐ It is occasionally located in the ear or occiput
- ☐ Conjunctival injection/lacrimation may be absent
- ☐ It may alternate sides in 20% of cases
- ☐ It is purely triggered in 2% of cases
- ☐ There may be associated epistaxis

Magnetic resonance imaging (MRI): features

- ☐ White matter lesions (WML)
- ☐ Causative lesions

Acronym

- ☐ SUNCT: Short-lasting unilateral neuralgiform headache attacks with conjunctival injection and tearing

SUNCT: TREATMENT

Drug treatments

- ☐ Lamotrigine: this is the best preventative drug
- ☐ Intravenous Lidocaine: this is used for short-term prevention
- ☐ Topiramate
- ☐ Gabapentin
- ☐ Carbamazepine
- ☐ Esclicarbazepine

Interventional treatments for refractory cases

- ☐ Occipital nerve stimulation (GONI)
- ☐ Deep brain stimulation (DBS): of the ventral tegmental hypothalamus
- ☐ Microvascular decompression of the trigeminal nerve

Acronym

- ☐ SUNCT: Short-lasting unilateral neuralgiform headache attacks with conjunctival injection and tearing

Intracranial pressure headaches

IDIOPATHIC INTRACRANIAL HYPERTENSION (IIH): TYPICAL CLINICAL FEATURES

Risk factors

- ☐ Obesity: this is usually in females
- ☐ Child-bearing years
- ☐ Binge eating disorder (BED)
- ☐ Systemic infections and inflammation

Headache features

- ☐ Headache is present in >90% of cases
- ☐ It is usually retro-orbital
- ☐ It is pressing or explosive
- ☐ It may be migrainous
- ☐ The headache severity does not correlate with the level of cerebrospinal fluid pressure
- ☐ It improves after lumbar puncture (LP) in 20% of cases
  - ○ But improvement after LP is not unique to IIH
- ☐ There may be associated pulsatile or non-pulsatile tinnitus

Neurological features

- ☐ Pulsatile intracranial noises
- ☐ Dizziness
- ☐ Nausea and vomiting
- ☐ Diplopia: due to abducens nerve palsy
- ☐ Olfactory impairment: this may be an early feature

Ophthalmic features

- ☐ Papilloedema: it may be asymmetrical or unilateral
- ☐ Visual obscurations
- ☐ Photophobia
- ☐ Retrobulbar pain
- ☐ Visual impairment
- ☐ Visual field loss
- ☐ Enlarged blind spot
- ☐ Optic atrophy
- ☐ Visual loss: the risk is higher in Blacks

Differential diagnoses of Papilloedema

- ☐ Drusen
- ☐ Tilted disc
- ☐ Hypotony
- ☐ Vitreous traction

Red flags against IIH

- ☐ Sudden onset and progression
- ☐ Abnormal clinical signs
- ☐ Abnormal cerebrospinal fluid (CSF)
- ☐ Atypical demographic profile
- ☐ Internuclear ophthalmoplegia (INO)
- ☐ Vertical gaze disorder

Synonym

- ☐ Primary pseudotumour cerebri syndrome (PTCS)

IDIOPATHIC INTRACRANIAL HYPERTENSION (IIH): VARIANT TYPES

IIH without Papilloedema (IIHWOP)

- ☐ This occurs in about 6% of IIH cases
- ☐ There are no associated visual fields defects
- ☐ There are no IIH risk factors
- ☐ Cerebrospinal fluid (CSF) opening pressures are lower than in typical IIH
- ☐ Most subjects are non-obese but obese cases have been reported
- ☐ Subjects may have bilateral transverse sinus thrombosis (BTSS)
- ☐ There is a good response to Topiramate

Fulminant IIH

- ☐ This is acute onset and severe IIH
- ☐ It results in severe visual loss within 4 weeks
- ☐ 50% are legally blind after treatment
- ☐ Repeated lumbar puncture and lumbar drain may be helpful temporising measures
- ☐ Intravenous steroids may also be used

Late onset IIH

- ☐ 64% are obese
- ☐ 36% are asymptomatic
- ☐ 29% are not idiopathic

IIH with normal CSF opening pressure

- ☐ There are rare case reports of IIH with normal CSF opening pressures
- ☐ They present with typical IIH clinical features
- ☐ They respond to Acetazolamide

IIH in men

- ☐ Men account for about 10% of people with IIH
- ☐ They are usually older and less obese than women with IIH
  - ○ But they are more obese than control subjects
- ☐ Visual loss occurs twice as often as in women
- ☐ They experience worse visual acuity and visual field impairment
- ☐ They have less headache at onset
- ☐ Obstructive sleep apnoea (OSA) occurs often
- ☐ Testosterone deficiency is frequent

Synonym

- ☐ Primary pseudotumour cerebri syndrome (PTCS)

DOI: 10.1201/9781003221258-45

IDIOPATHIC INTRACRANIAL HYPERTENSION (IIH): MEDICAL DIFFERENTIALS

Neurological

- ☐ Cerebral vein thrombosis (VCT)
- ☐ Jugular vein thrombosis
- ☐ Gliomatosis cerebri
- ☐ Brain tumours
- ☐ Leptomeningeal infiltration
- ☐ Behcet's disease
- ☐ Sarcoidosis
- ☐ Chiari malformation
- ☐ Craniosynostosis
- ☐ Lyme neuroborreliosis

Endocrine

- ☐ Addison's disease
- ☐ Hypothyroidism
- ☐ Hypoparathyroidism
- ☐ Cushing's disease

Respiratory

- ☐ Chronic obstructive pulmonary disease (COPD)
- ☐ Pulmonary hypertension
- ☐ Sleep apnoea
- ☐ Persistent coughing (Valsalva-triggered)

Chromosomal

- ☐ Down's syndrome
- ☐ Turner's syndrome

Rheumatological

- ☐ Systemic lupus erythematosus (SLE)
- ☐ Sjogren syndrome

Nutritional

- ☐ Iron deficiency anaemia
- ☐ Vitamin D deficiency
- ☐ Inflammatory bowel disease (IBD)

Other medical differentials

- ☐ Renal failure
- ☐ Polycystic ovarian syndrome (POC)
- ☐ Acquired aplastic anaemia
- ☐ Goldenhar's syndrome

Synonym

- ☐ Secondary pseudotumour cerebri syndrome (PTCS)

IDIOPATHIC INTRACRANIAL HYPERTENSION (IIH): DRUG DIFFERENTIALS

Antibiotics

- ☐ Tetracycline
- ☐ Doxycycline
- ☐ Minocycline
- ☐ Sulphonamides
- ☐ Nalidixic acid
- ☐ Ciprofloxacin

Hormones

- ☐ Oral contraceptive pills
- ☐ Growth hormone
- ☐ Thyroxine
- ☐ Tamoxifen
- ☐ Anabolic steroids

Drug withdrawal

- ☐ Steroids
- ☐ Lithium

Other drugs

- ☐ Hypervitaminosis A
- ☐ Lithium
- ☐ Mycophenolate

Synonym

- ☐ Secondary pseudotumour cerebri syndrome (PTCS)

IDIOPATHIC INTRACRANIAL HYPERTENSION (IIH): MRI FEATURES

Sella features

- ☐ Empty sella
- ☐ Partially empty sella
- ☐ Decreased pituitary height

Optic features

- ☐ Flattening of the posterior globes/sclera
- ☐ Optic nerve head intraocular protrusion
- ☐ Optic nerve sheath enlargement
- ☐ Tortuous optic nerve

Posterior fossa features

- ☐ Cerebellar tonsillar herniation
- ☐ Meningoceles

Venous sinus features

- ☐ Attenuation of the venous sinuses
- ☐ Bilateral transverse venous sinus stenosis (BTSS)
- ☐ Dominant transverse sinus stenosis

Other features

- ☐ Cerebrospinal fluid (CSF) leaks
- ☐ Increased number of arachnoid granulations
- ☐ Giant arachnoid granulations
- ☐ Prominent occipital emissary veins

IDIOPATHIC INTRACRANIAL HYPERTENSION (IIH): MEDICAL TREATMENT

Indications for treatment

- ☐ Impaired visual acuity
- ☐ Visual field loss
- ☐ Moderate to severe papilloedema
- ☐ Persistent headache

Non-drug treatments

- ☐ Weight loss of 5–10%
- ☐ Low calorie diet
- ☐ Low sodium diet: <100 mg/day
- ☐ Low tyramine
- ☐ Low Vitamin A

Acetazolamide: benefits and dosing

- ☐ This is a carbonic anhydrase inhibitor
- ☐ It is effective and improves quality of life
- ☐ The dose is 250–500 mg twice a day
- ☐ The safe maximum daily dose is 4g

Acetazolamide: side effects

- ☐ Diarrhoea
- ☐ Nausea and vomiting
- ☐ Dysgeusia (altered taste)
- ☐ Fatigue
- ☐ Paraesthesias
- ☐ Tinnitus
- ☐ Depression
- ☐ Renal stones

Non-evidenced drug treatments

- ☐ Topiramate: this is a carbonic anhydrase inhibitor: it may be more effective than Acetazolamide
- ☐ Zonisamide: this may be an alternative to Topiramate
- ☐ Methazolamide: this is a carbonic anhydrase inhibitor
- ☐ Furosemide: this is occasionally effective
- ☐ Intravenous Indomethacin
- ☐ Intravenous Methylprednisolone: in fulminant IIH awaiting surgery

Lumbar puncture (LP)

- ☐ This is indicated in fulminant IIH: to preserve vision whilst awaiting imminent surgery
- ☐ The benefit of LP is otherwise minimal and transient
  - ○ Some authors however report that LP may lead to permanent resolution of IIH
- ☐ There is a risk of exacerbation of headache after LP

Urgent treatments

- ☐ Lumbar drain
- ☐ Intravenous (IV) Acetazolamide/Steroids
- ☐ Urgent shunting
- ☐ Urgent optic nerve sheath fenestration (ONSF)

Emerging drug treatments

- ☐ Exendin-4: a glucagon-like peptide-1 (GLP-1) receptor agonist: this reduces CSF secretion
- ☐ 11Beta hydroxysteroid dehydrogenase type 1 (11β-HSD1) inhibitors: these regulate local cortisol

IDIOPATHIC INTRACRANIAL HYPERTENSION (IIH): SHUNTING

Indications

- ☐ Reduced visual acuity at onset
- ☐ Progressive visual loss
- ☐ Severe (high-grade) papilloedema
- ☐ Malignant IIH: this is IIH with rapid visual impairment
- ☐ Atrophic papilloedema
- ☐ Recent weight gain
- ☐ Hypertension
- ☐ Subretinal haemorrhage

Benefits

- ☐ Shunting improves medically intractable visual impairment
- ☐ It improves headaches in about 80% of cases within 2 years

Protocol

- ☐ Ventriculoperitoneal (VP) shunt is preferred to lumboperitoneal (LP)
- ☐ Neuro-navigation is used for shunt placement
- ☐ Adjustable valves with antigravity or anti-siphon devices are used

Complications

- ☐ Low pressure headache: this develops in just under 30% of cases
- ☐ Shunt failure: this is more frequent after VP shunts
- ☐ Shunt revision: this is required in 50% of cases after LP shunts
  - ○ 30% require multiple shunt revisions

IDIOPATHIC INTRACRANIAL HYPERTENSION (IIH): OTHER SURGICAL TREATMENTS

Dural venous sinus stenting (DVSS)

- ☐ This is an effective alternative to shunting in intractable cases
- ☐ Headaches improve or stabilize in all patients
- ☐ Visual function improves or stabilizes in more than 90% of cases
- ☐ It has better complication rates than shunting
- ☐ It may be complicated by restenosis: this is predicted by a high body mass index (BMI)
- ☐ The stent may fail: this is especially if the pre-stenting CSF pressure was very high

Optic nerve sheath fenestration (ONSF)

- ☐ Especially if visual symptoms occur without headache
- ☐ It improves visual loss and papilloedema in most cases
- ☐ The effect is bilateral even if done unilaterally

Bariatric surgery

- ☐ Bariatric surgery improves vision and resolves symptoms in the short term
- ☐ It is also more effective than community weight loss approaches in the long-term

SPONTANEOUS INTRACRANIAL HYPOTENSION (SIH): CLINICAL FEATURES

Types of spinal CSF leaks

- ☐ Type 1: dural tear: ventral or posterolateral
- ☐ Type 2: meningeal diverticula/dural ectasia: simple or complex
- ☐ Type 3: direct CSF-venous fistulas

Epidemiology

- ☐ Females are more frequently affected
- ☐ The peak incidence age is 40 years
- ☐ It could be familial
- ☐ There is a mechanical cause in a third of cases

Typical headache features

- ☐ The headache starts within 15 minutes of upright posture
- ☐ It is relieved within 15–30 minutes of lying down
- ☐ It is bilateral and pressure-like
- ☐ It is non-throbbing
- ☐ There is associated nausea and vertigo

Atypical headache features

- ☐ Headache when horizontal and relieved by standing up
- ☐ Headache relief only when lying on one side
- ☐ Headache induced by head shaking
- ☐ Non-posture related headache
- ☐ Exertional and thunderclap onset

Auditory features

- ☐ Hearing disturbance
- ☐ Tinnitus
- ☐ Ear fullness

Other associated features

- ☐ Visual disturbance
- ☐ Diplopia
- ☐ Facial numbness and pain
- ☐ Facial weakness and spasms
- ☐ Altered taste
- ☐ Hyperprolactinaemia or galactorrhoea: due to distortion of the pituitary stalk

Unusual presentations

- ☐ Older onset age: around 60 years
- ☐ Asymptomatic SIH
- ☐ Parkinsonism
- ☐ Ataxia
- ☐ Inter-scapular or low back pain
- ☐ Frontotemporal brain sagging syndrome (FBSS)
- ☐ Cognitive impairment
- ☐ Obtundation and coma

SPONTANEOUS INTRACRANIAL HYPOTENSION (SIH): MRI FEATURES

Fluid collections: locations

- ☐ Subdural: pseudo-subarachnoid haemorrhage
- ☐ Retrospinal: at C1-C2 level
- ☐ Extrathecal

Meningeal features

- ☐ Meningeal enhancement
- ☐ Meningeal diverticuli

Engorgements

- ☐ Engorged veins
- ☐ Pituitary engorgement
- ☐ Midbrain swelling
- ☐ Sagging brain with possible ventricular collapse
- ☐ Straight sinus distension

Spinal features

- ☐ Dinosaur tail sign: this appears as dorsal epidural hyperintensities on fat suppression T2 MRI (FST2WI)
- ☐ Syrinx

Other features

- ☐ Superficial siderosis: this appears as blooming on gradient echo MRI
- ☐ Narrow interpeduncular angle: between the cerebral peduncles
- ☐ The brain MRI is normal in about 20% of cases

MRI differentials

- ☐ Chiari malformation
- ☐ Subdural haematoma (SDH)
- ☐ Dural thickening
- ☐ Pituitary tumours
- ☐ Pituitary apoplexy

POST DURAL PUNCTURE HEADACHE (PDPH): CLINICAL FEATURES

Risk factors

- ☐ Use of traumatic needles: as against atraumatic needles
- ☐ Large needle size
- ☐ Inserting needle bevel perpendicular to the direction of the nerve fibers
- ☐ Non-replacement of stylet before needle withdrawal
- ☐ Repeated lumbar puncture (LP) attempts

Factors unrelated to risk of PDPH

- ☐ Volume of cerebrospinal fluid (CSF) drained
- ☐ Bed rest
- ☐ Position at LP

Clinical features

- ☐ The headaches are dull or throbbing
- ☐ They are bilateral
- ☐ They start frontally or occipitally
- ☐ They may radiate to the neck and shoulders
- ☐ They develop within 7 days of LP
- ☐ They resolve within 14 days
- ☐ They are worse within 15 minutes of getting upright
- ☐ They disappear or improve within 30 minutes of recumbency

Exacerbating features

- ☐ Head movements
- ☐ Valsalva manoeuvres
- ☐ Ocular compression

Associated features

- ☐ Neck stiffness
- ☐ Scalp paraesthesia
- ☐ Low back pain
- ☐ Nausea and vomiting
- ☐ Vertigo
- ☐ Tinnitus
- ☐ Diplopia
- ☐ Cortical blindness

Synonym

- ☐ Post lumbar puncture headache (PLPH)

POST DURAL PUNCTURE HEADACHE (PDPH): MANAGEMENT

Prevention

- ☐ Use smaller-sized needles
- ☐ Use non-cutting needles
- ☐ Insert bevel of cutting needle parallel to the dural fibers
- ☐ Replace stylet before needle withdrawal

Ineffective preventions

- ☐ Short duration of recumbency
- ☐ Small volume LP
- ☐ Increased fluid intake

Cerebrospinal fluid (CSF): features

- ☐ The CSF opening pressure is low
- ☐ There is mild CSF pleocytosis and lymphocytosis

Magnetic resonance imaging (MRI) features

- ☐ Dural enhancement
- ☐ Brain and brainstem descent
- ☐ Obliterated basilar cisterns
- ☐ Enlarged pituitary
- ☐ Dinosaur tail sign: dorsal epidural hyperintensities on fat suppression T2 MRI

Established treatments

- ☐ Epidural blood patch
- ☐ Caffeine
- ☐ Surgical closure

Emerging treatment

- ☐ Aminophylline

Treatments based on small trials and case reports

- ☐ Oral Prednisolone
- ☐ Intravenous Hydrocortisone

Synonym

- ☐ Post lumbar puncture headache (PLPH)

Other headache types

TENSION TYPE HEADACHE (TTH): CLINICAL FEATURES

Triggers

- ☐ Stress
- ☐ Irregular meals
- ☐ Coffee
- ☐ Caffeinated drinks
- ☐ Dehydration
- ☐ Sleep disorders
- ☐ Too much or too little sleep
- ☐ Low physical exercise

Clinical features

- ☐ The headache is bilateral and non-throbbing
- ☐ It is mild to moderate in severity
- ☐ It is not aggravated by physical activity
- ☐ There is no nausea or vomiting in episodic TTH
  - ○ There is mild nausea in chronic TTH
- ☐ There is either photophobia or phonophobia but not both
- ☐ There is pericranial muscle tenderness
- ☐ There are myofacial trigger points

Differential diagnosis

- ☐ New persistent daily headache (NPDH)
- ☐ Bilateral hemicrania continua (HC)
- ☐ Hypnic headache
- ☐ Giant cell arteritis (GCA)
- ☐ Intracranial neoplasms
- ☐ Idiopathic intracranial hypertension (IIH)
- ☐ Low pressure headache

TENSION TYPE HEADACHE (TTH): TREATMENT

Analgesics

- ☐ Aspirin 500–1000 mg PO
- ☐ Paracetamol 1000 mg PO
- ☐ Combination analgesics and caffeine

Non-steroidal anti-inflammatory drugs (NSAIDs)

- ☐ Ibuprofen 200–400 mg PO
- ☐ Naproxen sodium 375–550 mg PO
- ☐ Ketoprofen 25–50 mg PO
- ☐ Diclofenac potassium 50–100 mg PO

Prophylactic treatments

- ☐ Amitriptyline 75–150 mg daily PO
- ☐ Mirtazapine 30 mg daily PO
- ☐ Venlafaxine 37.5–300 mg daily PO
- ☐ Avoid opioids

Non-drug treatments

- ☐ Relaxation training
- ☐ Electromyogram (EMG) biofeedback
- ☐ Cognitive behaviour therapy (CBT)
- ☐ Physical therapy: this improves posture
- ☐ Exercise programs
- ☐ Hot and cold packs
- ☐ Ultrasound and electrical stimulation
- ☐ Acupuncture
- ☐ Combined tricyclic and stress management

Acronym

- ☐ PO: orally

DOI: 10.1201/9781003221258-46

MEDICATION OVERUSE HEADACHE (MOH): CLINICAL FEATURES

Diagnostic criteria

- ☐ Headache occurs on ≥15 days a month on Paracetamol, Aspirin, or NSAIDs
- ☐ Headache occurs on ≥10 days a month for Opiates, Triptans, or Ergotamine
- ☐ Regular analgesic use on ≥2 days a week for ≥3 months
- ☐ Headache develops or worsens during drug treatment of a primary headache
- ☐ Headache resolves or reverts within 2 months of drug discontinuation

Individual risk factors

- ☐ Age <50 years
- ☐ Female sex
- ☐ Low education level
- ☐ Obesity
- ☐ Smoking
- ☐ High caffeine use
- ☐ Physical inactivity
- ☐ Stress

Medical risk factors

- ☐ Migraine: this is the underlying primary headache in 80% of cases
- ☐ Anxiety
- ☐ Depression
- ☐ Chronic musculoskeletal complaints
- ☐ Chronic gastrointestinal complaints
- ☐ Regular tranquilizer use

Clinical features

- ☐ It typically develops on the background of chronic migraine
- ☐ It may develop on the background of tension type headache (TTH)
- ☐ It comes on after a predictable interval after analgesic intake
- ☐ It often awakens subjects from sleep
- ☐ It may lose its migrainous features
- ☐ The frequency increases over time
- ☐ There is increasing analgesic requirement

Differential diagnosis

- ☐ Intracranial hypertension
- ☐ Vasculitis
- ☐ Obstructive sleep apnoea
- ☐ Pituitary diseases
- ☐ Depression
- ☐ Chronic fatigue syndrome

Acronym

- ☐ NSAIDs: Non-steroidal anti-inflammatory drugs

MEDICATION OVERUSE HEADACHE (MOH): TREATMENT

Non-drug treatments

- ☐ Avoid triggers
- ☐ Mindfulness
- ☐ Cognitive behaviour therapy (CBT)
- ☐ Exercise
- ☐ Biofeedback

Drug treatments

- ☐ Topiramate
- ☐ Botulinum toxin
- ☐ Amitriptyline
- ☐ Prednisolone
- ☐ CGRP and CGRP-receptor monoclonal antibodies

Treatment of co-morbidities

- ☐ Anxiety
- ☐ Depression

Detoxification: benefits

- ☐ Detoxification is probably effective for opioid overuse
- ☐ Its role is however controversial
- ☐ It is used together with intravenous Lidocaine
- ☐ In-patient detoxification is probably not more effective than out-patient approaches

Detoxification: indications for in-patient care

- ☐ Withdrawal symptoms
- ☐ Psychological issues
- ☐ Medical comorbidities
- ☐ Previous failed withdrawal
- ☐ Overuse of Opioids, Barbiturates, or Benzodiazepines

Relapse: risk factors

- ☐ Long duration of headache
- ☐ Tension type headache rather than migraine as primary headache
- ☐ Use of >30 analgesic doses a month
- ☐ Smoking
- ☐ Alcohol
- ☐ Lack of improvement after 2 months

Relapse: prevention

- ☐ Continuous botulinum toxin
- ☐ Monitoring of drug intake
- ☐ Short-term psychotherapy

Patient education

- ☐ This may be sufficient alone for triptans and simple analgesics overuse
- ☐ It is most effective if there is no major psychiatric co-morbidity
- ☐ It is insufficient alone if there have been previous relapses

THUNDERCLAP HEADACHE (TCH)

Vascular causes

- ☐ Subarachnoid haemorrhage (SAH)
- ☐ Intracerebral haemorrhage (ICH)
- ☐ Spontaneous retroclival haematoma
- ☐ Cerebral vein thrombosis (CVT)
- ☐ Cervical artery dissection
- ☐ Reversible cerebral vasoconstriction syndrome (RCVS)
- ☐ Posterior reversible encephalopathy syndrome (PRES)
- ☐ Ischaemic stroke

Other neurological causes

- ☐ Pituitary apoplexy
- ☐ Posterior fossa tumours
- ☐ Third ventricle colloid cysts
- ☐ Aqueductal stenosis
- ☐ Chiari type 1 malformation
- ☐ Idiopathic benign TCH
- ☐ Spontaneous intracranial hypotension (SIH)

Medical causes

- ☐ Hypertensive crisis
- ☐ Acute sinusitis
- ☐ Temporal arteritis
- ☐ Cardiac cephalgia: from myocardial ischaemia
- ☐ Myocardial infarction
- ☐ Aortic dissection

Drug-induced

- ☐ Selective serotonin reuptake inhibitors (SSRIs)
- ☐ Triptans
- ☐ Ergot alkaloids
- ☐ Cannabis
- ☐ Cocaine
- ☐ Ecstasy
- ☐ Amphetamines

Triggers

- ☐ Valsalva manoeuvre
- ☐ Exertion
- ☐ Sexual activity
- ☐ Emotional stress
- ☐ Bathing or showering

Clinical features

- ☐ The onset is within a minute
- ☐ It is at least 7 on a 10-point severity scale
- ☐ It may be spontaneous or provoked

Assessment

- ☐ CT head imaging is indicated within 12 hours of onset
- ☐ Lumbar puncture (LP) is indicated if the CT is normal
  - ○ This is to exclude subarachnoid haemorrhage (SAH)

EXERTIONAL HEADACHE

Benign exertional headache

- ☐ The average onset age is 24 years
- ☐ Males comprise almost 90% of cases
- ☐ The headache is pulsating and never explosive
- ☐ There is associated nausea and photophobia
- ☐ About 50% of cases are bilateral
- ☐ The duration is minutes to 2 days
- ☐ It responds to Propranolol

Symptomatic exertional headache: causes

- ☐ Subarachnoid haemorrhage (SAH)
- ☐ Sinusitis
- ☐ Metastases
- ☐ Coronary artery disease
- ☐ Eagle syndrome (long styloid process)

Symptomatic exertional headache: clinical features

- ☐ The average onset age is about 40 years
- ☐ Males comprise about 40% of cases
- ☐ They have an explosive or pulsating quality
- ☐ There is associated nausea and vomiting
- ☐ Episodes last one day to a month
- ☐ Diplopia may develop
- ☐ There may be neck stiffness

SEXUAL HEADACHE

Causes

- ☐ Reversible cerebral vasoconstriction syndrome (RCVS): this accounts for two-thirds of cases
- ☐ Primary (idiopathic): this causes about a third of cases
- ☐ Subarachnoid haemorrhage (SAH)
- ☐ Basilar artery dissection

Clinical features

- ☐ The headache occurs during sex or masturbation
- ☐ It is pre-orgasmic or orgasmic
- ☐ It may have a thunderclap onset
- ☐ It is usually occipital and throbbing
- ☐ It is usually short lasting: mean duration is 30 minutes
- ☐ It usually resolves within 24 hours
- ☐ It does not occur with every sexual encounter
- ☐ It may be restricted to specific sexual practices
- ☐ It may be aborted by stopping sexual activity in some cases

Treatment

- ☐ Propranolol
- ☐ Indomethacin
- ☐ Greater occipital nerve injection (GONI): case report

NEW PERSISTENT DAILY HEADACHE (NPDH)

Clinical features

- ☐ This is sudden onset and non-remitting
- ☐ Subjects have an accurate recollection of its onset
- ☐ There is no preceding migraine or tension type headache (TTH)
- ☐ Some patients may have typical migraine features

Differential diagnosis

- ☐ Spontaneous intracranial hypotension (SIH)
- ☐ Cervical artery dissection
- ☐ Cerebral vein thrombosis (CVT)
- ☐ Chiari malformation
- ☐ Giant cell arteritis (GCA)
- ☐ Dual arteriovenous fistula (dAVF)
- ☐ Unruptured cerebral aneurysm
- ☐ Nutcracker syndrome: abdominal vein compression syndrome

Other causes of daily and near daily headaches

- ☐ Chronic or transformed migraine
- ☐ Chronic tension type headache (TTH)
- ☐ Hemicrania continua (HC)

Acute treatment

- ☐ Triptans: these may be effective in a third of cases even if the headache is not migrainous
- ☐ Intravenous Methylprednisolone
- ☐ Peripheral nerve blocks: of occipital, auriculotemporal, supraorbital, or supratrochlear nerves

Prophylaxis: evidence from small case series

- ☐ Nortriptyline
- ☐ Topiramate
- ☐ Clonazepam
- ☐ Botulinum toxin
- ☐ Mexiletene

CHAPTER 8

Vascular disorders

Ischaemic stroke features

TRANSIENT ISCHAEMIC ATTACKS (TIA): CLINICAL FEATURES

Ophthalmic features

- ☐ Amaurosis fugax: transient monocular blindness (TMB)
- ☐ Binocular visual disturbance
- ☐ Isolated diplopia
- ☐ Hemianopia

Focal limb deficits

- ☐ Unilateral weakness
- ☐ Unilateral numbness
- ☐ Hemisensory tingling
- ☐ Unilateral ataxia
- ☐ Limb shaking

Focal bulbar deficits

- ☐ Dysphagia
- ☐ Dysarthria

Cerebral features

- ☐ Transient confusion
- ☐ Amnesia
- ☐ Feeling unwell
- ☐ Positive visual phenomena
- ☐ Bilateral leg weakness
- ☐ Non-focal paraesthesias

Brainstem features

- ☐ Isolated vertigo
- ☐ Vertigo with non-focal symptoms
- ☐ Non-rotatory dizziness
- ☐ Unsteadiness
- ☐ Hearing impairment
- ☐ Tinnitus
- ☐ Fou rire prodromique: crying spells as TIAs
- ☐ Les folles larmes prodromique: crying spells preceding TIAs

Vegetative features

- ☐ Palpitations
- ☐ Sweating
- ☐ Nausea
- ☐ Vomiting

Up-going thumb sign

- ☐ This is hyperextension of the thumb
- ☐ It is tested with the arms extended and the palms facing each other
- ☐ It is a sensitive marker of TIA or minor stroke
- ☐ It helps differentiates TIAs from mimics

TRANSIENT ISCHAEMIC ATTACKS (TIA): INVESTIGATIONS

Magnetic resonance imaging (MRI) brain

- ☐ This is preferably done with diffusion weighted imaging (DWI)
- ☐ It should be done within 24 hours
- ☐ It is more urgent if the arterial territory or the cause are uncertain

Carotid doppler ultrasound

- ☐ The request should be made within 1 week
- ☐ The test should be carried out within 2 weeks

Intracranial vascular investigations

- ☐ Transcranial Doppler (TCD)
- ☐ Carotid doppler
- ☐ Magnetic resonance angiogram (MRA)
- ☐ Computed tomography angiogram (CTA)

Cardiac investigations

- ☐ Electrocardiogram (ECG)
- ☐ Prolonged cardiac monitoring if the cause remains unclear
- ☐ Echocardiogram (ECHO): if no cause is identified

Indications for transoesophageal ECHO (TOE)

- ☐ Atrial septal defect (ASD)
- ☐ Atrial septal aneurysm (ASA)
- ☐ Patent foramen ovale (PFO)
- ☐ Atrial thrombi
- ☐ Valvular heart disease
- ☐ Aortic arch atheroma

DOI: 10.1201/9781003221258-48

TRANSIENT ISCHAEMIC ATTACKS (TIA): TREATMENT

Antiplatelets

- ☐ Aspirin and Clopidogrel combination is recommended
- ☐ This is indicated if the ABCD2 score is >3 or with crescendo TIAs
- ☐ It is administered for 21 days

Other treatments

- ☐ Risk factor assessment and prevention
- ☐ Treat hypertension
- ☐ Cholesterol lowering diet/drugs
- ☐ Lifestyle advice

ISCHAEMIC STROKE: GENETIC RISK FACTORS

Connective tissue diseases

- ☐ Marfan's syndrome
- ☐ Ehlers Danlos syndrome IV (EDS IV)
- ☐ COL3A1 collagen type 3
- ☐ Osteogenesis imperfecta
- ☐ Pseudoxanthoma elasticum

Prothrombotic disorders

- ☐ Protein S deficiency
- ☐ Protein C deficiency
- ☐ Antithrombin III deficiency

Miscellaneous genetic disorders

- ☐ CADASIL
- ☐ CARASIL
- ☐ Sickle cell disease
- ☐ COL4A1 gene mutations
- ☐ Homocystinuria
- ☐ MELAS
- ☐ Fabry's disease
- ☐ Moyamoya disease: 10% are familial
- ☐ PLEKHG1 gene mutations

Genetics of sporadic stroke

- ☐ Factor V ArgGln506
- ☐ ACE/ID
- ☐ MTHFR C677T
- ☐ Prothrombin G20210A
- ☐ PAI-1 5G
- ☐ Glycoprotein IIIa Leu33Pro
- ☐ APOL1
- ☐ TSPAN2
- ☐ HDAC9
- ☐ ALDH2

Acronyms

- ☐ CADASIL: Cerebral autosomal dominant arteriopathy with subcortical infarcts and leukoencephalopathy
- ☐ CARASIL: Cerebral autosomal recessive arteriopathy with subcortical infarcts and leukoencephalopathy
- ☐ MELAS: Mitochondrial encephalomyopathy lactic acidosis and stroke-like episodes

ISCHAEMIC STROKE: MEDICAL RISK FACTORS

Cardiovascular risk factors

- [ ] Hypertension
- [ ] Cardiac disease: but not aortic valve calcification
- [ ] Congenital heart diseases, e.g. coarctation of the aorta
- [ ] Carotid stenosis
- [ ] Carotid artery web
- [ ] Intracranial arterial dolichoectasia (IADE): related to coronary and aortic artery ectasia

Contraceptives

- [ ] Highest risk is with combined oral contraceptives containing >35 μg ethinylestradiol
- [ ] There is no risk with progestogen-only or levonorgestrel-releasing intrauterine systems

Migraine with aura

- [ ] Migraine with aura is a stroke risk factor
- [ ] The risk is higher in smokers
- [ ] The risk is also higher in users of the combined oral contraceptives (OCPs)
- [ ] The risk is also increased following surgery

Medical co-morbidities

- [ ] Diabetes
- [ ] Trigeminal neuralgia
- [ ] Depression in middle age
- [ ] Sleep disordered breathing
- [ ] Sudden sensorineural hearing loss (SSNHL)
- [ ] Papillary fibroelastoma (PFE)
- [ ] Excessive daytime sleepiness (EDS)

Metabolic risk factors

- [ ] High potassium
- [ ] High sodium to potassium ratio
- [ ] High homocysteine
- [ ] β2 microglobulin: in women
- [ ] Hyperlipidemia
- [ ] Long-chain dicarboxylic acids: tetradecanedioate and hexadecanedioate
- [ ] Proteinuria

Infections

- [ ] Urinary tract infection
- [ ] Childhood infections
- [ ] Chronic periodontitis
- [ ] Chagas disease
- [ ] Herpes zoster
- [ ] Hepatitis B virus (HBV) infection is possibly protective
- [ ] Adult influenza vaccination is possibly protective

Other risk factors

- [ ] ECG p-wave abnormalities
- [ ] Retinal vein occlusion
- [ ] Initiation of α blocker therapy: in older people
- [ ] Eagle syndrome: elongated styloid bone
- [ ] Hypereosinophilic syndrome
- [ ] Raised vascular injury marker ICAM3

ISCHAEMIC STROKE: SOCIAL AND ENVIRONMENTAL RISK FACTORS

Individual risk factors

- [ ] Age
- [ ] Inadequate physical activity
- [ ] Obesity
- [ ] Childhood short stature

Smoking

- [ ] The risk is highest in women
- [ ] The risk is dose-dependent in young men and in women
- [ ] Second-hand smoking also increases the risk
- [ ] The risk may be genetically determined

Dietary

- [ ] Poor diet
- [ ] Alcohol
- [ ] Sugar
- [ ] Artificially sweetened beverages

Stress

- [ ] Long working hours
- [ ] High strain jobs
- [ ] Bereavement

Cocaine: mechanisms

- [ ] Vasospasm
- [ ] Cerebral vasculitis
- [ ] Hypertension
- [ ] Cardioembolism

Trauma

- [ ] This increases the risk of childhood stroke
- [ ] The risk is within 2 weeks of trauma

Environmental pollution

- [ ] Air pollution
- [ ] Fine particulate matter
- [ ] Residential proximity to motorways

Heavy metal exposure

- [ ] Cadmium exposure
- [ ] Arsenic exposure

Possible protective environmental factors

- [ ] Frequent sauna baths
- [ ] Vegetarian diet

ISCHAEMIC STROKE: DIFFERENTIAL DIAGNOSIS

Central neurological differentials

- [ ] Acute confusional state
- [ ] Alzheimer's disease (AD)
- [ ] Brachial artery embolism
- [ ] Cataplexy
- [ ] Contrast-induced encephalopathy
- [ ] Dementia
- [ ] Encephalitis
- [ ] Extradural or subdural haemorrhage
- [ ] Functional disorders
- [ ] Hemimeningitis
- [ ] Lyme neuroborreliosis
- [ ] Migraine
- [ ] Multiple sclerosis (MS)
- [ ] Myelopathy
- [ ] Parkinson's disease (PD)
- [ ] Primary progressive aphasia (PPA)
- [ ] Progressive supranuclear palsy (PSP)
- [ ] Re-expression of previous stroke symptoms
- [ ] Seizures
- [ ] Transient global amnesia (TGA)
- [ ] Wernicke's encephalopathy

Peripheral neurological differentials

- [ ] Acute mononeuropathy
- [ ] Miller Fisher syndrome (MFS)
- [ ] Motor neurone disease (MND)
- [ ] Myasthenia gravis (MG)
- [ ] Peripheral neuropathy (PN)

Systemic differentials

- [ ] Acute coronary syndrome
- [ ] Drugs and alcohol
- [ ] Giant cell arteritis (GCA)
- [ ] Granulomatosis with polyangiitis (GPA)
- [ ] Hypertensive emergency
- [ ] Hypoglycaemia
- [ ] Rheumatoid meningitis: this presents with stroke-like episodes
- [ ] Sepsis
- [ ] Somatisation
- [ ] Syncope
- [ ] Toxic-metabolic
- [ ] Vestibular neuronitis
- [ ] Whipple's disease

Radiological differentials

- [ ] Subdural haematoma (SDH)
- [ ] Abscess
- [ ] Trauma
- [ ] Brain tumours
- [ ] Central pontine myelinolysis (CPM)
- [ ] Progressive multifocal leukoencephalopathy (PML)

ISCHAEMIC STROKE COMPLICATIONS: CLASSIFICATION

Major stroke complications

- [ ] Haemorrhagic transformation
- [ ] Infarct growth
- [ ] Malignant brain oedema (MBE)
- [ ] Recurrent stroke
- [ ] Post-stroke seizures
- [ ] Post-stroke psychosis
- [ ] Stroke recurrence
- [ ] Stroke recrudescence
- [ ] Early neurological deterioration (END)

Neurological complications

- [ ] Perceptual impairments
- [ ] Bulbar impairment: dysphasia, dysarthria, dysphagia
- [ ] Dyspraxia
- [ ] Incontinence
- [ ] Contractures
- [ ] Spasticity
- [ ] Impaired mobility and falls
- [ ] Hemiplegic shoulder pain
- [ ] Central post-stroke pain
- [ ] Restless legs syndrome (RLS): especially with subcortical stroke
- [ ] Dementia

Post-stroke psychosis: types

- [ ] Delusional disorder
- [ ] Schizophrenia-like psychosis
- [ ] Mood disorder with psychotic features

Neuropsychiatric complications: others

- [ ] Anxiety
- [ ] Apathy
- [ ] Mania
- [ ] Emotional lability
- [ ] Personality disorder
- [ ] Post-stroke depression

Cardiorespiratory complications

- [ ] Myocardial infarction
- [ ] Takotsubo cardiomyopathy: stress-induced transient apical ventricular dysfunction
- [ ] Obstructive sleep apnoea (OSA) with sleep-disordered breathing

Systemic complications

- [ ] Post stroke fatigue: this is responsive to Modafinil
- [ ] Infection
- [ ] Malnutrition

CRYPTOGENIC STROKE: POTENTIAL CAUSES

Potential cardiac causes

- ☐ Occult paroxysmal atrial fibrillation
- ☐ Patent foramen ovale (PFO)
- ☐ Other right-to-left cardiac shunts
- ☐ Atrial cardiopathy
- ☐ Atrial septal aneurysm
- ☐ Aortic arch atheroma
- ☐ Substenotic atherosclerosis
- ☐ Arterial dissection
- ☐ Infective endocarditis

Potential systemic causes

- ☐ Antiphospholipid antibody syndrome
- ☐ Factor V Leiden deficiency
- ☐ Other hypercoagulable states
- ☐ Cancer
- ☐ Vasculitis: systemic lupus erythematosus, granulomatosis with polyangiitis (GPA)
- ☐ Viral infections: varicella-zoster, herpes simplex, cytomegalovirus
- ☐ Bacterial infections: syphilis, tuberculosis
- ☐ Genetic disorders: Fabry disease, mitochondrial diseases

Predictors of atrial fibrillation

- ☐ Age >60 years
- ☐ Previous cortical or cerebellar stroke
- ☐ Premature atrial contractions on initial ECG
- ☐ Prolonged PR interval
- ☐ Large left atrial diameter on echocardiogram: in males
- ☐ Higher thyroid stimulating hormone (TSH) levels

HAVOC AF prediction system

- ☐ Hypertension: 2 points
- ☐ Age ≥75 years: 2 points
- ☐ Peripheral vascular disease: 1 point
- ☐ Valvular heart disease: 2 points
- ☐ Obesity with body mass index >30: 1 point
- ☐ Coronary artery disease: 2 points
- ☐ Congestive heart failure: 4 points

HAVOC AF risk scoring

- ☐ Low risk: 0–4
- ☐ Medium risk: 5–9
- ☐ High risk: 10–14

EMBOLIC STROKE: RISK FACTORS

Major risk factors

- ☐ Atrial fibrillation (AF): the risk persists even after AF resolves
- ☐ Short-run atrial tachyarrhythmia
- ☐ Recent myocardial infarction
- ☐ Left atrial and ventricular thrombus
- ☐ Rheumatic mitral stenosis
- ☐ Infective endocarditis
- ☐ Nonbacterial thrombotic endocarditis
- ☐ Atrial myxoma
- ☐ Prosthetic mechanical valves
- ☐ Dilated cardiomyopathy
- ☐ Nonbacterial thrombotic endocarditis
- ☐ Dyskinetic/aneurysmal ventricular walls

Minor and uncertain risk factors

- ☐ Mitral valve prolapse (MVP)
- ☐ Mitral annular calcification
- ☐ Calcific aortic stenosis
- ☐ Mitral valve strands
- ☐ Atrial septal aneurysm (ASA)
- ☐ Patent foramen ovale (PFO)
- ☐ Aortic atheroma: causing retrograde embolism
  - ○ It appears as the aortic donut sign on CT angiogram
- ☐ Aortic dissection: this may be painless
- ☐ Giant Lambl's excrescences
- ☐ Left atrial spontaneous echo contrast
- ☐ Subaortic hypertrophic cardiomyopathy
- ☐ Congenital left ventricular diverticulum
- ☐ Cardiac surgery
- ☐ Catheter balloon angioplasty

EMBOLIC STROKE OF UNDETERMINED SOURCE (ESUS): POTENTIAL CAUSES

Conventional cardiac causes

- ☐ Arterial thromboembolism
- ☐ Paroxysmal atrial fibrillation (PAF)
- ☐ Patent foramen ovale (PFO)
- ☐ Congenital left ventricular diverticulum
- ☐ Cardiac structural abnormalities
- ☐ Atrial fibrosis
- ☐ Occult cardiomyopathy: consider cardiac MRI

Left atrial dysfunction

- ☐ High left atrial end-diastolic volume at rest
- ☐ Poor left atrial response to exercise
- ☐ Left atrial spherical remodelling

Atrial cardiopathy

- ☐ Serum N-terminal probrain natriuretic peptide (NT-proBNP) >250 pg/mL
- ☐ P-wave terminal force velocity in lead V1 (PTFV1) >5000 μV·ms
- ☐ Severe left atrial enlargement on echocardiogram

Carotid artery web

- ☐ This is the intimal variant of fibromuscular dysplasia
- ☐ It is diagnosed by CT angiography (CTA)

Potential systemic causes

- ☐ Varicella zoster virus (VZV)-related vasculopathy
- ☐ Hypercoagulable states
- ☐ Occult cancer (Trousseau syndrome)
- ☐ Migraine
- ☐ Fabry disease
- ☐ Hyperhomocystinaemia
- ☐ Susac syndrome
- ☐ Systemic autoimmune diseases
- ☐ May-Thurner syndrome (MTS)
  - ○ Compression of the left common iliac vein by the right common iliac artery
- ☐ Intravascular lymphoma

SPINAL CORD INFARCTION (SCI): RISK FACTORS AND CAUSES

Risk factors

- ☐ Hypertension
- ☐ Diabetes mellitus
- ☐ Dyslipidemia
- ☐ Atrial fibrillation (AF)
- ☐ Peripheral arterial disease
- ☐ Previous myocardial infarction (MI)
- ☐ Vascular risk factors are present in about 75% of cases

Procedural causes

- ☐ Aortic aneurysm repair
- ☐ Other aortic surgery
- ☐ Cardiac surgery
- ☐ Thoracic surgery
- ☐ Spinal decompression
- ☐ Epidural injection
- ☐ Angiography
- ☐ Nerve block
- ☐ Embolisation

Aortic causes

- ☐ Aneurysms
- ☐ Thrombosis
- ☐ Dissection

Embolic causes

- ☐ Cardioembolic
- ☐ Tumours
- ☐ Fibrocartilaginous (traumatised discs)

Vascular causes

- ☐ Vertebral atheroma
- ☐ Scapular artery occlusion
- ☐ Cervical artery dissection: this causes posterior spinal cord infarction
- ☐ Syphilitic arteritis
- ☐ Giant cell arteritis (GCA)

Other causes

- ☐ Chronic spinal disease
- ☐ Hypotension
- ☐ Thoracic trauma
- ☐ Cocaine abuse

Synonym

- ☐ Spinal stroke
- ☐ Ischaemic myelopathy

POSTERIOR CIRCULATION STROKE: CAUSES

Basilar artery stenosis

- ☐ This usually causes paramedian midbrain or pontine infarcts
- ☐ There are usually heralding signs before onset

Intracranial arterial dolichoectasia (IADE)

- ☐ These are dilated and elongated arteries
- ☐ 80% involve the basilar artery
- ☐ They are associated with dilated basal ganglia perivascular spaces
- ☐ There is a lesser association with lacunes and microbleeds

Other vascular causes

- ☐ Vertebral artery hypoplasia
- ☐ Giant cell arteritis
- ☐ Small vessel disease (SVD)
- ☐ Atherosclerosis
- ☐ Subclavian steal
- ☐ Cardiac embolism

Non-vascular causes

- ☐ Fabry's disease
- ☐ Migraine
- ☐ Bow Hunter's syndrome (BHS)

POSTERIOR CIRCULATION STROKE: CLINICAL FEATURES

Epidemiology

- ☐ This accounts for 20% of strokes
- ☐ It has a high risk of multiple transient ischaemic attacks (TIAs) at presentation
- ☐ It also has a high risk of recurrent stroke
- ☐ Mortality is high if there is ≥50% stenosis of the vertebrobasilar vessels

Anatomical supply of the posterior circulation

- ☐ Brainstem
- ☐ Cerebellum
- ☐ Medial and postero-lateral thalamus
- ☐ Occipital lobes
- ☐ Occasionally parts of medial temporal and parietal lobes

Features of impaired consciousness

- ☐ Disorientation
- ☐ Confusion
- ☐ Amnesia

Features of impaired vegetative functions

- ☐ Altered respiration
- ☐ Abnormal heart rate
- ☐ Blood pressure abnormalities

Features of weakness

- ☐ Bilateral or unilateral: weakness may alternate sides
- ☐ It may result in quadriparesis
- ☐ It may manifest as crossed syndromes

Unusual features

- ☐ Dental pain: from trigeminal nerve involvement
- ☐ Facial ulceration

Malignant cerebellar infarction

- ☐ Oedema
- ☐ Obstructive hydrocephalus
- ☐ Brainstem compression

Locked-in syndrome

- ☐ Oculomotor abnormalities
- ☐ Cardiorespiratory impairment
- ☐ Impaired consciousness
- ☐ Coma

Red flag presentations

- ☐ New onset vertigo
- ☐ New onset headaches
- ☐ Change in migraine character

Difficulties with clinical diagnosis

- ☐ FAST and ABCD scores are less sensitive here than in anterior circulation stroke
- ☐ Difficulty in diagnosis results in delayed thrombolysis

STROKE IN THE YOUNG: VASCULAR CAUSES

Vasculopathies

- [ ] Migraine with aura
- [ ] CADASIL
- [ ] Mitochondrial disease
- [ ] Reversible cerebral vasoconstriction syndrome (RCVS)
- [ ] Fabry disease
- [ ] COL4A1 mutations, e.g. HANAC
- [ ] HERNS: TREX1 gene mutation
- [ ] Hypertensive encephalopathy
- [ ] Primary angiitis of the central nervous system (PACNS)
- [ ] Pulmonary arteriovenous (AV) fistula
- [ ] Moyamoya disease
- [ ] Radiation vasculopathy

Prothrombotic conditions

- [ ] Factor V Leiden mutation
- [ ] Prothrombin gene mutation
- [ ] Protein C/S deficiency
- [ ] Antithrombin III deficiency
- [ ] Essential thrombocytosis

Acronyms

- [ ] CADASIL: Cerebral autosomal dominant arteriopathy, subcortical infarcts and leukoencephalopathy
- [ ] HANAC: Hereditary angiopathy, nephropathy, aneurysm, cramps
- [ ] HERNS: Hereditary endotheliopathy, retinopathy, nephropathy, stroke

STROKE IN THE YOUNG: SYSTEMIC CAUSES

Commonest cardioembolic causes

- [ ] Patent foramen ovale (PFO) with atrial septal aneurysm (ASA)
- [ ] Dilated cardiomyopathy
- [ ] Atrial fibrillation (AF)
- [ ] Recent myocardial infarction (MI)
- [ ] Infective endocarditis
- [ ] Mechanical aortic valve
- [ ] Congestive cardiac failure (CCF)
- [ ] Left ventricular thrombus
- [ ] Akinetic left ventricular segment
- [ ] Sick sinus syndrome
- [ ] Atrial myxoma

Low or uncertain cardioembolic risk

- [ ] Patent foramen ovale (PFO)
- [ ] Hypokinetic LV segment
- [ ] Mitral valve prolapse (MVP) and regurgitation
- [ ] Mitral annular calcification

Infective causes

- [ ] Lyme neuroborreliosis
- [ ] HIV
- [ ] Syphilis
- [ ] Tuberculosis (TB)
- [ ] Varicella zoster (VZV)
- [ ] Meningitis

Autoimmune causes

- [ ] Sjogren's syndrome
- [ ] Granulomatosis with polyangiitis (GPA)
- [ ] Eosinophilic granulomatosis with polyangiitis (EGPA)
- [ ] Takayasu arteritis
- [ ] Ulcerative colitis
- [ ] Antiphospholipid antibody (APL) syndrome
- [ ] Systemic lupus erythematosus (SLE)
- [ ] Sneddon's syndrome

Miscellaneous causes

- [ ] Malignancy
- [ ] Sepsis
- [ ] Disseminated intravascular coagulopathy (DIC)
- [ ] Hypoperfusion syndrome
- [ ] Nephrotic syndrome
- [ ] Pregnancy and puerperium
- [ ] Hyperthyroidism
- [ ] Oral contraceptive pills (OCPs)
- [ ] Recreational drugs

Stroke treatment

ISCHAEMIC STROKE: ACUTE TREATMENT OUTLINE

Antiplatelets

☐ Aspirin 160–325 mg within the first 24–48 hours: oral, rectal, or nasogastric
☐ Then dual therapy: Aspirin 75 mg and Clopidogrel 75 mg daily for 21 days

Thrombolysis

☐ This is administered within 4.5 hours of stroke onset
☐ It is given even if thrombectomy is being considered
☐ It may not confer additional benefit to thrombectomy

Mechanical thrombectomy

☐ This is now gold standard care

Anticoagulation

☐ This is started within 4–14 days for new atrial fibrillation
☐ It is reinstituted after 2 weeks of stroke for pre-existing atrial fibrillation (AF)
☐ It is reinstituted after 1 week for pre-existing prosthetic heart valves

Carotid endarterectomy (CEA)

☐ This is performed within 2 weeks of stroke onset

Management of malignant cerebral oedema (MBE)

☐ MBE is more likely with large hemispheric strokes
☐ The MBE score predicts its onset
☐ Treatment is with decompressive surgery
☐ Glyburide is an investigational treatment

Acute decompressive hemicraniectomy: indications

☐ Massive middle cerebral artery (MCA) stroke
  ○ The infarct size is at least 50% of the MCA territory on CT
☐ Significant cerebral oedema
☐ Age ≤60yrs
☐ NIHSS score >15
☐ Decreased consciousness

Treatment of silent brain infarcts

☐ Primary stroke prophylaxis is indicated

Emerging treatments for stroke

☐ Minocycline: it is potentially neuroprotective
☐ Peroxisome proliferator-activated receptor gamma agonists
☐ Glibenclamide

THROMBOLYSIS: CLINICAL USE

Timing

☐ Thrombolysis is effective up to 4.5 hours after stroke onset
☐ It is reportedly beneficial between 4.5 to 9 hours

Potentially beneficial but unconfirmed indications

☐ Wake up stroke
☐ Unknown time of onset stroke (UTOS)
☐ Lacunar strokes

Thrombolytic agents

☐ Alteplase 0.9 mg/kg
☐ Tenecteplase 0.25 mg/kg

Tenecteplase versus Alteplase

☐ Tenecteplase is an alternative to Alteplase
☐ It is as effective or more effective than Alteplase
☐ It is well-tolerated
☐ It may give better outcomes than Alteplase when used with thrombectomy
☐ There is a higher 90-day mortality than with Alteplase
☐ It is now recommended as an alternative to Alteplase

Thrombolysis and large strokes

☐ Thrombolysis is unlikely to be effective if the MCA territory clot is ≥ 8mm
☐ Consider intra-arterial thrombolysis or thrombectomy in this situation

Thrombolysis and seizures

☐ Seizures at onset of stroke do not contraindicate thrombolysis
☐ Thrombolysis reduces the risk of post-stroke seizures

Predictors of good outcome

☐ Age <80 years
☐ Female gender
☐ Recent smokers
☐ Cardioembolic stroke: compared to large vessel stroke
☐ Left hemisphere stroke
☐ Diffusion weighted imaging (DWI) ASPECTS score ≤5
☐ Smaller baseline diffusion weighted imaging (DWI) volume
☐ Absence of severe small vessel disease (SVD)
☐ Earlier institution of thrombolysis
☐ Successful recanalisation

Prediction scoring systems

☐ Glasgow coma scale (GCS) score
☐ Total health risks in vascular events (THRIVE) score

DOI: 10.1201/9781003221258-49

THROMBOLYSIS: CONTRAINDICATIONS

Bleeding related

- ☐ Intracranial haemorrhage (ICH)
- ☐ Subarachnoid haemorrhage (SAH)
- ☐ Active internal bleeding
- ☐ Arteriovenous malformations (AVMs)
- ☐ Aneurysms
- ☐ Some brain tumours
- ☐ Bleeding diathesis
- ☐ International normalised ratio (INR) >1.7
- ☐ Platelet count <100,000/cubic mm

Non-bleeding related

- ☐ Severe uncontrolled hypertension: blood pressure >180/105mmHg
- ☐ Within 3 months of intracranial or spinal surgery
- ☐ Within 3 months of serious head trauma

Additional European contraindications

- ☐ Age >80 years
- ☐ NIHSS >25
- ☐ Stroke involving >1/3 middle cerebral artery (MCA) territory
- ☐ Blood glucose 3–22 mmol/L
- ☐ Previous stroke
- ☐ Previous diabetes mellitus
- ☐ Mass effect on computed tomography (CT) head scan
- ☐ Alberta stroke programme early CT (ASPECT) score ≤7
- ☐ Any oral anticoagulant treatment
- ☐ NIHSS <6

THROMBECTOMY: CLINICAL USE

Key thrombectomy trials with <6-hour time window

- ☐ MR CLEAN
- ☐ ESCAPE
- ☐ EXTEND-1A
- ☐ SWIFT PRIME
- ☐ REVASCAT
- ☐ THRACE
- ☐ THERAPY
- ☐ HERMES

Key thrombectomy trials with >6-hour time window

- ☐ DAWN
- ☐ DEFUSE 3

Criteria for thrombectomy

- ☐ Large vessel occlusion (LVO)
  - ○ Internal carotid (ICA) or proximal middle cerebral artery (MCA)
- ☐ Pre-stroke mRS score of 0–1
- ☐ Age ≥ 18 years
- ☐ NIHSS score ≥ 6
- ☐ ASPECTS score ≥ 6

Timing

- ☐ Thrombolysis is first performed within 4.5 hours of stroke onset
- ☐ Thrombectomy is performed within 6 hours of stroke onset

Complications

- ☐ Recurrent stroke
- ☐ Arterial perforation/dissection
- ☐ Access site haematoma
- ☐ Intracranial haemorrhage (ICH)
- ☐ Subarachnoid haemorrhage (SAH)
- ☐ Vasospasm
- ☐ Visual loss
- ☐ Trapped thrombectomy device

SECONDARY STROKE PREVENTION

Antiplatelet therapy

- ☐ This reduces the risk of major stroke
- ☐ The benefit is highest in the first two weeks after stroke
- ☐ The benefit outweighs the risk of bleeding
- ☐ Clopidogrel may be used instead of Aspirin

Dual antiplatelet therapy

- ☐ Aspirin may be used with Clopidogrel or extended-release Dipyridamole
- ☐ F2R polymorphisms enhance the protective effect of dual therapy
- ☐ Dual therapy is not be better than Clopidogrel alone in the elderly
- ☐ The bleeding risk of antiplatelets is increased by dual therapy

Blood pressure reduction

- ☐ This is instituted after 24 hours
- ☐ The aim is to reduce blood pressure by 10/5mmHg
- ☐ Diuretics are used alone or with angiotensin converting enzyme inhibitors (ACEI)

Statin therapy

- ☐ This lowers the 10-year risk of stroke recurrence
- ☐ Target cholesterol level of <70 mg/dL or a 50% reduction
- ☐ Consider Niacin or Gemfibrozil if high density lipoprotein (HDL) is low

Smoking cessation: mechanisms

- ☐ Counselling
- ☐ Nicotine products
- ☐ Oral smoking cessation devices
- ☐ Avoid environmental tobacco smoke

Alcohol reduction

- ☐ Heavy drinkers should stop or reduce alcohol intake
- ☐ Alcohol should be restricted to 2 drinks/day in men and 1/day in women

Exercise

- ☐ Physical exercise prevents recurrent stroke in people with intracranial stenosis
- ☐ Moderate intensity aerobic exercise is done for ≥30 minutes 1–3 times weekly

Dietary control

- ☐ Salt restriction
- ☐ Weight loss
- ☐ Fruit/vegetable rich diet
- ☐ Low fat dairy diet

Treatment of atrial fibrillation

- ☐ Anticoagulation is preferred over antiplatelets
- ☐ Non-vitamin K antagonist oral anticoagulants are preferred

Other preventative measures

- ☐ Avoid hormone replacement therapy (HRT) after stroke or TIA

Investigational preventative measures

- ☐ Glucagon-like peptide 1 receptor agonists
- ☐ Colchicine: in people with coronary artery disease

STROKE REHABILITATION

Rehabilitation setting

- ☐ Rehabilitation is done in a dedicated stroke in-patient unit
- ☐ Rehabilitation is carried out by a core multidisciplinary team (MDT)

Goals

- ☐ Establish realistic rehabilitation goals
- ☐ Involve patients and carers early in rehabilitation
- ☐ Support caregivers

Assessments

- ☐ Assess level of disability
- ☐ Screen nutritional status
- ☐ Screen for disabilities and impairments
- ☐ Assess social care needs

Therapies

- ☐ Physical exercise: this prevents recurrent stroke
- ☐ Occupational therapy
- ☐ Cognitive rehabilitation
- ☐ Communication skills training

Investigational treatments

- ☐ CCR5 antagonists: these may aid stroke recovery
- ☐ CCR5 suppresses cortical plasticity

Discharge planning

- ☐ Consider early supported discharge for mild to moderate stroke
- ☐ Provide adequate information to patients, carers, and general practitioners

Post-discharge

- ☐ Aid return to work
- ☐ Provide interventions and adaptations to aid return to driving

Haemorrhagic stroke

INTRACEREBRAL HAEMORRHAGE (ICH): CAUSES AND RISK FACTORS

Vascular causes

- ☐ Hypertension
- ☐ Amyloid angiopathy
- ☐ Arteriovenous malformation (AVM)
- ☐ Cerebral aneurysm
- ☐ Cavernous malformation (cavernoma)
- ☐ Cerebral vein thrombosis (CVT)
- ☐ Dural arteriovenous fistula (dAVF)
- ☐ Vasculitis
- ☐ Small vessel disease (SVD)

Congenital heart diseases

- ☐ These cause an eight-fold increased risk of ICH
- ☐ The risk is higher with severe non-conotruncal defects
- ☐ The risk is also higher with coarctation of the aorta

Oral anticoagulants: predictors

- ☐ Advanced small vessel disease (SVD)
- ☐ Cerebral microbleeds
- ☐ Moderate to severe white matter hyperintensities

Genetic risk factors

- ☐ Familial cerebral amyloid angiopathy (CAA)
- ☐ Collagen 4A1 (COL4A1) gene
- ☐ Cholesteryl ester transfer protein (CETP) gene

Metabolic risk factors

- ☐ High potassium level
- ☐ High and low blood glucose
- ☐ Obesity
- ☐ Low LDL and low total cholesterol

Other risk factors

- ☐ Antiplatelets: they increase the risk of microbleed-related ICH
- ☐ Selective serotonin re-uptake inhibitors (SSRIs)
- ☐ Methamphetamines
- ☐ Heavy alcohol intake
- ☐ Brain tumours
- ☐ Traumatic brain injury (TBI)
- ☐ Infective endocarditis
- ☐ Liver cirrhosis
- ☐ Prolonged sleep
- ☐ Clotting factor deficiency
- ☐ Glial fibrillary acidic protein (GFAP)
- ☐ Statins: the evidence of risk is conflicting

INTRACEREBRAL HAEMORRHAGE (ICH): COMPLICATIONS

Early seizures

- ☐ These develop in about 15% of cases
- ☐ They occur within 7 days of stroke onset
- ☐ They are associated with cortical haemorrhages
- ☐ Status epilepticus develops in 1% of cases
- ☐ They do not influence outcome of ICH at 6 months

Delayed seizures: risk factors

- ☐ Cortical bleeds
- ☐ Subcortical bleeds
- ☐ Early seizures
- ☐ Pre-morbid dementia
- ☐ Prior multiple lobar haemorrhages
- ☐ Exclusively lobar microbleeds
- ☐ ≥1 APOE ε4 copies

Delayed seizures: CAVE predictive score

- ☐ Cortical involvement
- ☐ Age <65 years
- ☐ Volume >10 ml
- ☐ Early seizures

Intraventricular extension

- ☐ This occurs in 40% of cases
- ☐ It is graded by the Graeb score
- ☐ It may be complicated by acute hydrocephalus
- ☐ Surgical removal may improve outcome but the evidence for this is insufficient
- ☐ Intraventricular rtPA is an investigational treatment: it appears safe and effective

Hyperacute injury marker (HARM)

- ☐ This is a type of blood brain barrier disruption
- ☐ There is hyperintense signal in the fluid spaces on MRI
- ☐ This appears as contrast extravasation
- ☐ HARM may also occur in ischemic stroke

Recurrent haemorrhage: risk factors

- ☐ Lobar haemorrhage
- ☐ Older age
- ☐ Ongoing anticoagulation
- ☐ Apolipoprotein E epsilon2 or epsilon4 alleles
- ☐ Multiple microbleeds on MRI

Other neurological complications

- ☐ Late seizures
- ☐ Haematoma expansion
- ☐ Peri-haematomal oedema
- ☐ Dementia

DOI: 10.1201/9781003221258-50

Systemic complications

- [ ] Deep vein thrombosis (DVT)
- [ ] Pulmonary embolism
- [ ] Fever
- [ ] Hyperglycaemia
- [ ] Hypertension

INTRACEREBRAL HAEMORRHAGE (ICH): ACUTE MEDICAL TREATMENT

Reverse anticoagulation

- [ ] Prothrombin complex concentrate (PCC)
- [ ] Intravenous vitamin K
- [ ] Selective antidotes for new oral anticoagulants (NOACs)

Monitor intracranial pressure (ICP): indications

- [ ] Glasgow coma scale (GCS) score ≤ 8
- [ ] Transtentorial herniation
- [ ] Significant intraventricular haemorrhage (IVH)
- [ ] Significant hydrocephalus

Intracranial pressure (ICP): management

- [ ] 30° head-up position in bed
- [ ] Sedation
- [ ] Optimize cerebral perfusion pressure: target is 70–110mmHh
- [ ] Osmotherapy: Mannitol or hypertonic saline
- [ ] Controlled hyperventilation: target pCO2 is 26–30mmHg
- [ ] High dose Pentobarbital therapy
- [ ] Hypothermia: core body temperature is kept at 32–33°C

Blood pressure management

- [ ] Begin as soon as possible after onset of ICH
- [ ] Aim for mean systolic BP of 130–139mmHg in the first 24 hours
- [ ] Long term aim is blood pressure <130/80mmHg
- [ ] Agents: Labetolol, Esmolol, Nicardipine, Enalaprilat, Fenoldopam

Seizure management

- [ ] Avoid prophylactic anticonvulsants
- [ ] Treat visible and electroencephalogram (EEG) seizures: treat for 1 month
- [ ] Continuous EEG monitoring: if mental status is disproportionately depressed
- [ ] Agents: Lorazepam, Phenytoin, Phosphenytoin, Levetiracetam

Prevent deep vein thrombosis (DVT)

- [ ] Intermittent pneumatic compression and elastic stockings
- [ ] Low molecular weight (LMWH) or unfractionated (UFH) heparin
- [ ] Use Heparin after the 2nd day if the patient is immobile
- [ ] Continue Heparin for 1–4 days after bleeding stops

Other treatments

- [ ] Intensive care unit (ICU) for initial monitoring and management
- [ ] Screen for myocardial ischaemia or infarction: ECG and cardiac enzymes
- [ ] Maintain normoglycaemia
- [ ] Early enteral feeding within the first 48 hours: this reduces the risk of pneumonia
- [ ] Treat fever
- [ ] Multidisciplinary rehabilitation

Precautions

- ☐ Avoid hemostatic therapy for acute ICH: unless ICH is secondary to antithrombotic drugs
- ☐ Avoid graduated compression stockings
- ☐ Avoid glucose-potassium-insulin regime to treat early hyperglycaemia

Investigational treatments

- ☐ Minocycline: this may be neuroprotective

SUBARACHNOID HAEMORRHAGE (SAH): CAUSES

Vascular malformations

- ☐ Cerebral aneurysms
- ☐ Arteriovenous malformations (AVMs)
- ☐ Cavernomas
- ☐ Lower cervical spine dural arteriovenous fistula (dAVF)

Vasculopathies

- ☐ Cerebral amyloid angiopathy
- ☐ Reversible cerebral vasoconstriction syndrome (RCVS)
- ☐ Posterior reversible encephalopathy syndrome (PRES)

Vascular disorders

- ☐ Cervical artery dissection (CAD)
- ☐ Segmental arterial mediolysis (SAM)
- ☐ High grade carotid stenosis
- ☐ Cerebral vein thrombosis (CVT)
- ☐ Paraneoplastic cerebral vasculitis
- ☐ Idiopathic: long term follow-up is not required

Brain lesions

- ☐ Abscesses
- ☐ Brain tumours

Systemic causes

- ☐ Vasculitis
- ☐ Coagulation disorders
- ☐ Infective endocarditis
- ☐ HELLP syndrome with idiopathic thrombocytopaenic purpura (ITP)

Aspirin

- ☐ Short-term Aspirin use increases the risk of SAH
- ☐ Long term use may reduce the risk

SUBARACHNOID HAEMORRHAGE (SAH): CLINICAL FEATURES

Headache

- ☐ Headache occurs in about 60% of cases
- ☐ It is severe in about 45% of cases
- ☐ It is typically sudden onset (thunderclap)
- ☐ It is often occipital and stabbing
- ☐ It may be dull in convexity SAH
- ☐ The headache resolves within 48 hours in 10% of patients

Loss of consciousness

- ☐ This may be the initial presentation of SAH
- ☐ It is a poor prognostic feature

Sudden death: predictors

- ☐ Smoking >5 cigarettes a day
- ☐ High blood pressure
- ☐ Age >50 years

Terson's syndrome

- ☐ This is vitreous (subhyaloid) haemorrhage
- ☐ It is a poor prognostic sign

Other clinical features

- ☐ Periorbital ecchymoses: raccoon eyes
- ☐ Lethargy
- ☐ Acute confusional state
- ☐ Vomiting
- ☐ Neck stiffness
- ☐ Seizures
- ☐ Transient motor and sensory deficits
- ☐ Recurrent aphasia
- ☐ Cranial nerve palsies: these are secondary to aneurysms and dissection

SUBARACHNOID HAEMORRHAGE (SAH): MEDICAL TREATMENT

General medical treatment

- ☐ Bed rest in a quiet room
- ☐ Head of bed elevated to 30 degrees
- ☐ Analgesia
- ☐ Antiemetics
- ☐ Fluid management
- ☐ Stool softeners to prevent constipation
- ☐ Antacid treatment
- ☐ Deep vein thrombosis (DVT) prophylaxis

Blood pressure control

- ☐ Use titratable agent before surgery
- ☐ Keep systolic blood pressure <160mmHg

Seizure control

- ☐ Consider prophylactic anticonvulsants in immediate post-bleed period

Indications for long-term antiepileptic drug (AED) treatment

- ☐ Prior seizure
- ☐ Intracerebral haematoma
- ☐ Intractable hypertension
- ☐ Infarction
- ☐ Middle cerebral artery (MCA) aneurysm

Nimodipine

- ☐ Nimodipine is indicated for all patients
- ☐ It improves neurological outcomes but not vasospasm
- ☐ Intraventricular sustained-release Nimodipine is promising in trials

Other treatments

- ☐ Early identification and treatment of heparin-induced thrombocytopenia (HIT)
- ☐ Valproate is being investigated: it may reduce the risk of respiratory failure

Vascular malformations

CEREBRAL ANEURYSMS: RISK FACTORS FOR FORMATION

Acquired risk factors

- ☐ Smoking
- ☐ Hypertension
- ☐ Alcohol
- ☐ Possibly oral contraceptive pills (OCPs)
- ☐ Previous aneurysm: especially in women and familial aneurysms
- ☐ Hypothyroidism
- ☐ HIV associated vasculopathy: with multiple aneurysms
- ☐ Cervical artery tortuosity
- ☐ Coronary artery disease seems protective
- ☐ Low bone mineral density

Familial risk factors

- ☐ Family history of subarachnoid haemorrhage (SAH)
  - ○ Especially with ≥ 2 first degree family members
  - ○ Siblings are more important than parents or children
- ☐ Family history of cerebral aneurysms
- ☐ Family history of adult polycystic kidney disease (ADCKD)

Adult polycystic kidney disease (APCKD)

- ☐ Aneurysms occur in 11% of cases
- ☐ There is a high risk of multiple aneurysms
- ☐ Rupture occurs at a younger age than in other aneurysms
- ☐ Smaller aneurysms are more liable to rupture than with other aneurysm risk factors
- ☐ Screening for aneurysms is recommended at diagnosis and at 2–10 yearly intervals

Other connective tissue disorders

- ☐ Loeys–Dietz syndrome
- ☐ Ehlers–Danlos syndrome type IV (EDS IV)
- ☐ Marfan's syndrome
- ☐ Neurofibromatosis type 1 (NF1)
- ☐ Osteogenesis imperfecta

Candidate genes

- ☐ Collagen genes: COL3A1 and COL1A2
- ☐ Lysyl oxidase (LOX)
- ☐ Fibrillin 2 (FBN2)
- ☐ Alpha1 anti trypsin
- ☐ Matrix metalloproteinases (MMPs)
- ☐ TOMPs
- ☐ Kallikreins

Risk factors for multiple aneurysms

- ☐ Female sex
- ☐ Older age
- ☐ Hypertension
- ☐ Smoking
- ☐ Familial aneurysms
- ☐ Low bone mineral density
- ☐ Adult polycystic kidney disease (APKD)

CEREBRAL ANEURYSMS: CLINICAL FEATURES

Features of familial aneurysms

- ☐ Younger age
- ☐ Larger size aneurysms
- ☐ Multiple lesions
- ☐ Higher rupture risk
- ☐ Familial tendency to occur at the same site and bleed in the same decade

Complications of cerebral aneurysms

- ☐ Aneurysm rupture with subarachnoid haemorrhage (SAH)
- ☐ Pseudoaneurysm formation
- ☐ Giant serpentine aneurysms

Cranial nerve impairment

- ☐ Oculomotor nerve compression: this is the commonest cranial nerve involved
- ☐ Optic nerve compression: this may cause visual loss

TIA and stroke

- ☐ These are usually caused by emboli arising from the aneurysm
- ☐ They may also result from thrombus extension
- ☐ The thrombus may occur proximal or distal to the aneurysm

Prognosis of ruptured aneurysms

- ☐ The median survival is 20 days
- ☐ The one-year mortality rate is 65%

DOI: 10.1201/9781003221258-51

CEREBRAL ANEURYSMS: SCREENING

Indications for aneurysm screening

- ☐ ≥2 first degree relatives with subarachnoid haemorrhage (SAH)
- ☐ Subject <40 years with one affected first degree relative
- ☐ Anxious subject with one affected first degree relative
- ☐ History of subarachnoid haemorrhage (SAH) in a twin
- ☐ Family history of adult polycystic kidney disease (APCKD)
- ☐ Bicuspid aortic valve

Screening frequency

- ☐ Start after age 20 years: aneurysms are rare under this age
- ☐ Screen every 5–7 years afterwards: this is cost-effective
  - ○ Screen 2 yearly if there is a family history of rupture developing within 5 years
- ☐ Continue screening until age 70–80 years

Counselling points

- ☐ Risk of aneurysm rupture
- ☐ Treatment
- ☐ Follow up
- ☐ Effect on driving/flying licence
- ☐ Effect on life insurance
- ☐ Implication of negative screen
- ☐ Smoking advice
- ☐ Blood pressure monitoring advice

Screening after aneurysm surgery

- ☐ Imaging after surgery is recommended: to document aneurysm obliteration
- ☐ Consider long-term follow up: there is a risk of aneurysm formation and recurrence

CEREBRAL ANEURYSMS: TREATMENTS

Coil embolisation: risks

- ☐ Incomplete aneurysm occlusion
- ☐ Aneurysm recurrence
- ☐ Aneurysm re-rupture
- ☐ Delayed leukoencephalopathy
- ☐ Intra-procedural re-rupture (IPR): this increases the risks of hydrocephalus and vasospasm

Coil embolisation: predictors for acute re-rupture (within 3 days)

- ☐ Incomplete occlusion of initial aneurysm
- ☐ Hematoma adjacent to ruptured aneurysm
- ☐ Associated aneurysmal outpouching
- ☐ Poor Hunt and Hess grade at the time of treatment
- ☐ Anterior communicating artery aneurysm
- ☐ Aneurysm dome-to-neck ratio <2

Surgical clipping

- ☐ Complete aneurysm occlusion is achieved in 82–100% of cases
- ☐ The aneurysm recurrence rate is about 3%
- ☐ Anterior communicating artery aneurysms are most likely to recur

Surgical clipping compared to coiling

- ☐ Clipping leads to better recovery of third cranial nerve function
- ☐ It has a higher incidence of complete occlusion than coiling
- ☐ The outcomes of clipping are however poorer than coiling
  - ○ There are more post-operative complications
- ☐ Both have similar mortality and re-bleeding rates

Woven Endobridge (WEB) device

- ☐ This is an alternative to coiling
- ☐ It is usually indicated for wide-necked aneurysms
- ☐ It may be useful for recurrent aneurysms
- ☐ It is reportedly very safe and effective

Preventative measures against rupture

- ☐ Treat high blood pressure
- ☐ Avoid alcohol and tobacco
- ☐ High vegetable diet
- ☐ Screening of familial SAH
- ☐ Investigate for co-existing aneurysms after SAH
- ☐ Immediate imaging post-repair of ruptured aneurysm
- ☐ Counsel on risk factors of aneurysm growth and rupture
- ☐ Monitor for aneurysm growth and rupture with intermittent imaging

Acronyms

- ☐ PCOM: posterior communicating artery
- ☐ ACOM: anterior communicating artery

ARTERIOVENOUS MALFORMATIONS (AVM): CLINICAL FEATURES

Epidemiology

- ☐ The incidence is 1:100,000 per year
- ☐ The prevalence is 18:100,000
- ☐ The annual risk of first haemorrhage is 2%
- ☐ The recurrent haemorrhage risk in the first year is 18%
- ☐ Most cases are congenital but some arise de novo

Risk factors for de novo (acquired) AVMs

- ☐ Ischaemic stroke
- ☐ Intracerebral haemorrhage (ICH)
- ☐ Traumatic brain injury (TBI)
- ☐ Neuroinflammation
- ☐ Intracranial aneurysms
- ☐ Cavernous malformation (cavernoma)
- ☐ Brain surgery
- ☐ Radiotherapy
- ☐ Sickle cell disease
- ☐ Hereditary haemorrhagic telangiectasia (HHT)
- ☐ Some are incidental with no risk factors

Associated disorders

- ☐ Wyburn-Mason syndrome: Retinoencephalofacial angiomatosis
- ☐ Blue rubber bleb naevus syndrome

Presentations

- ☐ Subarachnoid haemorrhage (SAH)
- ☐ Intracerebral haemorrhage (ICH)
- ☐ Ischaemic stroke: AVMs cause 3% of young strokes
- ☐ Seizures
- ☐ Spinal claudication with spinal AVMs

Risk factors for haemorrhage

- ☐ Older age
- ☐ Female sex
- ☐ Deep location: basal ganglia, thalamus, brainstem
- ☐ Initial presentation with haemorrhage
- ☐ Exclusive deep venous drainage
- ☐ Associated aneurysms
- ☐ Pregnancy does not seem to increase the risk of haemorrhage

Risk factors for seizures

- ☐ Males
- ☐ Superficial venous drainage
- ☐ Increasing size
- ☐ Frontal lobe location
- ☐ Arterial border zone location

AVM rupture risk grading systems

- ☐ Spetzler-Martin grading system: grades I-VI
  - ○ It uses AVM size, eloquence of affected brain, and venous drainage
- ☐ A simplified 3-tier grading system has been proposed: Classes A-C

SPINAL DURAL ARTERIOVENOUS FISTULA (DAVF): CLINICAL FEATURES

Pathology

- ☐ They are classified as type 1 spinal arteriovenous malformations (AVMs)
- ☐ They develop between the radicular artery and vein
- ☐ They are either extradural or intradural
- ☐ They cause congestion of venous outflow and ischaemia of the spinal cord
- ☐ Myelopathy develops from venous hypertension
  - ○ Not from steal, compression, or haemorrhage
- ☐ They are usually thoracolumbar: 2% are cervical and 4% are sacral

Risk factors

- ☐ Hereditary haemorrhagic telangiectasias (HHT)
  - ○ This is caused by ACVRL gene mutations
- ☐ Capillary malformation-arteriovenous malformation (CM-AVM)
  - ○ This is caused by RASA1 gene mutations
- ☐ Neural tube defects

Clinical features

- ☐ They typically occur in middle aged men: mean age is 55–60 years
- ☐ The onset is acute in 5–18% of cases
- ☐ They present with gait difficulty
- ☐ There is progressive myelopathy with ascending sensory and motor symptoms
- ☐ There is radicular pain
- ☐ There are associated bowel, bladder, and sexual impairments
- ☐ There are combined upper and lower motor neurone signs

Triggers of symptoms

- ☐ Exercise
- ☐ Upright posture
- ☐ Ambulation
- ☐ Pregnancy
- ☐ Menstruation
- ☐ Singing

Differential diagnosis: peripheral neuropathy (PN)

- ☐ There is usually no upper limb involvement in dAVF: unlike in PN
- ☐ Urinary symptoms occur in 80% of spinal dAVF: these are unusual in PN
- ☐ Onset is asymmetric in dAVF: this is unusual in PN

Differential diagnosis: other spinal vascular malformations

- ☐ Spinal arteriovenous malformations (AVMs)
- ☐ Spinal haemangiomas
- ☐ Spinal cavernous angiomas
- ☐ Spinal aneurysms
- ☐ Spinal epidural arteriovenous fistula (SE-AVF)

Differential diagnosis: others

- ☐ Polyradiculopathy
- ☐ Motor neurone disease (MND)

SPINAL DURAL ARTERIOVENOUS FISTULA (DAVF): MANAGEMENT

Magnetic resonance imaging (MRI): features

- [ ] Spinal cord swelling
- [ ] Central hyperintense T2 signal over 5–7 segments
- [ ] Hypointense tortuous flow voids: these are dorsal to the spinal cord
- [ ] Contrast enhancement of spinal cord: this shows as the missing piece sign
  - ○ It appears 40–45 minutes after contrast injection
- [ ] Serpentine peri-medullary structures: these are seen on magnetic resonance angiogram (MRA)

Spinal catheter angiography

- [ ] This is the gold standard test
- [ ] It is performed if there are T2 hyperintensities or flow voids on MRI
  - ○ The absence of both excludes the diagnosis

Endovascular embolisation therapy

- [ ] This uses liquid polymers: particles are more likely to lead to recurrence
- [ ] It is contraindicated if the feeder is a segmental medullary artery
- [ ] It is successful in 46% of cases

Microsurgical occlusion

- [ ] Ligation/clipping is the most definitive treatment
- [ ] It is successful in 98–100% of cases

Precaution

- [ ] Avoid intravenous Methylprednisolone: it may cause irreversible clinical deterioration

Vasculopathies

CERVICAL ARTERY DISSECTION (CAD): CAUSES AND RISK FACTORS

Physiological risk factors

- ☐ Male gender:
  - ○ Females are younger and prone to multiple dissections
- ☐ Older age
- ☐ Low body weight

Metabolic risk factors

- ☐ Low cholesterol
- ☐ Hyperhomocystinaemia
- ☐ Low α1 anti-trypsin
- ☐ Methylenetetrahydrofolate reductase (MTHFR) deficiency
  - ○ The 677TT genotype is associated with high homocysteine
- ☐ ICAM-1 E469K polymorphism

Vascular risk factors

- ☐ Fibromuscular dysplasia
- ☐ Segmental arterial mediolysis (SAM)
- ☐ Vascular Ehlers–Danlos syndrome (EDS)
- ☐ Hypertension
- ☐ Tortuous cervical vessels
- ☐ Juvenile polyposis syndrome (JPS)

Environmental risk factors

- ☐ Recent infection
- ☐ Winter time: this is possibly due to infection
- ☐ Use of Fluoroquinolones

Direct causes

- ☐ Trauma: head, neck, and thoracic
- ☐ Cerebral angiography
- ☐ Spinal manipulation
- ☐ Eagle syndrome: the styloid process is >3cm long
- ☐ Severe coughing
- ☐ Violent sneezing
- ☐ Whiplash

Other causes

- ☐ Migraine: with and without aura
- ☐ Viral meningitis
- ☐ Thyrotoxicosis
- ☐ Aortic root diameter >34mm
- ☐ >18% change in the common carotid diameter during the cardiac cycle
- ☐ Kabuki syndrome: this is a congenital disorder with craniofacial anomalies
- ☐ Pregnancy

Familial CAD (fCAD): genetic variants

- ☐ COL3A1
- ☐ COL4: COL4A1, COL4A3, COL4A4
- ☐ COL5: COL5A1, COL5A2
- ☐ FBN1
- ☐ TGFBR2
- ☐ Suggestive variants: ABCC6, COL3A1, COL5A2, MEF2A, RNF213

DOI: 10.1201/9781003221258-52

CERVICAL ARTERY DISSECTION (CAD): CLINICAL FEATURES

Headache

- [ ] The headache occurs before the onset of stroke
- [ ] It is often non-specific but it may present as migraine or cluster headache
- [ ] It may also present as hemicrania continua

Neck pain

- [ ] Neck pain is in the upper anterior neck with internal carotid artery dissection
- [ ] It is in the posterior neck in vertebral artery dissection
- [ ] It is often absent in patients ≥ 60 years old

Stroke

- [ ] CAD accounts for 10–20% of stroke in young adults
- [ ] Stroke risk is restricted to the first two weeks after dissection

Global orbital infarction syndrome

- [ ] Progressive visual impairment
- [ ] Ophthalmoparesis
- [ ] Mydriasis
- [ ] Ptosis
- [ ] Proptosis
- [ ] Chemosis

Other features

- [ ] Pathologic laughter on swallowing: with basilar artery dissection

Features of familial CAD (fCAD)

- [ ] CAD is familial in 1% of cases
- [ ] The mean onset age is younger than in non-familial cases
- [ ] Multiple and recurrent dissections are more likely
- [ ] The affected vessels are similar within families
- [ ] The age at onset is similar within families

Differential diagnosis of headaches preceding stroke

- [ ] Cerebral vein thrombosis (CVT)
- [ ] Vasculitis
- [ ] Reversible cerebral vasoconstriction syndrome (RCVS)

Recurrent cervical artery dissection

- [ ] There is a familial predisposition to recurrent dissection
- [ ] Associated connective tissue disorders may predispose to recurrence
- [ ] Early recurrence (within 4 weeks) occurs in about 10% of cases
- [ ] Late recurrence (after 4 weeks) occurs in about 7% of cases
- [ ] Multiple recurrences occur in about 2% of cases
- [ ] The presentation is the same as with non-recurrent cases
- [ ] Recurrence may affect multiple cervical arteries sequentially
- [ ] Treatment is with antiplatelets rather than with Warfarin

Prognosis

- [ ] Pulsatile tinnitus predicts a good outcome
- [ ] Dissected artery occlusion (DAO) predicts a poor outcome

CEREBRAL AMYLOID ANGIOPATHY (CAA): CLINICAL FEATURES

Pathology

- [ ] There are β-amyloid deposits in the cortical and leptomeningeal arteries
- [ ] These cause an inflammatory vasculopathy
- [ ] Sporadic cases may be associated with APOE ε4 gene mutations
- [ ] It usually affects older adults

Hereditary CAA: types

- [ ] Piedmont type
  - ○ This is caused by Leu705Val amyloid precursor protein (APP) mutations
- [ ] Dutch type: HCHWA-D

Transient focal neurological episodes (TFNE, amyloid spells): types

- [ ] Paraesthesias
- [ ] Numbness
- [ ] Limb jerking
- [ ] Migraine-like visual symptoms

Transient focal neurological episodes (TFNE, amyloid spells): features

- [ ] The attacks are brief and stereotyped
- [ ] They are responsive to antiepileptic drugs (AEDs)
- [ ] They predict early symptomatic intracerebral haemorrhage (ICH)

Intracerebral haemorrhage (ICH): predictive features

- [ ] Associated subarachnoid haemorrhage (SAH)
- [ ] ICH with finger-like projections on CT scan
- [ ] Associated APOE ε4 genotype

Subarachnoid haemorrhage (SAH)

- [ ] This is atraumatic
- [ ] There is bleeding into several adjacent sulci: unlike in aneurysmal SAH

Cognitive impairment

- [ ] Mild cognitive impairment is prevalent
- [ ] Dementia may develop

Other clinical features

- [ ] Headache
- [ ] Seizures
- [ ] Weakness
- [ ] Dysphasia
- [ ] Behavioural change
- [ ] Early onset age: reported after cadaveric dural graft
- [ ] CAA related inflammation (CAAri)

Boston criteria for probable CAA

- ☐ Age ≥55 years
- ☐ Multiple haemorrhages: lobar, cortical, or subcortical
- ☐ Superficial siderosis
- ☐ No other cause of cerebral haemorrhage

Acronym

- ☐ HCHWA-D: hereditary cerebral haemorrhage with amyloidosis-Dutch type

CEREBRAL AMYLOID ANGIOPATHY (CAA): RADIOLOGICAL FEATURES

Microbleeds

- ☐ They are located in lobar, cortical, and subcortical areas
- ☐ They are <5mm in size
- ☐ Their number correlates with bleeding risk and cognition
- ☐ They are hypointense on T2-weighted magnetic resonance imaging (MRI)
- ☐ They are best seen on gradient echo sequences
- ☐ They are found in 3–5% of normal people

Haemorrhage types

- ☐ Convexity subarachnoid haemorrhage (cSAH)
  - ○ This predicts a high risk of intracerebral haemorrhage
- ☐ Intracerebral haemorrhage (ICH): this is peripheral, cortical, or subcortical
- ☐ Intraventricular haemorrhage (IVH)
- ☐ Subdural haemorrhage (SDH)

Superficial siderosis (SS)

- ☐ This is cortical in location
  - ○ Unlike other forms of SS which are in the brainstem and posterior fossa
- ☐ It results from convexity subarachnoid haemorrhage (cSAH)
- ☐ It is usually disseminated
- ☐ It presents with transient focal neurological deficits
- ☐ It predicts an increased risk of recurrent lobar haemorrhage

Ischaemic features

- ☐ Multiple subcortical white matter hyperintensities (WMH)
  - ○ Unlike peri-basal ganglia pattern in hypertensive WMH
- ☐ Silent acute ischaemic lesions
- ☐ Small vessel disease (SVD)
- ☐ Lobar lacunes: unlike deep lacunes of hypertension

Other MRI features

- ☐ Pseudotumour: these are non-enhancing lesions
  - ○ They are assessed by perfusion MRI or MR spectroscopy
- ☐ Dilated hemispheric perivascular spaces (PVSs)
  - ○ Hypertensive PVSs are in the basal ganglia
- ☐ Cortical and white matter atrophy
- ☐ Possible leptomeningeal or parenchymal enhancement

Amyloid PET scan features

- ☐ This is ^{18}F-florbetapir-PET scan: a PET amyloid tracer
- ☐ It has about 80% sensitivity and specificity for CAA
- ☐ It has about 90% sensitivity for CAA related intracerebral haemorrhage (ICH)
- ☐ The diagnostic value is unclear: it does not easily distinguish Alzheimer's disease (AD)

Differential diagnosis of microhaemorrhages

- ☐ Cerebral cavernous malformations (cavernomas)
- ☐ CADASIL: Cerebral autosomal dominant arteriopathy with subcortical infarcts and leukoencephalopathy
- ☐ Primary angiitis of the central nervous system (PACNS)

REVERSIBLE CEREBRAL VASOCONSTRICTION SYNDROME (RCVS): CAUSES

Antidepressants

☐ Selective serotonin reuptake inhibitors (SSRIs): these account for about 20% of cases

Nasal decongestants

☐ Ephedrine
☐ Pseudoephedrine

Migraine drugs

☐ Ergotamine
☐ Sumatriptan

Cytotoxic agents

☐ Cyclophosphamide
☐ Methotrexate
☐ Tacrolimus

Other drugs

☐ Interferon alpha (INFα)
☐ Intravenous immunoglobulins (IVIg)
☐ Erythropoeitin
☐ Red cell transfusion
☐ Bromocriptine
☐ Cabergoline
☐ Nicotine patches
☐ Intramuscular Adrenaline
☐ Oral contraceptive pills (OCPs)

Drugs of abuse

☐ Cannabis
☐ Cocaine
☐ Ecstasy
☐ Amphetamines
☐ Lysergic acid diethylamine (LSD)
☐ Alcohol binge in cannabis users

Medical causes

☐ Phaeochromocytoma
☐ Bronchial carcinoid
☐ Hypercalcaemia
☐ Porphyria
☐ Carotid glomus tumour

Neurosurgical causes

☐ Head trauma
☐ Spinal subdural haematoma (SDH)
☐ Post carotid endarterectomy
☐ Post neurosurgery

Other causes

☐ It is spontaneous in 37% of cases
☐ Postpartum cases account for 12% of cases

REVERSIBLE CEREBRAL VASOCONSTRICTION SYNDROME (RCVS): CLINICAL FEATURES

Demographic features

☐ The mean onset age is 42 years
☐ Women are more frequently affected
☐ Affected women are usually older than affected men

Headache features

☐ RCVS presents with multiple thunderclap headaches
☐ The headaches occur over one to three weeks
☐ They may be triggered by exertion, sexual intercourse, or emotions

Other features

☐ Nausea
☐ Vomiting
☐ Photophobia
☐ Confusion
☐ Blurred vision
☐ Focal deficits: these occur in about 25% of cases
☐ Hypertension: this occurs in a third of cases
☐ Seizures

RCVS$_2$ diagnostic scoring system (-2 to +10)

☐ Thunderclap headache
☐ Carotid artery involvement
☐ Vasoconstrictive trigger
☐ Female gender
☐ Subarachnoid haemorrhage (SAH)
☐ Highest sensitivity is with score ≥5
☐ A score of ≤2 is strongly against RCVS

Complications

☐ Transient ischaemic attacks (TIAs)
☐ Ischaemic stroke
☐ Cortical subarachnoid haemorrhage (SAH)
☐ Intracerebral haemorrhage (ICH)
☐ Posterior reversible encephalopathy syndrome (PRES)
☐ Vertebral artery dissection

Course

☐ It usually resolves in 1–3 months
☐ There are no relapses
☐ Progression may be associated with the use of steroids

PRIMARY ANGIITIS OF THE CENTRAL NERVOUS SYSTEM (PACNS): CLINICAL FEATURES

Classification

- ☐ Granulomatous angiitis: this affects small-sized vessels
- ☐ Lymphocytic PACNS
- ☐ Angiographically defined PACNS: this affects medium-sized vessels
- ☐ Mass or tumour-like lesions
- ☐ Amyloid beta related cerebral angiitis
- ☐ Haemorrhagic PACNS: this is associated with sympathomimetic drug use
- ☐ Isolated spinal cord PACNS
- ☐ Unilateral hemispheric PACNS: this may be relapsing

Risk factors

- ☐ Mycoplasma
- ☐ Herpes zoster
- ☐ Tuberculosis (TB)
- ☐ Syphilis
- ☐ Fungal infections
- ☐ Hodgkin's lymphoma
- ☐ IgA deficiency
- ☐ HIV
- ☐ Phenylpropanolamine
- ☐ Amphetamine abuse
- ☐ Cocaine

Demographic features

- ☐ The mean onset age is 50 years
- ☐ Men are affected twice as frequently as women
- ☐ Younger people are more likely to manifest with mass or tumour-like lesions

Headache

- ☐ Headache occurs in most cases
- ☐ It is subacute or chronic

Stroke and transient ischaemic attacks (TIAs)

- ☐ These occur in 30–50% of cases
- ☐ They affect different vascular territories
- ☐ Single stroke presentation is uncommon

Other clinical features

- ☐ Seizures: these are less frequent with tumour-like cases
- ☐ Recurrent intracranial haemorrhage (ICH)
- ☐ Cognitive impairment
- ☐ Chronic meningitis
- ☐ Cranial nerve dysfunction
- ☐ Myelopathy
- ☐ Ataxia
- ☐ Psychosis

PRIMARY ANGIITIS OF THE CENTRAL NERVOUS SYSTEM (PACNS): RADIOLOGICAL DIFFERENTIALS

Vascular differentials

- ☐ Arteriovenous malformations (AVM)
- ☐ Cerebral amyloid angiopathy (CAA)
- ☐ Posterior reversible encephalopathy syndrome (PRES)
- ☐ CADASIL
- ☐ Susac's syndrome
- ☐ Hereditary endotheliopathy with retinopathy, nephropathy, and stroke (HERNS)

Haemorrhagic differentials

- ☐ Intracerebral haemorrhage (ICH)
- ☐ Subarachnoid haemorrhage (SAH)
- ☐ Spinal subdural haematoma

Infectious differentials

- ☐ Central nervous system (CNS) infections
- ☐ Tuberculosis
- ☐ Fungal
- ☐ Parasitosis

Neoplastic differentials

- ☐ Degos disease: malignant atrophic papulosis
  - ○ This is a multi-organ thromboproliferative disorder
- ☐ Intravascular lymphoma
- ☐ Gliomatosis cerebri
- ☐ Brain tumours

Inflammatory differentials

- ☐ Acute disseminated encephalomyelitis (ADEM)
- ☐ Multiple sclerosis (MS)
- ☐ Progressive multifocal leukoencephalopathy (PML)

Angiographic differentials

- ☐ Fibromuscular dysplasia
- ☐ Lymphoproliferative disorders: angiotropic or intravascular
- ☐ Moyamoya disease
- ☐ Radiation vasculopathy
- ☐ Reversible cerebral vasoconstriction syndrome (RCVS)

Acronym

- ☐ CADASIL: Cerebral autosomal dominant arteriopathy, subcortical infarcts and leukoencephalopathy

CADASIL: CLINICAL FEATURES

Stroke

- ☐ Stroke develops in 85% of patients
- ☐ It typically occurs in the 4th decade
- ☐ It is almost always lacunar
- ☐ The risk is increased by hypertension, smoking, and microbleeds
- ☐ Smoking leads to an earlier onset age of stroke

Migraine

- ☐ This is atypical and prolonged
- ☐ Auras occur in 40% of cases
- ☐ Confusion occurs: usually after attacks of migraine with aura

Cognitive features

- ☐ Cognitive disturbance occurs in 50% of cases
- ☐ This usually develops in the 5th decade

Psychiatric features

- ☐ Mood disturbance occurs in 40% of cases
- ☐ Apathy occurs in more than 50% of cases

Other features

- ☐ Reversible encephalopathy
- ☐ Coma
- ☐ Pseudobulbar palsy
- ☐ Spastic paraparesis
- ☐ Parkinsonism
- ☐ Seizures
- ☐ Retinal vascular changes

Atypical manifestations

- ☐ Intracerebral haemorrhages
- ☐ Visual disturbances
- ☐ Absent family history
- ☐ Spinal cord involvement

Acronym

- ☐ CADASIL: Cerebral autosomal dominant arteriopathy subcortical infarcts and leukoencephalopathy

CADASIL: MANAGEMENT

Magnetic resonance imaging (MRI): features

- ☐ High signal changes in the anterior temporal poles
- ☐ Diffuse white matter high signal changes
- ☐ Microbleeds: these are usually in the thalamus

Cerebrospinal fluid (CSF) analysis

- ☐ Mild elevation of protein level
- ☐ Oligoclonal bands (OCB) may be present

Other investigations

- ☐ Skin biopsy: granular osmophilic material (GOM)
- ☐ Visual evoked responses (VERs): abnormalities may be delayed
- ☐ NOTCH 3 gene mutation: this is negative in 80% of suspected cases

Treatment

- ☐ Aspirin
- ☐ Statins
- ☐ Caution with anticoagulants
- ☐ Smoking cessation: smoking is a risk factor for progression

Acronym

- ☐ CADASIL: Cerebral autosomal dominant arteriopathy subcortical infarcts and leukoencephalopathy

Venous disorders

CEREBRAL VEIN THROMBOSIS (CVT): HAEMATOLOGICAL RISK FACTORS

Thrombophilia

- ☐ Antithrombin III deficiency
- ☐ Protein C/S deficiency
- ☐ Factor V Leiden mutation
- ☐ Prothrombin gene mutation
- ☐ Antiphospholipid antibodies
- ☐ Hyperhomocysteinemia
- ☐ Antiphospholipid/anticardiolipin antibodies
- ☐ Resistance to activated protein C
- ☐ Factor II G20210A mutation
- ☐ Elevated factor VIII (FVIII) level

Blood disorders

- ☐ Polycythaemia
- ☐ Essential thrombocytosis
- ☐ Paroxysmal nocturnal haemoglobinuria

Other haematological disorders

- ☐ Iron deficiency anaemia
- ☐ Nephrotic syndrome
- ☐ Polycythaemia
- ☐ Thrombocytopenia

Synonym

- ☐ Venous sinus thrombosis (VST)

CEREBRAL VEIN THROMBOSIS (CVT): NON-HAEMATOLOGICAL RISK FACTORS

Medical conditions

- ☐ Homocystinuria
- ☐ Otolaryngological infections
- ☐ Meningitis
- ☐ Systemic infections
- ☐ Nephrotic syndrome
- ☐ Thyroid disease
- ☐ Cancer
- ☐ Pregnancy/postpartum
- ☐ Head injury
- ☐ Cerebral sinus injuries
- ☐ Spontaneous intracranial hypotension (SIH)
- ☐ Obese women on oral contraceptive pills

Immunological conditions

- ☐ Vasculitis
- ☐ Inflammatory bowel disease (IBD)
- ☐ Systemic lupus erythematosus (SLE)
- ☐ Behcet's disease
- ☐ Sarcoidosis

Procedures

- ☐ Jugular vein cannulation
- ☐ Neurosurgery
- ☐ Lumbar puncture
- ☐ Epidural blood patch

Drugs

- ☐ Oral contraceptive pills (OCPs)
- ☐ Hormone replacement therapy (HRT)
- ☐ Androgen
- ☐ Danazol
- ☐ Lithium
- ☐ Vitamin A
- ☐ Intravenous immunoglobulins (IVIg)
- ☐ Ecstasy
- ☐ Tamoxifen
- ☐ L-Asparaginase
- ☐ Idaricuzimab

High altitude

- ☐ The risk of CVT is related to underlying hypercoagulable states

Synonym

- ☐ Venous sinus thrombosis (VST)

DOI: 10.1201/9781003221258-53

CEREBRAL VEIN THROMBOSIS (CVT): CLINICAL FEATURES

Distribution of CVT

- ☐ Transverse sinus in >80%
- ☐ Superior sagittal sinus in about 35%
- ☐ Straight sinus in 35%
- ☐ Sigmoid sinus in about 2%
- ☐ Internal jugular vein in10%
- ☐ Cortical veins in 3%

Usual presentations

- ☐ Headache
- ☐ Encephalopathy
- ☐ Dilated scalp veins
- ☐ Focal neurological deficits
- ☐ Raised cerebrospinal fluid (CSF) opening pressure

Other presentations

- ☐ Thunderclap headache (TCH)
- ☐ Migraine with aura
- ☐ Transient ischaemic attacks (TIAs)
- ☐ Isolated psychiatric features
- ☐ Isolated cranial nerve palsy

Complications

- ☐ Venous infarcts: these develop in half of cases
  - ○ 30–40% of these are haemorrhagic
- ☐ Raised intracranial pressure (ICP): this could be an isolated finding
- ☐ Intracranial hypotension: this is due to spontaneous or iatrogenic CSF leak
- ☐ Late seizures: these develop in 10% of cases
- ☐ Hydrocephalus: this is probably from foramen of Monroe obstruction
- ☐ Hyperglycaemia: this predicts a poor outcome

Risk factors for recurrent CVT

- ☐ Male gender
- ☐ Within the first year
- ☐ Previous venous thrombosis
- ☐ Myeloproliferative disorders
- ☐ Polycythaemia
- ☐ Thrombocythaemia

Predictors of good outcome

- ☐ Age <50 years
- ☐ Isolated superior sagittal sinus thrombosis
- ☐ Complete recanalisation

Synonym

- ☐ Venous sinus thrombosis (VST)

CEREBRAL VEIN THROMBOSIS (CVT): INVESTIGATIONS

Thrombophilia tests: indications

- ☐ A previous history of venous thrombosis
- ☐ A family history of venous thrombosis
- ☐ Young age at presentation of CVT
- ☐ CVT without any risk factors

Thrombophilia tests: screening

- ☐ Screen at least 3 months after VST
- ☐ It is positive in 75% of cases: this is usually a high plasma Factor VIII

D-dimer

- ☐ Check D-dimer before imaging
- ☐ A normal D-dimer indicates a low probability of VST
- ☐ It is raised in 76% of those tested
- ☐ It is falsely positive in about 10%
- ☐ It is falsely negative in about 25%

Magnetic resonance imaging (MRV): features

- ☐ Venous occlusion
- ☐ Haemorrhagic and non-haemorrhagic ischaemia
- ☐ Intracerebral haemorrhage (ICH)
- ☐ Subarachnoid haemorrhage (SAH)

Computed tomography venogram (CTV): benefits

- ☐ CTV is the recommended imaging of choice if MRV is not available
- ☐ It is most useful in subacute and chronic cases

Computed tomography venogram (CTV): diagnostic signs

- ☐ Cord sign: this is due to hyperdense venous sinuses or cortical veins
- ☐ Empty delta sign: this is a filling defect in the superior sagittal sinus
- ☐ Intracranial venous collaterals

Paramagnetic-sensitive MRI sequences

- ☐ These show a positive brush sign (BS)
- ☐ This is an abnormal accentuation of signal drop in subependymal and deep medullary veins
- ☐ It correlates with severity of CVT

Other imaging techniques

- ☐ MRI arterial spin labelling perfusion weighted imaging (ASL-PWI)
  - ○ This shows a bright sinus appearance
- ☐ Magnetic resonance black-blood thrombus imaging (MRBTI): this is promising
- ☐ Cerebral angiography: this is indicated if other imaging modalities are negative

Radiological differential

- ☐ Congenital variant

Synonym

- ☐ Venous sinus thrombosis (VST)

CEREBRAL VEIN THROMBOSIS (CVT): ANTICOAGULANT TREATMENT

Acute anticoagulation

☐ Unfractionated heparin
☐ Low molecular weight heparin (LMWH)

Longer term anticoagulation

☐ Vitamin K antagonists
☐ New oral anticoagulants (NOACs): Dabigatran, Apixaban, Rivaroxaban
   ○ Dabigatran is as effective as Warfarin
☐ Avoid direct oral anticoagulants: Factor Xa and thrombin inhibitors

Short-term anticoagulation (3–6 months): indications

☐ Trauma-provoked CVT
☐ Infection-provoked CVT

Chronic anticoagulation (6–12 months): indications

☐ Unprovoked CVT
☐ Thrombotic disorders
☐ Malignancy
☐ Lupus anticoagulant

Indefinite anticoagulation: indications

☐ Persistent risk factors
☐ Recurrent CVT
☐ Venous thromboembolism developing after CVT
☐ Severe thrombophilia

Follow-up imaging

☐ Perform an MR venogram (MRV) 3–6 months after starting treatment
☐ This is to assess for recanalisation

Synonym

☐ Venous sinus thrombosis (VST)

CAVERNOUS SINUS SYNDROME (CSS)

Contents of the cavernous sinus

☐ Carotid artery
☐ Cavernous sinus
☐ Cranial nerves: oculomotor, trochlear, abducens, trigeminal (first and second divisions)
☐ Sympathetic fibers

Causes

☐ Trauma
☐ Carotid aneurysms
☐ Carotid-cavernous fistula
☐ Cavernous sinus tumours
☐ Cavernous sinus thrombosis
☐ Sarcoidosis
☐ Midline granuloma
☐ Infection
☐ Herpes zoster

Clinical features

☐ Ophthalmoplegia
☐ Orbital congestion
☐ Proptosis
☐ Trigeminal sensory loss
☐ Horner's syndrome

CHAPTER 9

Cranial nerves

Optic nerve

OPTIC NEUROPATHY: MEDICAL CAUSES

Autoimmune

- ☐ Optic neuritis (ON)
- ☐ Chronic relapsing inflammatory optic neuropathy (CRION)
- ☐ Neuromyelitis optica (NMO)
- ☐ Acute demyelinating encephalomyelitis (ADEM)
- ☐ Schilder's disease
- ☐ Anti-MOG antibody disease

Connective tissue diseases

- ☐ Sarcoidosis
- ☐ Systemic lupus erythematosus (SLE)
- ☐ Sjogren's syndrome
- ☐ Antiphospholipid antibody (APL) syndrome
- ☐ Wegener's granulomatosis
- ☐ Behcet's disease
- ☐ Giant cell arteritis (GCA)

Inflammatory

- ☐ Post vaccination
- ☐ Neuroretinitis
- ☐ Tolosa-Hunt syndrome (THS)

Compressive

- ☐ Primary tumours
- ☐ Metastases
- ☐ Thyroid ophthalmopathy
- ☐ Aneurysms
- ☐ Sinus mucoceles

Hereditary

- ☐ Leber hereditary optic neuropathy (LHON)
- ☐ Autosomal dominant optic neuropathy
- ☐ Kjer autosomal dominant optic atrophy
- ☐ Charcot–Marie–Tooth disease (CMT)
- ☐ Friedreich's ataxia (FA)

Ischaemic

- ☐ Anterior ischaemic optic neuropathy (AION)
- ☐ Posterior ischaemic optic neuropathy (PION)
- ☐ Diabetic papillopathy

Miscellaneous causes

- ☐ Vitamin B12 deficiency
- ☐ Trauma
- ☐ Radiation
- ☐ Paraneoplastic
- ☐ Influenza vaccination

OPTIC NEUROPATHY: INFECTIOUS CAUSES

Viral causes

- ☐ Adenovirus
- ☐ Coxsackie virus
- ☐ Dengue fever
- ☐ Measles
- ☐ Mumps
- ☐ Rubella
- ☐ Chickungunya virus
- ☐ West Nile virus
- ☐ Varicella zoster virus (VZV)
- ☐ Hepatitis B virus (HBV)
- ☐ Rabies

Bacterial causes

- ☐ Lyme neuroborreliosis
- ☐ Tuberculosis (TB)
- ☐ Brucellosis
- ☐ Haemolytic streptococcal infection
- ☐ Meningococcal infection
- ☐ Typhoid fever
- ☐ Tetanus
- ☐ Anthrax
- ☐ Toxoplasmosis
- ☐ Syphilis
- ☐ Leptospirosis
- ☐ Cat scratch disease
- ☐ Whipple's disease

DOI: 10.1201/9781003221258-55

OPTIC NEUROPATHY: TOXIC AND DRUG-INDUCED

Toxic causes

- ☐ Tobacco-alcohol amblyopia
- ☐ Methanol intoxication
- ☐ Carbon monoxide
- ☐ Ethylene glycol
- ☐ Perchloroethylene
- ☐ Arsenic toxicity
- ☐ Cobalt

Drug-induced

- ☐ Ethambutol
- ☐ Isoniazid
- ☐ Linezolid
- ☐ Metronidazole
- ☐ Amiodarone
- ☐ Phosphodiesterase inhibitors, e.g. Sildenafil
- ☐ Methotrexate
- ☐ Vincristine
- ☐ Cisplatin
- ☐ Carboplatin
- ☐ Paclitaxel
- ☐ Infliximab
- ☐ Oxymetazoline
- ☐ Clioquinol
- ☐ Quinine

OPTIC NEUROPATHY: CLINICAL FEATURES

Major features

- ☐ Painful eye movements: with inflammatory causes
- ☐ Reduced visual acuity
- ☐ Impaired colour vision
- ☐ Abnormal visual fields
- ☐ Relative afferent pupillary defect (RAPD)

Uhthoff's phenomenon

- ☐ Reduced vision when the body temperature rises
- ☐ It occurs with inflammation, LHON, and sarcoidosis

Fundoscopy features

- ☐ The optic disc is swollen in the early stages
- ☐ Disc pallor sets in after 4–6 weeks

Differential diagnoses

- ☐ Optic nerve drusen
- ☐ Optic nerve hypoplasia
- ☐ Optic nerve coloboma
- ☐ Morning-glory disc anomaly
- ☐ Maculopathy
- ☐ Papilloedema

Acronym

- ☐ LHON: Leber hereditary optic neuropathy

OPTIC NEURITIS: CLINICAL FEATURES

Onset and progression

- ☐ The onset age is usually <50 years
- ☐ There is subacute unilateral visual impairment
- ☐ It is progressive over days
- ☐ Improvement occurs after 2–3 weeks

Features of eye pain

- ☐ The pain may occur before or with the visual loss
- ☐ It is peri-ocular
- ☐ It is worse with eye movements

Other symptoms

- ☐ Vision worsens in bright light
- ☐ Phosphenes or photopsias: spontaneous flashes of light in vision
  - ○ They are provoked by eye movements

Relative apparent pupillary defect (RAPD)

- ☐ The affected pupil only constricts when light is shone in the contralateral eye
- ☐ This may be absent in bilateral ON
- ☐ It is subjectively reported as a difference in brightness between the two eyes

Uhthoff's phenomenon

- ☐ Vision worsens with exercise or heat
- ☐ This develops on recovery
- ☐ It is also seen in other conditions
  - ○ Leber hereditary optic neuropathy (LHON)
  - ○ Sarcoidosis

Pulfrich phenomenon

- ☐ This is misperception of the direction of movement of an object
- ☐ It develops on recovery

Fundoscopy

- ☐ This is normal with retrobulbar ON: this accounts for 65% of cases
- ☐ The disc is swollen, pale or anomalous: the swelling is not severe
- ☐ The macula and peripheral retina are normal
- ☐ There are no haemorrhages

Other features

- ☐ Visual field defects
- ☐ Dyschromatopsia: red colour desaturation
- ☐ Contrast sensitivity

Optical coherence tomography (OCT)

- ☐ This is very sensitive for optic neuritis

OPTIC NEURITIS: DIFFERENTIAL DIAGNOSIS

Differential diagnosis of optic neuritis

- ☐ Neuromyelitis optica (NMO)
- ☐ Sarcoidosis
- ☐ Chronic relapsing inflammatory optic neuropathy (CRION)
- ☐ Anterior ischaemic optic neuropathy (AION)
- ☐ Neuroretinitis
- ☐ Leber hereditary optic neuropathy (LHON)
- ☐ Central serous chorioretinopathy
- ☐ Other causes of optic neuropathy

Differential diagnosis of optic nerve head oedema (ONHE)

- ☐ Optic neuritis
- ☐ Idiopathic intracranial hypertension (IIH)
- ☐ CSF shunt malfunction or infection

OPTIC ATROPHY: GENETIC CAUSES

Nutritional and metabolic

- [ ] Cobalamin C disease (cbIC)
- [ ] Vitamin B6 deficiency
- [ ] Acute intermittent porphyria (AIP)
- [ ] Propionic academia
- [ ] Costeff optic atrophy syndrome
  - ○ 3-Methylglutaconic aciduria (MGA) type 3
- [ ] Mucopolysaccharidoses
- [ ] Wolfram syndrome (DIDMOAD)

Mitochondrial

- [ ] Leber hereditary optic neuropathy (LHON)
- [ ] Dominant optic atrophy (DOA)
- [ ] POLG mutations
- [ ] Autosomal dominant optic atrophy and cataract (ADOAC)
- [ ] Combined oxidative phosphorylation deficiency type 7 (COXPD7)
- [ ] Bosch-Boonstra-Schaaf optic atrophy syndrome (BBSOAS)

Genetic neuropathy

- [ ] Charcot–Marie–Tooth disease type 6 (CMT6)
- [ ] Familial dysautonomia
- [ ] Giant axonal neuropathy (GAN)

Neurodegenerative

- [ ] Friedreich's ataxia (FA)
- [ ] Spinocerebellar ataxia 7 (SCA7)
- [ ] Pantethonate kinase associated neurodegeneration (PKAN)
- [ ] Leber congenital amaurosis

Dystonic

- [ ] Deafness-dystonia-optic atrophy syndrome
- [ ] Paroxysmal exercise-induced dystonia

Miscellaneous causes

- [ ] Osteopetrosis
- [ ] PEHO syndrome
- [ ] SPOAN syndrome
- [ ] AARS2 (alanyl-tRNA synthetase 2) syndrome
- [ ] CAPOS syndrome
- [ ] SLC25A46 gene mutations
- [ ] Crouzon syndrome: craniosynostosis with midfacial hypoplasia

Acronyms

- [ ] CAPOS: Cerebellar ataxia, areflexia, pes cavus, optic atrophy, and sensorineural hearing loss
- [ ] DIDMOAD: diabetes insipidus, diabetes mellitus, optic atrophy, and deafness
- [ ] PEHO: Progressive encephalopathy, oedema, hypsarrhythmia, optic atrophy
- [ ] SPOAN: Spastic paraplegia, optic atrophy, neuropathy

OPTIC ATROPHY: NON-GENETIC CAUSES

Neoplastic

- [ ] Meningioma
- [ ] Glioma
- [ ] Pituitary adenoma
- [ ] Craniopharyngioma

Infectious

- [ ] Tuberculous meningitis
- [ ] Viral meningoencephalitis
- [ ] Syphilis
- [ ] Creutzfeldt-Jakob disease (CJD)
- [ ] Subacute sclerosing pan-encephalitis (SSPE)
- [ ] Endemic typhus
- [ ] Ophthalmomyiasis

Autoimmune and inflammatory

- [ ] Multiples sclerosis (MS)
- [ ] Neuro-Behcet's disease
- [ ] Neuromyelitis optica (NMO)
- [ ] Systemic lupus erythematosus (SLE)
- [ ] Antiphospholipid antibody syndrome (APS)
- [ ] Adrenoleukodystrophy (ALD)

Vascular

- [ ] Hypoxic ischaemic encephalopathy
- [ ] Anterior ischaemic optic neuropathy (AION)

Toxic and drug-induced

- [ ] Methanol poisoning
- [ ] Lead
- [ ] Methyl bromide
- [ ] Sildenafil

Ocular

- [ ] Glaucoma
- [ ] Chronic papilloedema
- [ ] Intravitreal surgery for diabetic proliferative retinopathy

Miscellaneous causes

- [ ] Traumatic brain injury (TBI)
- [ ] Hydrocephalus

Trigeminal nerve

TRIGEMINAL NEUROPATHY: CAUSES

Neoplastic

- [ ] Meningioma
- [ ] Schwannoma
- [ ] Nasopharyngeal cancer
- [ ] Lymphoma
- [ ] Metastases
- [ ] Carcinomatous meningitis

Infective

- [ ] Leprosy
- [ ] Lyme neuroborreliosis
- [ ] Syphilis
- [ ] Actinomycosis
- [ ] Varicella zoster virus (VZV)
- [ ] Herpes simplex virus (HSV)
- [ ] Sinusitis

Drug-induced

- [ ] Stilbamide
- [ ] Trichloroethylene
- [ ] Oxaliplatin

Neurological

- [ ] X-linked bulbar and spinal muscular atrophy (BSMA; Kennedy disease)
- [ ] Isolated trigeminal neuropathy: Spillane's neuropathy
- [ ] Idiopathic intracranial hypertension (IIH)
- [ ] Paraneoplastic sensory neuronopathy
- [ ] Sjogren's syndrome sensory neuronopathy
- [ ] Skull base anomalies
- [ ] Congenital trigeminal anaesthesia
  - ○ With or without Goldenhar-Gorlin or Mobius syndrome

Medical causes

- [ ] Diabetes mellitus
- [ ] Amyloidosis
- [ ] Impacted third molar
- [ ] Otitis media: Gradenigo's syndrome
- [ ] Traumatic/surgical
- [ ] Connective tissue disease
- [ ] Ischaemic
- [ ] Vascular malformation
- [ ] Facial morphoea profunda

TRIGEMINAL NEURALGIA (TN): CLINICAL FEATURES

Triggers

- [ ] Light touch
- [ ] Light wind
- [ ] Brushing the teeth
- [ ] Shaving
- [ ] Eating and drinking
- [ ] Talking
- [ ] Smiling
- [ ] Washing the face
- [ ] Vibrations from walking

Trigger zones

- [ ] Mid-face
- [ ] Oral cavity
- [ ] Around the mouth
- [ ] Around the nose

Pain features

- [ ] TN is a sharp shooting or stabbing electric-like pain
- [ ] It is stimulus-evoked in most cases
  - ○ Exclusively spontaneous pain is unusual
- [ ] It has a rapid onset and termination
- [ ] It is moderate to severe in intensity
- [ ] It typically lasts 1–60 seconds
- [ ] It is relieved by keeping still
- [ ] It may be a mild ache lasting up to 30 minutes in atypical cases
- [ ] There may be a concomitant continuous pain
  - ○ This is associated with trigeminal nerve root atrophy
- [ ] There are no associated autonomic symptoms

Other features

- [ ] Subtle sensory abnormalities: these are found on quantitative sensory tests
- [ ] Depression: this is common
- [ ] Trigeminal neurotrophic ulcers

DOI: 10.1201/9781003221258-56

TRIGEMINAL NEURALGIA (TN): MANAGEMENT

Head imaging

- ☐ Magnetic resonance tomoangiography (MRTA)
  - ○ This is 3D T2-weighted, TOF-MRA and T1-Gad
  - ○ It shows the relationship of the nerve to the blood vessels
- ☐ 3D constructive interference in steady-state (3D-CISS)
  - ○ This may be superior to MRTA
- ☐ High resolution MRI: to demonstrate neurovascular compression
  - ○ There is insufficient evidence for this

Trigeminal nerve evoked potentials

- ☐ This is indicated if MRI is contraindicated or not available

First line drug treatments

- ☐ Carbamazepine 200–1,200 mg daily: level A evidence
- ☐ Oxcarbazepine 300–1,800 mg daily: level B evidence

Second line or add-on drug treatments

- ☐ Baclofen: level C evidence
- ☐ Lamotrigine: level C evidence
- ☐ Gabapentin
- ☐ Botulinum toxin type A
- ☐ Pregabalin
- ☐ Phenytoin

Insufficient-evidenced treatment

- ☐ Clonazepam
- ☐ Tizanidine
- ☐ Sodium valproate
- ☐ Topical Capsaicin
- ☐ Amlodipine-responsive TN: one case report

Microvascular decompression

- ☐ This is the first line surgery for classical TN
- ☐ It is indicated for medically refractory or medication-intolerant TN
- ☐ It provides longer lasting pain control than neuroablative treatments

Gasserian ganglion neuroablative treatments

- ☐ Gamma knife stereotactic radiosurgery (GKS)
- ☐ Radiofrequency thermocoagulation (RFTC)
- ☐ Glycerol rhizolysis
- ☐ Balloon compression
- ☐ Partial sensory rhizotomy
- ☐ Internal neurolysis

Treatments of refractory cases

- ☐ Extended pulsed radiofrequency
- ☐ Botulinum toxin
- ☐ Lamotrigine-Pregabalin combination: case report
- ☐ Nursing and psychological support

Investigational treatments

- ☐ CNV1014802: a $Na_v1.7$ sodium channel blocker
- ☐ Transcranial direct-current stimulation
- ☐ Repetitive transcranial magnetic stimulation

Facial nerve

BELL'S PALSY: CLINICAL FEATURES

Facial weakness

- [ ] The weakness affects the upper and lower parts of the face
- [ ] There is drooping of the brow and the angle of the mouth
- [ ] There is incomplete eyelid and mouth closure

Associated features

- [ ] Bell's phenomenon
  - ○ This is the visible upward eyeball movement on attempted eyelid closure
- [ ] Dry eye
- [ ] Hyperacusis
- [ ] Impaired taste
- [ ] Pain around the ear
- [ ] Loss of the ability to wiggle the ear
- [ ] Sucking candy sign
  - ○ The tongue is pigmented contralaterally after sucking coloured sweets
  - ○ This is due to loss of taste sensation ipsilaterally

Features of aberrant renervation

- [ ] Syndrome of crocodile tears
  - ○ This is tearing whilst salivating
- [ ] Marcus Gunn jaw winking phenomenon (MGJWP)
  - ○ This is eyelid elevation on pterygoid muscle contraction
- [ ] Marin-Amat syndrome
  - ○ This is involuntary eye closure on jaw opening

House–Brackmann grading system

- [ ] I: Normal facial function
- [ ] II: Mild dysfunction
- [ ] III: Moderate dysfunction
- [ ] IV: Moderately severe dysfunction
- [ ] V: Severe dysfunction
- [ ] VI: Total paralysis

Other grading systems

- [ ] Sydney
- [ ] Sunnybrook
- [ ] Yanaghira
- [ ] Adour-Swanson
- [ ] Burres-Fisch

Poor prognostic factors

- [ ] Complete nerve paralysis
- [ ] Poor recovery after 3 weeks
- [ ] Age >60 years
- [ ] Severe pain
- [ ] Compound muscle action potential (CMAP) reduction >50%

Synonyms

- [ ] Seventh cranial nerve
- [ ] 7th cranial nerve
- [ ] Cranial nerve VII

BELL'S PALSY: DIFFERENTIAL DIAGNOSIS

Infectious differentials

- [ ] Varicella zoster (VZV)
- [ ] Lyme neuroborreliosis

Parry–Romberg syndrome

- [ ] This is progressive hemifacial atrophy (PHA)
- [ ] It is probably a type of scleroderma
- [ ] It may present with seizures and headaches
- [ ] There are white matter changes and calcifications on MRI brain

Stroke

- [ ] Pontine infarct
- [ ] Contralateral precentral gyrus infarct

Foville syndrome

- [ ] Facial nerve palsy
- [ ] Ipsilateral abducens palsy
- [ ] Contralateral hemiparesis

Millard-Gubler syndrome

- [ ] Facial nerve palsy
- [ ] Ipsilateral abducens nerve palsy
- [ ] Contralateral limb weakness

Cerebellopontine angle syndrome

- [ ] Facial nerve palsy
- [ ] Trigeminal nerve palsy
- [ ] Vestibulocochlear nerve palsy
- [ ] Glossopharyngeal nerve palsy
- [ ] Vagus nerve palsy
- [ ] Ipsilateral loss of corneal reflex

Other neurological differentials

- [ ] Guillain–Barre syndrome (GBS)
- [ ] Sarcoidosis

DOI: 10.1201/9781003221258-57

BELL'S PALSY: MANAGEMENT

Investigations

- ☐ Facial nerve imaging
- ☐ Nerve conduction studies (NCS)
- ☐ Electroneuromyography
- ☐ Transcranial magnetic stimulation (TMS): this localizes the site of the lesion
- ☐ Audiometry
- ☐ Electronystagmography
- ☐ Videonystagmography
- ☐ Videooculoscopy

Tests to exclude differentials

- ☐ Polymerase chain reaction (PCR)
- ☐ Serology
- ☐ Cerebrospinal fluid analysis (CSF) analysis

Antiviral and steroid treatment

- ☐ Prednisolone within 72 hours of onset: 60 mg daily tapering over 10 days
- ☐ Acyclovir 400 mg 5 times daily for 7 days or
- ☐ Valacyclovir 1g tid for 7 days
- ☐ Antivirals should not be administered without steroids

Eye protection

- ☐ Taping the eyelid
- ☐ Corneal lubrication
- ☐ Scleral contact lenses

Facial re-animation

- ☐ Nerve-to-nerve transfer
- ☐ Free tissue transfer

Treatment of facial and eyelid weakness

- ☐ Gold weight implants
- ☐ Palpebral spring
- ☐ Tarsorrhaphy
- ☐ Transcutaneous electrical stimulation
- ☐ Subperiostal facial suspension (face lifting)
- ☐ Facial nerve cable grafting

Treatment of synkinesis

- ☐ Physiotherapy
- ☐ Botulinum toxin

Other treatments

- ☐ Oral care
- ☐ Assistance with feeding

Synonyms

- ☐ Seventh cranial nerve
- ☐ 7th cranial nerve
- ☐ Cranial nerve VII

RAMSAY HUNT SYNDROME (RHS)

Pathology

- ☐ This is varicella zoster virus (VZV) infection of the geniculate ganglion
- ☐ It may involve cranial nerves V-XI
- ☐ It may rarely involve the cervical nerves

Classic triad

- ☐ Facial nerve paralysis
- ☐ Ipsilateral rash: ear, tongue, palate
- ☐ Ear pain (otalgia)

Clinical features: others

- ☐ Tinnitus
- ☐ Hearing impairment or hyperacusis
- ☐ Vomiting
- ☐ Vertigo
- ☐ Nystagmus
- ☐ Laryngitis
- ☐ Dysphagia
- ☐ Cerebellar ataxia
- ☐ Zoster sine herpete: this is zoster without an accompanying skin rash

Differential diagnosis: Bell's palsy

- ☐ Bell's palsy is less severe than RSH
- ☐ There is more complete recovery with Bell's palsy than with RHS

Investigations

- ☐ Rising titres of VZV antibodies

Antiviral treatment

- ☐ Acyclovir: it has better results when used with steroids
- ☐ Valacyclovir
- ☐ Famciclovir: it is probably more effective than Acyclovir

Other treatments

- ☐ Systemic steroids
- ☐ Intratympanic Dexamethasone: this improves outcomes
- ☐ Analgesics
- ☐ Herpes zoster vaccine for people >60 years

Other Ramsay Hunt syndromes

- ☐ Dyssynergia cellebellaris progressiva
- ☐ Carotid artery occlusion
- ☐ Deep palmar median nerve compression

Synonym

- ☐ Herpes zoster oticus

POST HERPETIC NEURALGIA (PHN)

Definition

- ☐ This is persistence of herpes zoster pain for >3 months after resolution of the rash
- ☐ It occurs in 10–15% of cases

Risk factors

- ☐ Older age
- ☐ Females
- ☐ Presence of a prodrome
- ☐ Severe rash
- ☐ Severity of acute pain
- ☐ Severe immunosuppression
- ☐ Autoimmune diseases
- ☐ Smoking
- ☐ Overweight and underweight
- ☐ Late treatment of herpes zoster

Treatment

- ☐ Tricyclics
- ☐ Gabapentin
- ☐ Pregabalin
- ☐ Opioids: Morphine, Levorpharnol, Tramadol
- ☐ Topical Capsaicin
- ☐ Lidocaine patches
- ☐ Intrathecal Methylprednisolone: this is indicated if nothing else works
- ☐ Carbamazepine: the evidence for this is inconclusive

Other cranial nerves

ANOSMIA: CAUSES

Rhinological causes

- [ ] Cigarette smoking
- [ ] Rhinitis
- [ ] Upper respiratory tract infections
- [ ] Intranasal zinc

Parkinson's disease (PD)

- [ ] Genetic PD: PARK 1, 2, 8: minimally in PARK 6
- [ ] X-linked recessive dystonia-parkinsonism (Lubag)
- [ ] Parkinson's disease (PD) complex of Guam
- [ ] Glucocerebrosidase (GBA) Parkinsonism

Other neurodegenerative diseases

- [ ] Alzheimer's disease (AD)
- [ ] Dementia with Lewy bodies (DLB)
- [ ] Multiple system atrophy (MSA)
- [ ] Pure autonomic failure
- [ ] Accelerated cognitive decline

Other neurological causes

- [ ] Multiple sclerosis (MS)
- [ ] Motor neurone disease (MND): not confirmed in some studies
- [ ] Myasthenia gravis (MG)
- [ ] Traumatic brain injury (TBI)
- [ ] Craniotomy
- [ ] Subarachnoid haemorrhage (SAH)
- [ ] Olfactory groove meningioma
- [ ] Neurosarcoidosis

Systemic causes

- [ ] Kallman syndrome
- [ ] Schizophrenia
- [ ] Chagas disease
- [ ] Hypothyroidism
- [ ] Mulga snake venom

Drug-induced

- [ ] Midodrine
- [ ] Lithium
- [ ] Pegylated interferon

Nutritional causes

- [ ] Vitamin A deficiency
- [ ] Zinc deficiency

OCULOMOTOR NERVE PALSY: CLINICAL FEATURES

Muscles innervated by the oculomotor nerve

- [ ] The extraocular muscles: except the lateral rectus and superior oblique
- [ ] The levator palpebrae superioris: the eyelid elevators
- [ ] The ciliary muscles: the iris constrictors

Clinical features

- [ ] Diplopia
- [ ] Ptosis
- [ ] Mydriasis (large pupil)
- [ ] Impaired contralateral lid elevation: this is a feature of nuclear lesions
- [ ] It may present as isolated ptosis
- [ ] Some cases are pupil sparing

Syndromes of oculomotor nucleus palsy

- [ ] Weber's syndrome: this is associated with contralateral hemiparesis
- [ ] Nothnagel syndrome: this is associated with contralateral ataxia
  - ( ) There is superior cerebellar peduncle involvement
- [ ] Claude's syndrome: this is associated with contralateral ataxia
  - ( ) There is red nucleus involvement
- [ ] Reverse Claude's syndrome: this is associated with ipsilateral ataxia
- [ ] Benedikt's syndrome: this is associated with contralateral hemiparesis
  - ( ) There is also contralateral tremor and involuntary movements

Features of aberrant regeneration of the oculomotor nerve

- [ ] Sector contractions of the iris sphincter: this is in response to light and eye movements
- [ ] Abnormal pupillary unrest (pupillary size fluctuations)
- [ ] Pupillary constriction on downgaze
- [ ] Tonic pupils
- [ ] Lagophthalmos: this is the inability to completely shut the eyelids
- [ ] Paradoxical eye movements
- [ ] Neuromyotonia

Synonyms for oculomotor nerve

- [ ] Third cranial nerve
- [ ] 3rd cranial nerve
- [ ] Cranial nerve III

Synonyms for aberrant regeneration

- [ ] Acquired oculomotor synkinesis
- [ ] Ocular misdirection

DOI: 10.1201/9781003221258-58

TROCHLEAR NERVE PALSY: CAUSES

Neurological causes

- [ ] Multiple sclerosis (MS)
- [ ] Idiopathic intracranial hypertension (IIH)
- [ ] Intracranial hypotension
- [ ] Tolosa-Hunt syndrome
- [ ] Traumatic brain injury (TBI)
- [ ] Congenital trochlear nerve agenesis

Vascular causes

- [ ] Midbrain haemorrhage
- [ ] Microvascular ischaemia
- [ ] Dorsal midbrain stroke
- [ ] Systemic vasculitis
- [ ] Basilar artery dolichoectasia
- [ ] Carotico-cavernous sinus fistula
- [ ] Cavernous carotid aneurysm
- [ ] Superior cerebellar artery aneurysm
- [ ] Perimesencephalic subarachnoid haemorrhage (SAH)

Neoplastic causes

- [ ] Trochlear nerve schwannoma or meningioma
- [ ] Pilocytic astrocytoma
- [ ] Cavernous sinus meningioma
- [ ] Intracranial dermoid cyst
- [ ] Tectal plate germinoma
- [ ] Pituitary macroadenoma
- [ ] Polycythaemia rubra vera

Infective causes

- [ ] Tuberculous meningitis
- [ ] Herpes zoster ophthalmicus
- [ ] Neurosyphilis
- [ ] HIV infection
- [ ] Ehrlichiosis
- [ ] Sphenoethmoidal mucocele

Iatrogenic causes

- [ ] Botulinum toxin injection
- [ ] Endoscopic sinus surgery
- [ ] Temporal lobectomy
- [ ] Percutaneous balloon compression for trigeminal neuralgia
- [ ] Anaesthesia: spinal and dental

Synonyms

- [ ] Fourth cranial nerve
- [ ] 4th cranial nerve
- [ ] IV cranial nerve

ABDUCENS NERVE PALSY: NEUROLOGICAL CAUSES

Traumatic and iatrogenic causes

- [ ] Traumatic brain injury (TBI)
- [ ] Microvascular decompression for hemifacial spasm
- [ ] Dural puncture

Intracranial vascular causes

- [ ] Pontine stroke
- [ ] Carotid artery dolichoectasia
- [ ] Vertebral artery dolichoectasia
- [ ] Internal carotid artery (ICA) aneurysm
- [ ] Anterior inferior cerebellar artery (AICA) aneurysm
- [ ] Cavernous sinus thrombosis

Inflammatory and immune causes

- [ ] Multiple sclerosis (MS)
- [ ] Neurosarcoidosis

Neoplastic causes

- [ ] Schwannoma of the abducens nerve
- [ ] Pituitary adenoma
- [ ] Trigeminal nerve sheath tumour
- [ ] Lumbar spinal ependymoma: associated with subarachnoid haemorrhage (SAH)

Other neurological causes

- [ ] Ophthalmoplegic migraine: MRI may show reversible enhancement of the nerve
- [ ] Spontaneous intracranial hypotension (SIH)
- [ ] Pituitary apoplexy
- [ ] Pachymeningitis
- [ ] Preeclampsia

Synonyms

- [ ] Sixth cranial nerve
- [ ] 6th cranial nerve
- [ ] Cranial nerve VI

ABDUCENS NERVE PALSY: SYSTEMIC CAUSES

Vascular risk factors

- [ ] Diabetes
- [ ] Hypertension
- [ ] Arteriosclerosis
- [ ] Giant cell arteritis (GCA)
- [ ] Anaemia
- [ ] Hyperhomocystinaemia

Viral causes

- [ ] Varicella zoster virus (VZV)
- [ ] Cytomegalovirus (CMV)

Bacterial infections

- [ ] Sellar and parasellar region infections
- [ ] Tick paralysis
- [ ] Leprosy
- [ ] Maxillary sinusitis
- [ ] Mycoplasma pneumonia

Fungal infections

- [ ] Cryptococcal meningitis
- [ ] Fungal sphenoid sinusitis

Medical causes

- [ ] Systemic lupus erythematosus (SLE)
- [ ] Haemolytic uraemic syndrome (HUS)
- [ ] Multiple myeloma
- [ ] Leukaemia
- [ ] Langerhans' cell histiocytosis

Drug-induced

- [ ] Vincristine neurotoxicity
- [ ] Vitamin A
- [ ] Retinoic acid therapy
- [ ] Intravitreal Ranibizumab
- [ ] Intravitreal Bevacizumab
- [ ] Lithium toxicity

Synonyms

- [ ] Sixth cranial nerve
- [ ] 6th cranial nerve
- [ ] Cranial nerve VI

ABDUCENS NERVE PALSY: BRAINSTEM SYNDROMES

Raymond's syndrome

- [ ] Ipsilateral abducens nerve palsy
- [ ] Contralateral hemiparesis

Millard-Gublar syndrome

- [ ] Ipsilateral abducens nerve palsy
- [ ] Ipsilateral facial nerve palsy
- [ ] Contralateral hemiparesis

Foville syndrome

- [ ] Ipsilateral abducens nerve palsy
- [ ] Horizontal conjugate gaze palsy
- [ ] Ipsilateral trigeminal nerve palsy
- [ ] Ipsilateral facial nerve palsy
- [ ] Ipsilateral vestibulocochlear nerve palsy
- [ ] Ipsilateral Horner's syndrome

Godtfredsen (eye twist and tongue twist) syndrome

- [ ] Ipsilateral abducens nerve palsy
- [ ] Ipsilateral hypoglossal nerve palsy
- [ ] It is often associated with trigeminal neuralgia (TN)
- [ ] It is caused by nasopharyngeal carcinoma or clival metastases

Synonyms

- [ ] Sixth cranial nerve
- [ ] 6th cranial nerve
- [ ] Cranial nerve VI

VAGUS NERVE PALSY: CAUSES

Intracranial causes

- ☐ Vascular
- ☐ Dissection
- ☐ Meningeal disease

Neoplastic causes

- ☐ Breast cancer: this is associated with Horner's syndrome and phrenic nerve palsy
  - ○ The combination is known as Rowland Payne syndrome
- ☐ Lung tumour: this causes left recurrent laryngeal nerve palsy
- ☐ Mediastinal tumours

Cardiovascular causes

- ☐ Aortic arch aneurysms
- ☐ Large left atrium
- ☐ Subclavian artery disease

Thoracic causes

- ☐ Mediastinal lymphadenopathy
- ☐ Tracheobronchial nodes
- ☐ Thyroidectomy

Other neurological causes

- ☐ Hereditary neuropathy with liability to pressure palsy (HNPP)
- ☐ Spinocerebellar ataxia 1 (SCA 1)

Systemic causes

- ☐ Systemic lupus erythematosus (SLE)

Synonyms

- ☐ 10th cranial nerve
- ☐ Cranial nerve X
- ☐ Tenth cranial nerve

VAGUS NERVE PALSY: CLINICAL FEATURES

Clinical features

- ☐ Dysphonia: this manifests as a hoarse, nasal voice
- ☐ The soft palate droops ipsilaterally: it does not rise with phonation
- ☐ The uvula deviates to the normal side on phonation
- ☐ There is loss of the gag reflex ipsilaterally
- ☐ There is a curtain movement of the lateral pharyngeal wall
- ☐ There is a midway vocal cord ipsilaterally (cadaveric position)
  - ○ It is between adduction and abduction
- ☐ It may present with sensory neuropathic cough

Sensory neuropathic cough

- ☐ This is a sensory neuropathy of the recurrent laryngeal nerve
- ☐ It may result from upper airway pathology: infection, inflammation, or allergy
- ☐ It presents as chronic cough
- ☐ It is likely caused by cough reflex hyper-responsiveness
- ☐ Coughing bouts are triggered by mild physical or chemical stimuli
- ☐ It is responsive to Amitriptyline and Gabapentin

Synonyms

- ☐ 10th cranial nerve
- ☐ Cranial nerve X
- ☐ Tenth cranial nerve

DYSPHONIA: CAUSES

Neurological causes

- [ ] Parkinson's disease (PD)
- [ ] Multiple system atrophy (MSA)
- [ ] Spasmodic dysphonia
- [ ] Vocal tremor
- [ ] Vocal cord paralysis
- [ ] Stroke
- [ ] Myasthenia gravis (MG)
- [ ] Multiple sclerosis (MS)
- [ ] Motor neurone disease (MND)
- [ ] Hereditary whispering dystonia (DYT4)

Occupational causes

- [ ] Singers
- [ ] Telemarketers
- [ ] Aerobics instructors
- [ ] Teachers

Laryngeal causes

- [ ] Laryngitis
- [ ] Foreign body
- [ ] Vocal fold nodules
- [ ] Vocal cord haematoma from anticoagulants
- [ ] Laryngeal trauma and cancer
- [ ] Recent endotracheal intubation
- [ ] Age-related: presbyphonia

Head and neck causes

- [ ] Neck trauma, surgery, and radiation
- [ ] Thyroid cancer
- [ ] Craniofacial anomalies
- [ ] Thoracic aortic aneurysm: affecting the recurrent laryngeal nerve

Medical causes

- [ ] Testosterone deficiency
- [ ] Hypothyroidism
- [ ] Reflux oesophagitis
- [ ] Sjogren's syndrome
- [ ] Alcohol and smoking
- [ ] Anxiety and functional hoarseness
- [ ] Relapsing polychondritis

Drug-induced

- [ ] Antipsychotics
- [ ] Angiotensin converting enzyme inhibitors (ACEI)
- [ ] Bisphosphonates causing chemical laryngitis
- [ ] Danocrine
- [ ] Inhaled steroids
- [ ] Testosterone
- [ ] Antihistamines
- [ ] Diuretics
- [ ] Anticholinergics

DEAFNESS: GENETIC CAUSES

Genetic causes of deafness

- [ ] Usher syndrome
- [ ] Treacher Collins syndrome
- [ ] Pendred syndrome
- [ ] Alport syndrome
- [ ] Waardenburg syndrome
- [ ] Neurofibromatosis type 2 (NF2)
- [ ] Mucopolysaccharidoses
- [ ] Refsum's disease
- [ ] Mohr-Tranebjaerg syndrome (MTS)
- [ ] Woodhouse–Sakati syndrome
- [ ] Mitochondrial disorders
- [ ] Absent cochlear nerves: with MASP1 gene mutations

DEAFNESS: ACQUIRED CAUSES

Intracranial

- [ ] Cortical deafness
- [ ] Vertebro-basilar insufficiency
- [ ] Pontine infarction
- [ ] Cerebellopontine angle meningiomas
- [ ] Cerebellopontine angle schwannomas
- [ ] Neurosarcoidosis
- [ ] Susac's syndrome
- [ ] Superficial siderosis
- [ ] Carbon monoxide poisoning
- [ ] Multiple sclerosis

Infective

- [ ] Bacterial
- [ ] Tuberculosis (TB)
- [ ] Herpes zoster
- [ ] Neurosyphilis
- [ ] Lyme neuroborreliosis

Drug-induced

- [ ] Aminoglycosides
- [ ] Macrolides
- [ ] Anti-tuberculosis (TB) drugs
- [ ] Aspirin
- [ ] Non-steroidal anti-inflammatory drugs (NSAIDs)
- [ ] Loop diuretics
- [ ] Quinine
- [ ] Cytotoxics
- [ ] Valproate

Otologic

- [ ] Cochlear ischaemia
- [ ] Trauma
- [ ] Meniere's disease
- [ ] Presbyacusis
- [ ] Paget's disease

Autoimmune

- [ ] Cogan's syndrome
- [ ] Granulomatosis with polyangiitis (GPA)
- [ ] Polyarteritis nodosa
- [ ] Systemic lupus erythematosus (SLE)
- [ ] Sjogren's syndrome

HYPOGLOSSAL NERVE PALSY: CAUSES

Vascular causes

- [ ] Stroke
- [ ] Aneurysms: carotid and vertebral
- [ ] Dural arteriovenous fistula (DAVF)
- [ ] Cervical artery dissection
- [ ] Internal carotid artery vasculitis
- [ ] Godtfredsen (clival) syndrome: retroclival subdural haematoma

Hypoglossal nerve tumours

- [ ] Schwannoma
- [ ] Paraganglioma
- [ ] Chondroid chordoma

Other neurological causes

- [ ] Pontine tumours
- [ ] Metastases to the base of the skull
- [ ] Motor neurone disease (MND)
- [ ] Multiple sclerosis (MS)
- [ ] Guillain–Barre syndrome (GBS)
- [ ] Cervical spondylosis
- [ ] Behcet's syndrome

Orthopaedic causes

- [ ] Fracture of the base of the skull
- [ ] C1 vertebral dislocation
- [ ] Atlanto-occipital joint synovial cyst
- [ ] Eagle syndrome (long styloid process)

Iatrogenic causes

- [ ] Radiation
- [ ] Carotid endarterectomy (CEA)
- [ ] Anterior cervical spine surgery
- [ ] Airway management for general anaesthesia
- [ ] Intrascalene brachial plexus block

Other causes

- [ ] Infectious mononucleosis
- [ ] Tuberculosis
- [ ] Infected impacted tooth
- [ ] Idiopathic
- [ ] Trauma
- [ ] Dental caries
- [ ] Chiari malformation
- [ ] Functional
- [ ] Nasopharyngeal carcinoma

Synonyms

- [ ] 12th cranial nerve
- [ ] Cranial nerve XII
- [ ] Twelfth cranial nerve

HYPOGLOSSAL NERVE PALSY: CLINICAL FEATURES

Clinical features

- ☐ Dysarthria
- ☐ Dysphagia
- ☐ Inability to indent the cheek or lick the upper lip
- ☐ Tongue fasciculations and myokymia
- ☐ Tongue hemi-atrophy
- ☐ Tongue deviation: this is to the contralateral side at rest and to the ipsilateral side on protrusion

Collet Sicard syndrome

- ☐ Hypoglossal nerve palsy
- ☐ Glossopharyngeal nerve palsy
- ☐ Vagus nerve palsy
- ☐ Accessory nerve palsy

Jugular foramen syndrome

- ☐ Hypoglossal nerve palsy
- ☐ Glossopharyngeal nerve palsy
- ☐ Vagus nerve palsy
- ☐ Accessory nerve palsy

Schmidt syndrome

- ☐ Hypoglossal nerve palsy
- ☐ Glossopharyngeal nerve palsy
- ☐ Vagus nerve palsy
- ☐ Accessory nerve palsy
- ☐ Contralateral hemiparesis

Villaret's syndrome

- ☐ Hypoglossal nerve palsy
- ☐ Glossopharyngeal nerve palsy
- ☐ Vagus nerve palsy
- ☐ Accessory nerve palsy
- ☐ Ipsilateral Horner's syndrome

Jackson syndrome

- ☐ Hypoglossal nerve palsy
- ☐ Contralateral hemiplegia

Opalski syndrome

- ☐ Hypoglossal nerve palsy
- ☐ Ipsilateral hemiparesis and lemniscal sensory loss

Dejerine syndrome

- ☐ Hypoglossal nerve palsy
- ☐ Contralateral hemiplegia and impaired proprioception

Tapia syndrome

- ☐ Hypoglossal nerve palsy: it may be bilateral
- ☐ Ipsilateral recurrent laryngeal nerve palsy

Synonyms

- ☐ 12th cranial nerve
- ☐ Cranial nerve XII
- ☐ Twelfth cranial nerve

Cranial nerve associated disorders

PAINFUL OPHTHALMOPLEGIA: CAUSES

Aneurysms

- ☐ Posterior communicating artery (PCOM)
- ☐ Basilar
- ☐ Carotid

Tumours

- ☐ Metastases
- ☐ Lymphoma
- ☐ Leukaemia

Cavernous sinus lesions

- ☐ Cavernous sinus thrombosis
- ☐ Carotico-cavernous fistula
- ☐ Pericavernous meningioma
- ☐ Cavernous sinus inflammation

Inflammatory and infective causes

- ☐ Giant cell arteritis (GCA)
- ☐ Sarcoidosis
- ☐ Gummatous periostitis at orbital fissures
- ☐ Meningovascular syphilis
- ☐ Contiguous sinusitis
- ☐ Mucormycosis
- ☐ Herpes zoster

Orbital lesions

- ☐ Tolosa–Hunt syndrome
- ☐ Orbital myositis

Pituitary lesions

- ☐ Pituitary adenoma
- ☐ Pituitary apoplexy

Other causes

- ☐ Arteriovenous malformations (AVM)
- ☐ Dilated carotid artery
- ☐ Parasellar lesions
- ☐ Ophthalmoplegic migraine
- ☐ Diabetic ophthalmoplegia

SUPRANUCLEAR GAZE PALSY: CAUSES

Parkinsonian causes

- ☐ Progressive supranuclear palsy (PSP)
- ☐ Dementia with Lewy bodies (DLB)
- ☐ Corticobasal degeneration (CBD)
- ☐ Vascular parkinsonism

Infective causes

- ☐ Creutzfeldt–Jakob disease (CJD)
- ☐ Whipple's disease

Other neurological causes

- ☐ Variant Alzheimer's disease (AD)
- ☐ Niemann–Pick Type C (NPC)
- ☐ Pantothenate kinase-associated neurodegeneration (PKAN)
- ☐ Progressive encephalomyelitis with rigidity and myoclonus (PERM)

Iatrogenic causes

- ☐ Deep brain stimulation (DBS)

DOI: 10.1201/9781003221258-59

CHAPTER 10

Spinal cord disorders

Myelopathy

ACUTE TRANSVERSE MYELITIS (ATM): INFECTIOUS AND INFLAMMATORY CAUSES

Inflammatory

- ☐ Idiopathic: possible familial risk with VPS37A gene variant
- ☐ Multiple sclerosis (MS)
- ☐ Neuromyelitis optica (NMO)
- ☐ Acute demyelinating encephalomyelitis (ADEM)
- ☐ Neurosarcoidosis
- ☐ Behcet's disease

Viral

- ☐ HIV
- ☐ Human T cell leukaemia virus (HTLV)
- ☐ Varicella zoster (VZV)
- ☐ Herpes simplex type 2 (HSV2)
- ☐ Cytomegalovirus (CMV)
- ☐ Hepatitis E virus (HEV)
- ☐ Hepatitis A virus (HAV)
- ☐ Measles virus
- ☐ Epstein Barr virus (EBV)
- ☐ Dengue virus
- ☐ Enterovirus D68 (EV-D68)

Bacterial

- ☐ Tuberculosis
- ☐ Neurosyphilis
- ☐ Lyme neuroborreliosis
- ☐ Mycoplasma pneumoniae
- ☐ Staphylococcus aureus
- ☐ Salmonella bacteraemia

Parasitic and fungal

- ☐ Schistosomiasis
- ☐ Trypanosomiasis
- ☐ Psittacosis
- ☐ Aspergillosis

Vaccinations

- ☐ Hepatitis B
- ☐ Typhoid
- ☐ Oral polio
- ☐ Rabies
- ☐ Influenza

ACUTE TRANSVERSE MYELITIS (ATM): OTHER CAUSES

Vascular and ischaemic

- ☐ Spinal cord infarction
- ☐ Dural arteriovenous fistula (dAVF)
- ☐ Fibrocartilaginous emboli
- ☐ Surfer's myelopathy: this is a non-traumatic myelopathy in novice surfers
  - ○ It results from prolonged spinal hyperextension

Autoimmune and paraneoplastic

- ☐ Neuromyelitis optica (NMO): aquaporin 4 antibodies
- ☐ Anti-MOG antibody myelopathy
- ☐ Anti-CRMP5 (collapsin response-mediator protein 5) related myelopathy
- ☐ Anti amphiphysin antibody myelopathy
- ☐ Systemic lupus erythematosus (SLE)
- ☐ Sjogren's syndrome
- ☐ Antiphospholipid antibody syndrome (APS)
- ☐ Vogt-Koyanagi-Harada disease

Neoplastic

- ☐ Intrinsic cord tumours
- ☐ Leptomeningeal carcinomatosis

Nutritional

- ☐ Subacute combined degeneration (vitamin B12 deficiency)
- ☐ Copper deficiency

Drug-induced

- ☐ Methotrexate
- ☐ Intramuscular Benzathine Penicillin
- ☐ Intrathecal chemotherapy
- ☐ TNF α inhibitors

Other causes

- ☐ Thymic hyperplasia
- ☐ Spinal anaesthesia
- ☐ Heroin
- ☐ Leukaemia

DOI: 10.1201/9781003221258-61

CERVICAL COMPRESSIVE MYELOPATHY: CLINICAL FEATURES

Causes

- ☐ Degenerative spondylosis
- ☐ Trauma
- ☐ Neoplastic
- ☐ Rheumatoid arthritis
- ☐ Spinal infections: abscesses
- ☐ Haematoma
- ☐ Fluorosis

Symptoms

- ☐ Non-dermatomal paraesthesias
- ☐ Impaired fine motor function
- ☐ Gait and balance difficulty: these are often the first features
- ☐ Bowel and bladder dysfunction: these are uncommon
- ☐ Spinal claudication
- ☐ Associated mild radicular neck pain

Clinical signs

- ☐ Hoffman's sign
- ☐ Lhermitte's sign
- ☐ Clonus
- ☐ Babinski reflex
- ☐ Finger escape sign
- ☐ Inverted supinator jerk

Myelopathy hand

- ☐ This is difficulty with adduction and extension of the ulnar fingers
- ☐ This impairs their smooth movements during grip and release cycles
- ☐ This is the grip-and-release sign

Magnetic resonance imaging (MRI) spine: features

- ☐ This shows pancake-like intramedullary gadolinium enhancement
- ☐ This is caused by focal blood-brain barrier disruption
- ☐ It may persist post-operatively
- ☐ It is an indicator of a poor prognosis

Predictors of poor progression

- ☐ Abnormal somatosensory evoked potentials
- ☐ High signal on magnetic resonance imaging (MRI) spine
- ☐ Symptomatic radiculopathy

Synonym

- ☐ Cervical cord compression

NON-COMPRESSIVE MYELOPATHY: NEUROLOGICAL CAUSES

Inflammatory and vasculitic causes

- ☐ Primary progressive multiple sclerosis (PPMS)
- ☐ Neuromyelitis optica (NMO)
- ☐ Eale's disease
- ☐ Subacute necrotising myelitis
- ☐ Neurosarcoidosis
- ☐ Systemic lupus erythematosus (SLE)
- ☐ Sjögren's syndrome

Degenerative causes

- ☐ Primary lateral sclerosis (PLS)
- ☐ Hereditary spastic paraparesis (HSP)
- ☐ Spinocerebellar ataxia (SCA)
- ☐ Iron neurodegeneration
- ☐ Friedreich's ataxia (FA)

Other causes

- ☐ Spinal stroke
- ☐ Surfer's myelopathy
- ☐ Intracranial dural arteriovenous fistula (dAVF)
- ☐ Arterial thrombosis

MYELOPATHY WITH NORMAL MRI SCAN

Neurodegenerative causes

☐ Friedreich's ataxia (FA)
☐ Motor neurone disease (MND)
☐ Hereditary spastic paraparesis (HSP)

Metabolic causes

☐ Vitamin B12 deficiency
☐ Folate deficiency
☐ Copper deficiency
☐ Adrenomyeloneuropathy (AMN)
☐ Krabbe disease

Infective causes

☐ HIV
☐ Tropical spastic paraparesis (TSP): HTLV1

Other causes

☐ Epidural lipomatosis
☐ The convalescent period of myelitis

Misdiagnosis

☐ Guillain–Barré syndrome (GBS)

Spastic paraparesis

SPASTIC PARAPARESIS: CAUSES

Neurodegenerative

- ☐ Hereditary spastic paraparesis (HSP)
- ☐ Dopa-responsive dystonia (DRD)
- ☐ Primary lateral sclerosis (PLS)
- ☐ Spinocerebellar ataxia (SCA)
- ☐ Friedreich's ataxia (FA)

Inflammatory and infective

- ☐ Multiple sclerosis (MS)
- ☐ Neurosarcoidosis
- ☐ HIV myelopathy
- ☐ Human T cell leukaemia virus (HTLV 1)
- ☐ Stiff person syndrome (SPS)
- ☐ Syphilis
- ☐ Schistosomiasis
- ☐ Brucellosis
- ☐ Arginase deficiency
- ☐ Abetalipoproteinaemia

Nutritional and metabolic

- ☐ Vitamin B12 deficiency
- ☐ Vitamin E deficiency
- ☐ Folate deficiency
- ☐ Copper deficiency
- ☐ Lathyrism
- ☐ Nitrous oxide toxicity
- ☐ Adrenoleukodystrophy (ALD)
- ☐ Adrenomyeloneuropathy (AMN)
- ☐ Krabbe disease
- ☐ CADASIL
- ☐ Phenylketonuria

Structural and vascular

- ☐ Parasagittal tumours
- ☐ Spinal tumours
- ☐ Cervical compressive myelopathy
- ☐ Chiari malformation
- ☐ Cerebral vasculitis
- ☐ Dural arteriovenous fistula (dAVF)
- ☐ Cerebral palsy (CP)
- ☐ Cerebrotendinous xanthomatosis (CTX)

Other causes

- ☐ Radiation myelopathy

Acronym

- ☐ CADASIL: Cerebral autosomal dominant arteriopathy with subcortical infarcts and leukoencephalopathy

SPASTIC PARAPARESIS: INVESTIGATIONS

Biochemistry tests

- ☐ Vitamin B12
- ☐ Vitamin E
- ☐ Very long chain fatty acids (VLCFA)
- ☐ White cell enzymes
- ☐ Plasma amino acids
- ☐ Lipoproteins
- ☐ Copper and ceruloplasmin

Microbiology

- ☐ Syphilis serology
- ☐ HIV screen
- ☐ Human T cell leukaemia virus (HTLV)

Genetics

- ☐ SPG mutation: for hereditary spastic paraparesis (HSP)
- ☐ ABCD1 mutations: for adrenomyeloneuropathy (AMN)

Neurophysiology

- ☐ Electromyogram (EMG)
- ☐ Nerve conduction studies (NCS)
- ☐ Somatosensory evoked potentials

Other tests

- ☐ Magnetic resonance imaging (MRI): brain and spinal cord
- ☐ Cerebrospinal fluid (CSF)

DOI: 10.1201/9781003221258-62

Spinal cord tumours

SPINAL CORD TUMOURS: CLASSIFICATION

Intramedullary

- [ ] Astrocytomas
- [ ] Dermoid cyst
- [ ] Ependymomas
- [ ] Epidermoid cyst
- [ ] Ganglioglioma
- [ ] Germinoma
- [ ] Glioblastoma
- [ ] Hamartomas
- [ ] Haemangioblastoma
- [ ] Lipomas
- [ ] Lymphoma
- [ ] Maxillopapillary ependymoma
- [ ] Paraganglioglioma
- [ ] Pilocytic astrocytoma
- [ ] Primary spinal cord melanoma
- [ ] Primitive neuroectodermal tumour (PNET)
- [ ] Subependymoma
- [ ] Teratomas

Intradural extramedullary

- [ ] Lipomas
- [ ] Meningiomas
- [ ] Metastases
- [ ] Neurofibromas
- [ ] Paragangliomas
- [ ] Sarcomas
- [ ] Schwannomas
- [ ] Spinal nerve sheath myxomas
- [ ] Vascular tumours

Extradural

- [ ] Metastases
- [ ] Extension of haemangioblastoma
- [ ] Paraspinal aggregoma: this is a light chain deposition disease (LCDD)
  - ○ It is a form of primary CNS lymphoma (PCNSL)

SPINAL CORD TUMOURS: CLINICAL FEATURES AND MANAGEMENT

Symptoms

- [ ] Limb weakness: paraparesis or quadriparesis
- [ ] Limb numbness
- [ ] Hand incoordination
- [ ] Burning dysaesthesias
- [ ] Urinary incontinence
- [ ] Radicular back pain
- [ ] Gait difficulty

Clinical signs

- [ ] Pyramidal signs
- [ ] Sensory level
- [ ] Hydrocephalus: this develops in about 1% of cases
- [ ] Papilloedema

Causes of papilloedema with spinal cord tumours

- [ ] Neoplastic arachnoiditis: this results from early intracranial metastases
- [ ] Occlusion of the subarachnoid pathways: this is by tumour cysts
- [ ] Increased cerebrospinal fluid (CSF) fibrinogen
- [ ] Subarachnoid haemorrhage (SAH): this is due to bleeding from the tumour
- [ ] Reduced spinal compliance: this is the water hammer effect
  - ○ It is due to CSF obstruction
- [ ] It is not likely due to increased CSF viscosity from high CSF protein

Differentials of intramedullary spinal tumours

- [ ] Multiple sclerosis (MS)
- [ ] Spinal cord infarction
- [ ] Transverse myelitis (TM)
- [ ] Arteriovenous fistula (AVF)
- [ ] Cavernoma
- [ ] Syringomyelia
- [ ] Vitamin B12 deficiency

Magnetic resonance imaging (MRI): features

- [ ] Tumours show cord expansion and oedema
- [ ] MRI does not distinguish between ependymoma and astrocytoma
- [ ] Associated cysts do not enhance

Treatment

- [ ] Surgery
- [ ] Avoid shunting before surgery if there is associated hydrocephalus

DOI: 10.1201/9781003221258-63

METASTATIC CORD COMPRESSION

Commonest primary sites

- ☐ Breast
- ☐ Lung
- ☐ Kidney
- ☐ Prostate
- ☐ Thyroid
- ☐ Melanoma
- ☐ Myeloma
- ☐ Lymphoma
- ☐ Colorectal

Clinical features

- ☐ Local pain
- ☐ Mechanical pain
- ☐ Radicular pain
- ☐ Myelopathy

Surgical treatment: decompression

- ☐ This is indicated if life expectancy is >3 months
- ☐ It is done only for spinal stability or pain control if onset of paraplegia is >24 hours

Radiotherapy

- ☐ This is done within 24 hours if the patient is unsuitable for surgery
- ☐ It is not indicated for painless complete weakness lasting >24 hours

Bisphosphonates: indications

- ☐ Myeloma primary
- ☐ Breast primary
- ☐ Prostate primary if analgesia fails

Other treatments

- ☐ Dexamethasone 16 mg daily loading dose
- ☐ Deep vein thrombosis (DVT) prophylaxis
- ☐ Nursing in neutral spine alignment
- ☐ Log roll every 2–3 hours if on bed rest

Poor prognostic factors

- ☐ Untreatable tumour
- ☐ Rapid tumour growth
- ☐ Bone destruction
- ☐ Multiple metastases
- ☐ Bony metastases
- ☐ Visceral metastases
- ☐ Presence of paralysis
- ☐ Low life expectancy
- ☐ Poor Karnofsky performance status

Spinal canal stenosis

SPINAL CANAL STENOSIS: CLINICAL FEATURES AND MANAGEMENT

Pain characteristics

- ☐ The pain is radicular and non-cramping
- ☐ It is located in the buttock, thigh, or leg
- ☐ It is usually bilateral
- ☐ It develops before numbness and weakness

Provoking factors

- ☐ Standing upright
- ☐ Walking (claudication)
- ☐ It is not provoked by cycling, exercising, or Valsalva manoeuvre, e.g. coughing and straining

Relieving factors

- ☐ Stooping
- ☐ Bending forward
- ☐ Sitting
- ☐ Squatting
- ☐ Walking uphill: patients may walk down the stairs backwards
- ☐ Relief takes 5–15 minutes
  - ○ The pain does not immediately resolve after stopping exercise or standing still

Sensory and autonomic symptoms

- ☐ Paraesthesias
- ☐ Numbness
- ☐ Incontinence
- ☐ Priapism (erection) on walking
- ☐ Vespers curse (restless legs)
- ☐ Tenderness: lumbar, paraspinal, and gluteal

Stance and gait difficulty

- ☐ Simian stance: the hips and knees are slightly flexed and the trunk is stooped forward
- ☐ Trendelenburg gait: this is a waddling gait caused by a drooping pelvis
- ☐ There is progressive reduction in walking distance
- ☐ There is difficulty toe walking with S1 root involvement
- ☐ There is difficulty heel walking with L4 or L5 root involvement

Clinical assessments

- ☐ Straight-leg raising test
  - ○ This is often negative: it may even improve the pain
  - ○ It may be falsely positive because of tight hamstrings
- ☐ Bicycle test of van Gelderen
  - ○ Cycling does not provoke spinal claudication as the trunk is flexed forward
  - ○ Cycling however increases the pain of vascular claudication
- ☐ Lumbar extension test
  - ○ This is done with the patient standing and hyperextending the lumbar spine for 30 to 60 seconds
  - ○ This provokes pain in the buttock or leg

Magnetic resonance imaging (MRI)

- ☐ Waist- or hourglass-shaped spinal canal: this is seen on sagittal images
- ☐ Trefoil-shaped spinal canal: this is seen on axial images

Treatment

- ☐ Decompression surgery is indicated
- ☐ Best outcomes are achieved if there is >50% reduction in the spinal canal area

DOI: 10.1201/9781003221258-64

SPINAL CANAL STENOSIS: DIFFERENTIAL DIAGNOSIS

Vascular claudication

- ☐ There is usually no history of back pain or injury with vascular claudication
- ☐ Pain is in the calf: it is in the buttock, thigh or leg in spinal claudication
- ☐ It is worse walking uphill: it is better going uphill with spinal claudication
- ☐ Cycling provokes pain unlike with spinal claudication
- ☐ Pain is relieved by standing still or stopping exercise: spinal claudication is provoked by standing
- ☐ Relief of pain occurs within 15 seconds of resting: it takes 5–15 minutes with spinal claudication
- ☐ The claudication distance is constant: it is variable in spinal claudication
- ☐ There is a stocking sensory loss: it is segmental in spinal claudication
- ☐ It is not provoked by Valsalva: unlike with spinal claudication
- ☐ There are abnormal foot pulses in vascular claudication
- ☐ There are arterial bruits in vascular claudication

Lateral disc prolapse

- ☐ Patients with this are usually younger than those with canal stenosis
  - ○ The mean age is 41 years v 65 years in canal stenosis
- ☐ The pain is in a specific dermatomal pattern
- ☐ The pain is often at rest and at night
- ☐ It is worse with the Valsalva manoeuvre

Other differentials

- ☐ Cauda equina tumours
- ☐ Spinal arteriovenous malformations (AVM)

CHAPTER 11

Anterior horn cell disorders

Motor neurone disease

MOTOR NEURONE DISEASE (MND): MAJOR GENETIC RISK FACTORS

SOD-1 gene mutations

- [ ] This is the copper/zinc superoxide-dismutase-1 (SOD-1) gene mutation
- [ ] It is present in 20% of familial cases
- [ ] More than 135 mutations have been described
- [ ] It is also seen in some sporadic MND cases
- [ ] CNTF gene mutations may modify SOD 1 and confer an earlier onset age of MND

C9orf72 gene mutation

- [ ] This is on chromosome 9p21
- [ ] It shows genetic anticipation

Multisystem proteinopathy gene mutations

- [ ] VCP
- [ ] hnRNPA1
- [ ] hnRNPA2B1
- [ ] Matrin 3 (MATR3)
- [ ] SQSTM1

ALS gene mutations

- [ ] ALS 2 (Alsin)
- [ ] ALS 6 (FUS)
- [ ] ALS 4 (SETX)
- [ ] ALS 5 (SPG11)
- [ ] ALS 8 (VAPB)
- [ ] ALS 9 (ANG)
- [ ] ALS 10 (TARDBP)
- [ ] ALS 11 (FIG 4)
- [ ] ALS 12 (OPTN)
- [ ] ALS 14 (VCP)
- [ ] ALS 15 (UBQLN2)
- [ ] ALS 16 (SIGMAR 1)

CHCHD10 gene mutations: features

- [ ] MND
- [ ] Ataxia
- [ ] Parkinsonism
- [ ] Sensorineural hearing loss
- [ ] Mitochondrial myopathy

TBK1 gene mutations

- [ ] This is TANK-binding kinase 1 (TBK1)
- [ ] It confers a risk of MND with frontotemporal dementia (FTD)
- [ ] It causes severe hypermetabolism with reduced appetite
- [ ] There is hypothalamic and widespread brain atrophy on imaging

MOTOR NEURONE DISEASE (MND): NON-GENETIC RISK FACTORS

Individual risk factors

- [ ] High physical fitness and activity
- [ ] Head trauma: especially between ages 35 to 54 years
- [ ] High total cholesterol
- [ ] High LDL cholesterol
- [ ] Repeated antibiotic use
- [ ] Low body weight or body mass index (BMI)

Human endogenous retrovirus (HERV-K)

- [ ] This is possibly associated with HIV-related MND

Heavy metals

- [ ] Lead
- [ ] Mercury
- [ ] Silica

Possible occupational risk factors

- [ ] Formaldehyde exposure
- [ ] Professional football
- [ ] Farming
- [ ] Glass work
- [ ] Pottery
- [ ] Tile work
- [ ] Precision-tool manufacturing
- [ ] Extremely low frequency magnetic fields (ELF-MF)
- [ ] Military service

Uncertain risk factor: smoking

- [ ] The risk of MND from smoking appears to be small
- [ ] Two major papers found no causative association

DOI: 10.1201/9781003221258-66

MOTOR NEURONE DISEASE (MND): NEUROMUSCULAR FEATURES

Onset

- ☐ The onset is relatively abrupt
- ☐ Diabetes may delay the onset by 4 years

Major MND subtypes

- ☐ Amyotrophic lateral sclerosis (ALS): upper and lower motor neurone features
- ☐ Progressive muscular atrophy (PMA): lower motor neurone features only
- ☐ Primary lateral sclerosis (PLS): upper motor neurone features only
- ☐ Progressive bulbar palsy (PBP): bulbar features only

Signs of muscle weakness

- ☐ Dropping objects
- ☐ Difficulty turning keys
- ☐ Poor handwriting
- ☐ Difficulty opening bottles
- ☐ Foot drop and tendency to trip
- ☐ Difficulty rising from low chairs
- ☐ Difficulty climbing stairs
- ☐ Plateaus and reversals: these occur in the early stages

Bulbar and pseudobulbar features

- ☐ Dysphagia
- ☐ Dysarthria
- ☐ Inability to shout or sing
- ☐ Tongue fasciculations
- ☐ Pseudobulbar signs: inappropriate laughter and crying
- ☐ Absent gag reflex
- ☐ Positive jaw jerk

Split signs

- ☐ Split hand sign: the lateral half of the hand is more wasted than the medial
- ☐ Split hand plus sign: the abductor pollicis brevis is weaker than the flexor pollicis longus
- ☐ Split elbow sign: the biceps is weaker than the triceps
- ☐ Split leg sign: the dorsiflexors are weaker than the plantar flexors
- ☐ Split finger sign: the first flexor digitorum profundus muscle is weaker than the fourth

Tongue features

- ☐ The tongue is usually spastic and wasted
- ☐ There may occasionally be pseudohypertrophy with fatty replacement
- ☐ This develops in advanced cases: it is possibly due to overfeeding

Other neuromuscular features

- ☐ Easy fatigue
- ☐ Cramps
- ☐ Fasciculations
- ☐ Head drop
- ☐ Respiratory difficulties
- ☐ Spasticity
- ☐ Hyperreflexia
- ☐ Bilateral diaphragmatic paralysis: this may be the initial presentation

MOTOR NEURONE DISEASE (MND): OTHER FEATURES

Sleep disorders

- ☐ Insomnia
- ☐ Fragmented sleep
- ☐ Periodic limb movements of sleep (PLMS)

Cognitive impairments

- ☐ Fluency
- ☐ Social cognition
- ☐ Executive function
- ☐ Verbal memory

Neuropsychiatric features

- ☐ Depression: this may precede MND diagnosis by years
- ☐ Apathy
- ☐ Frontotemporal dementia (FTD)

Autonomic features

- ☐ Spastic bladder: in primary lateral sclerosis (PLS)
- ☐ Sialorrhoea

Pain

- ☐ Pain may precede motor symptoms
- ☐ It predicts morbidity and mortality

Movement disorders

- ☐ Action tremor: this is centrally mediated
- ☐ Left hand dystonia: this was reported in one family with the C9orf72 mutation

Risk of cancer

- ☐ There are some reports of increased risk of testicular and salivary gland cancer
- ☐ Other studies report no association with cancer
- ☐ Some studies report reduced cancer risk

Other features

- ☐ Insulin resistance
- ☐ Persistent bitter taste (dysgeusia)
- ☐ Polycythaemia: case report

Behavioural assessment tools

- ☐ Beaumont Behavioural Inventory (BBI)
- ☐ Amyotrophic Lateral Sclerosis-Frontotemporal Dementia-Questionnaire (ALS FTD-Q)
- ☐ Edinburgh Cognitive and Behavioural ALS Screen (ECAS)

MOTOR NEURONE DISEASE (MND): DIAGNOSTIC CRITERIA

Diagnostic classification systems

- ☐ Awaji
- ☐ Revised El Escorial

Neurophysiological requirements

- ☐ Signs of lower motor neurone degeneration in one or more limb
- ☐ Evidence of lower motor neurone loss: this shows as a reduced interference pattern
- ☐ Evidence of renervation: this shows as large amplitude long duration motor units
- ☐ Fibrillations and sharp waves or fasciculation potentials

Clinical requirements

- ☐ Signs of lower motor neurone degeneration in one or more limb
- ☐ Signs of upper motor neurone degeneration in one or more limbs
- ☐ Progressive spread of signs within the limb or to other limbs
- ☐ Absence of other disease processes that could explain the findings

Definite ALS

- ☐ Upper and lower motor neurone signs in bulbar and ≥2 spinal regions or
- ☐ Upper and lower motor neurone signs in 3 spinal regions

Probable ALS

- ☐ Upper and lower motor neurone signs in 2 spinal regions and
- ☐ Some lower motor neurone signs rostral to upper motor neurone signs

Probable ALS-laboratory supported

- ☐ Clinical upper and lower motor neurone signs in 1 region and
- ☐ Neurophysiological lower motor neurone signs in ≥2 regions

Possible ALS

- ☐ Upper and lower motor neurone signs in 1 spinal region or
- ☐ Upper motor neurone signs in ≥2 regions or
- ☐ Lower motor neurone signs rostral to upper motor neurone signs

MOTOR NEURONE DISEASE (MND): DIFFERENTIAL DIAGNOSIS

Peripheral differentials: multifocal motor neuropathy (MMN)

- [ ] MMN is the closest differential diagnosis of MND
- [ ] Imaging of the ulnar and median nerves may help to differentiate them
- [ ] The cross-sectional areas (CSA) of the nerves are larger in MMN

Peripheral differentials: others

- [ ] Spinal muscular atrophy (SMA)
- [ ] Spinal and bulbar muscular atrophy (SBMA, Kennedy disease)
- [ ] Post-polio syndrome (PPS)
- [ ] Pancoast syndrome
- [ ] Myasthenia gravis (MG): especially anti MUSK
- [ ] Adult polyglucosan body disease
- [ ] Inclusion body myositis (IBM)
- [ ] Transthyretin familial amyloid neuropathy: this may cause tongue fasciculations and atrophy
- [ ] Radiation-induced radiculopathy
- [ ] Brachial neuritis (neuralgic amyotrophy)
- [ ] Benign fasciculations syndrome

Central differentials

- [ ] Multiple sclerosis (MS)
- [ ] Cervical myelopathy
- [ ] Hereditary spastic paraparesis (HSP)
- [ ] Chorea-acanthocytosis
- [ ] Syringomyelia
- [ ] Vitamin B 12 deficiency
- [ ] Copper deficiency
- [ ] Adrenomyeloneuropathy (AMN)
- [ ] Anti IgLON5 antibody disease

SOD 1 deficiency

- [ ] This is caused by the homozygous truncating variant c.335dupG (p.C112Wfs*11)
- [ ] It results in total absence of SOD1 enzyme activity
- [ ] It causes spastic quadriparesis and hyperekplexia-like symptoms
- [ ] The brain MRI shows mild cerebellar atrophy

Non-neurological differentials

- [ ] Hyperthyroidism
- [ ] Hypoparathyroidism
- [ ] Lyme neuroborreliosis
- [ ] Eosinophilic fasciitis
- [ ] Triple A syndrome: achalasia, alacrima, and adrenal insufficiency
- [ ] HIV infection

ALS differential diagnostic index (ALSDI)

- [ ] This is a score that differentiates MND from other mimics
- [ ] It is especially helpful if it is ≥4

Split hand (SI) differential diagnostic index

- [ ] This is a neurophysiological index
- [ ] It estimates the difference between hand muscle CMAP values
- [ ] It compares the first dorsal interosseous and the abductor pollicis brevis with the abductor digiti minimi

PRIMARY LATERAL SCLEROSIS (PLS): CLINICAL FEATURES

Demographic features

- [ ] PLS accounts for 1–3% of MND
- [ ] The onset is usually from the 5th decade
- [ ] There is no family history

Features of spasticity

- [ ] The onset is with insidious spastic paraparesis
- [ ] The presentation is with symmetrical pyramidal features
- [ ] Spasticity is exacerbated by stress or noise

Other features

- [ ] Dysuria
- [ ] Urgency
- [ ] Bulbar features
- [ ] Pseudobulbar features
- [ ] Cramps
- [ ] Fasciculations

Occasional features

- [ ] A Parkinsonian presentation has been reported

Diagnostic inclusion criteria

- [ ] Age ≥25 years
- [ ] Progressive upper motor neuron (UMN) symptoms for ≥2 years
- [ ] Signs of UMN dysfunction in at least two of three regions
  - ○ Lower extremity, upper extremity, and bulbar

Diagnostic exclusion criteria

- [ ] Sensory symptoms unexplained by comorbid conditions
- [ ] Active lower motor neuron (LMN) degeneration
- [ ] An alternative diagnosis on investigations

Progression

- [ ] It is gradually progressive over >3 years
- [ ] The diagnosis of PLS is only made after 4 years without lower motor neurone signs
- [ ] This is because lower motor neurone signs develop within 4 years in most cases
- [ ] The diagnosis in the first 4 years is therefore upper motor neurone-dominant ALS

Predictors of progression to ALS

- [ ] Focal muscle weakness
- [ ] Weight loss
- [ ] Reduced forced vital capacity (FVC)

PROGRESSIVE MUSCULAR ATROPHY (PMA)

Demographic features

- [ ] Males are more frequently affected
- [ ] The onset age is older than in amyotrophic lateral sclerosis (ALS)
- [ ] About a fifth of patients develop upper motor neurone signs within 5 years
- [ ] Familial forms have been reported with the SOD1 gene mutation

Pathology

- [ ] Upper motor neurone pathology is seen in 50–80% of cases
- [ ] Ubiquinated inclusions are present in 95% of cases
- [ ] TAR DNA-binding protein (TDP-43) pathology is seen in 85% of cases
  - ○ It is present in 100% of ALS cases
- [ ] Fused-in-sarcoma (FUS)-positive inclusions are seen in 15% of cases

Clinical features

- [ ] The onset may be in the upper limb, lower limb, or axial muscles
- [ ] There is rapid progression in about 95% of cases
- [ ] The prognosis is similar to that of ALS
- [ ] The worst outcome is with axial onset

Differential diagnosis

- [ ] Slowly progressive spinal muscular atrophy
- [ ] Distal spinal muscular atrophy
- [ ] Segmental distal spinal muscular atrophy
- [ ] Segmental proximal spinal muscular atrophy
- [ ] Hereditary lower motor neurone diseases (LMND)
- [ ] Adult onset spinal muscular atrophy (SMA)
- [ ] X-linked spinal and bulbar muscular atrophy (SBMA, Kennedy disease)
- [ ] Post radiation lower motor neurone syndrome (PRLMNS)

FLAIL ARM SYNDROME (FAS) VARIANT MOTOR NEURONE DISEASE (MND)

Demographic features

- ☐ This accounts for about 10% of cases of MND
- ☐ The male to female ratio is about 4 to 9
- ☐ A flail leg variant is seen in 6% of cases

Genetics

- ☐ The hnRNPA1 gene mutation increases the risk
- ☐ A TARDBP mutation has been reported

Onset features

- ☐ The onset age is younger than in typical MND
- ☐ The onset is asymmetrical but it eventually becomes symmetrical
- ☐ The onset may be in distal or in both distal and proximal muscles

Clinical features

- ☐ It is a predominantly lower motor neuron upper limb syndrome
- ☐ There is profound wasting and weakness
- ☐ Lower limb upper motor neurone signs are often present
- ☐ Bulbar signs may develop on follow up
- ☐ Other body regions are functionally intact at presentation
- ☐ There is prolonged survival compared to limb onset MND

Differential diagnosis

- ☐ X-linked spinal and bulbar muscular atrophy (SBMA, Kennedy disease)
- ☐ Spinal muscular atrophy (SMA)
- ☐ Multifocal motor neuropathy (MMN)

Investigations

- ☐ Electromyography (EMG): the split hand pattern of hand involvement is absent
- ☐ Magnetic resonance imaging (MRI): this shows the owl's eye sign on axial spinal images

Pathology

- ☐ Motor neuronal loss in the brainstem and cervical spinal cord
- ☐ Bilateral pyramidal tract degeneration
- ☐ Inclusions: Bunina bodies, Lewy body-like, and skein-like
- ☐ Cytoplasmic vacuoles in the lumbar anterior horn motor neurons

Synonym

- ☐ Vulpian-Bernhart syndrome

C9ORF72 VARIANT MOTOR NEURONE DISEASE (MND): CLINICAL FEATURES

Epidemiology

- ☐ This accounts for about 50% of familial MND
- ☐ It causes 20% of sporadic MND
- ☐ It has an equal gender ratio
- ☐ There is no difference in age, race, or site of onset compared to sporadic ALS
- ☐ There is more frequent dementia in family members

Onset features

- ☐ The onset age is earlier than in sporadic MND
- ☐ Bulbar onset is more frequent in females
- ☐ Bulbar onset is more frequent than in other familial MND variants
- ☐ Spinal onset is more frequent in males

Cognitive features

- ☐ Dementia occurs more frequently than in other familial MND variants
- ☐ Dementia is also more frequent than in sporadic MND
- ☐ There is co-morbid frontotemporal dementia (FTD) in about 15% of cases
- ☐ Cognitive impairments are also present in pre-symptomatic carriers
- ☐ Pre-symptomatic mutation carriers have impaired verbal fluency

Neurological features

- ☐ Familial left-hand dystonia: case report
- ☐ Accelerated respiratory decline

Psychiatric features

- ☐ Disinhibition
- ☐ Apathy
- ☐ Psychosis with delusions and hallucinations
- ☐ Kindred have increased risk of psychosis, suicide, and autism

Cancer risk

- ☐ There is a possible increased risk of melanoma

Predictors of poor prognosis

- ☐ Older age at onset
- ☐ Shorter interval to diagnosis
- ☐ Bulbar onset
- ☐ Males with spinal onset
- ☐ CSF phosphorylated neurofilament heavy chain (pNFH)
- ☐ The prognosis is worse than with sporadic MND

C9ORF72 VARIANT MOTOR NEURONE DISEASE (MND): INVESTIGATIONS

Genetics

- ☐ The C9orf72 gene mutation is on chromosome 9p21: on open reading frame 72
- ☐ It is a G_4C_2 (GGGGCC) hexanucleotide repeat expansion disease
- ☐ The repeat size correlates with age
- ☐ ≥24 repeats may be pathogenic
- ☐ It demonstrates genetic anticipation by about 7 years
- ☐ The transmission is autosomal dominant

Pathology

- ☐ The C9orf72 protein plays a role in cellular traffic
- ☐ The pathology shows TDP-43 aggregation: this is especially in the thalamus and cerebellum
- ☐ There is early involvement of von Economo neurones (VENs)

Magnetic resonance imaging (MRI) brain: features

- ☐ Early focal atrophy of the left supramarginal gyrus
- ☐ Focal thalamic atrophy
- ☐ Later diffuse atrophy

Pre-symptomatic MRI markers

- ☐ Abnormally low cortical gyrification
- ☐ Cervical spinal cord white matter atrophy

Cerebrospinal fluid (CSF): features

- ☐ Elevated neurofilament medium polypeptide (NEFM)
- ☐ Elevated chitotriosidase-1 (CHIT1)
- ☐ Elevated phosphorylated neurofilament heavy chain (pNFH)
- ☐ Decreased neuronal pentraxin receptor (NPTXR)

MicroRNAs

- ☐ Over-expressed: miR-34a-5p and miR-345–5p
- ☐ Under-expressed: miR-200c-3p and miR-10a-3p

RILUZOLE

Pharmacology

- ☐ Riluzole is a benzothiazole derivative
- ☐ It inhibits presynaptic glutamate release
- ☐ It is indicated for both ALS and PMA

Benefits

- ☐ It slows progression of muscle weakness
- ☐ It slows deterioration in muscle strength
- ☐ It improves survival by about 3 months

Dosing and administration

- ☐ The dose is 50 mg bid orally
- ☐ A liquid form is available
- ☐ Intrathecal administration is under review

Monitoring

- ☐ Monitor liver function tests 4 weekly in the first three months: then 3-monthly
- ☐ Stop treatment if serum transaminases rise >3 times normal

Side effects

- ☐ Fatigue
- ☐ Nausea
- ☐ Headache
- ☐ Raised liver enzymes levels
- ☐ Recurrent acute pancreatitis
- ☐ Severe neutropenia occasionally
- ☐ Hypersensitivity pneumonitis
- ☐ Interstitial lung disease
- ☐ Hypertension

Acronyms

- ☐ ALS: amyotrophic lateral sclerosis
- ☐ PMA: progressive muscular atrophy

EDARAVONE

Pharmacology and benefits

- ☐ Edaravone has antioxidant properties
- ☐ It mainly improves pinch strength
- ☐ It may delay progression of motor neurone disease (MND)

Dosing

- ☐ The initial cycle dose is 60 mg by intravenous infusion over 6 minutes
  - ○ This is administered daily for 14 days
- ☐ The dose for subsequent cycles is 60 mg daily for 10 days out of 14 days
- ☐ There are 14-day drug-free intervals between treatment cycles

Side effects

- ☐ Hypersensitivity
- ☐ Allergic reactions
- ☐ Bruising
- ☐ Gait impairment
- ☐ Headache
- ☐ Dermatitis

MOTOR NEURONE DISEASE (MND): NEUROLOGICAL SYMPTOMATIC TREATMENTS

Spasticity

- ☐ Baclofen 10–80 mg daily
  - ○ It may also be administered intrathecally
- ☐ Tizanidine 6–24 mg daily
- ☐ Dantrolene 25–100 mg daily
- ☐ Memantine 10–60 mg daily
- ☐ Nabiximols: investigational

Cramps

- ☐ Quinine sulphate 200 mg twice daily
- ☐ Mexiletine 150 mg bid
- ☐ Carbamazepine
- ☐ Diazepam
- ☐ Phenytoin

Labile emotions

- ☐ Dextromethorphan
- ☐ Quinidine
- ☐ Amitriptyline
- ☐ Imipramine
- ☐ Levodopa

Pain

- ☐ Comfortable seating and sleeping positions
- ☐ Simple analgesics
- ☐ Non-steroidal anti-inflammatory drugs (NSAIDS)
- ☐ Opiates
- ☐ Antidepressants
- ☐ Gabapentin

Anxiety

- ☐ Lorazepam sublingual or orally
- ☐ Diazepam suppositories
- ☐ Midazolam

Fatigue

- ☐ Modafinil
- ☐ Pyridostigmine

Insomnia

- ☐ Amitriptyline
- ☐ Zolpidem

MOTOR NEURONE DISEASE (MND): SYSTEMIC SYMPTOMATIC TREATMENTS

Sialorrhoea and drooling

- ☐ Atropine tablets or liquid: 0.25–0.75 mg three times daily
- ☐ Atropine eye drops sublingually
- ☐ Benztropine tablets or liquid
- ☐ Benzhexol tablets
- ☐ Hyoscine tablets or transdermal patches
- ☐ Amitriptyline tablets or liquid
- ☐ Glycopyrrolate liquid: subcutaneous, intramuscular, or via gastrostomy
- ☐ Home suction device
- ☐ Carbocisteine for thick sputum: 250–750 mg syrup tid orally or via gastrostomy

Refractory sialorrhoea and drooling

- ☐ Botulinum toxin injection of the salivary glands
- ☐ Salivary gland irradiation: this is probably better than botulinum toxin
- ☐ Trans-tympanic neurectomy

Dyspnoea

- ☐ Sublingual Lorazepam: for acute attacks of dyspnoea or laryngospasm
- ☐ Morphine: for end-stage respiratory impairment
- ☐ Chest physiotherapy

Laryngospasm

- ☐ Upright positioning of the trunk
- ☐ Appropriate spacing of meals
- ☐ Avoid late-night meals
- ☐ Avoid medications that increase gastric acid secretion

Constipation

- ☐ Ispaghula
- ☐ Methyl cellulose
- ☐ Lactulose
- ☐ Glycerine suppositories

Anxiety

- ☐ Lorazepam sublingual or orally
- ☐ Diazepam suppositories
- ☐ Midazolam

Other symptomatic treatments

- ☐ Excessive yawning: Baclofen
- ☐ Poor quality of life: meditation training

MOTOR NEURONE DISEASE (MND): SUPPORTIVE CARE

Measures to improve swallow

- ☐ Head back tilt: for tongue weakness
- ☐ Chin tuck: for pharyngeal weakness
- ☐ Manual lip sealing: for buccal weakness
- ☐ Supraglottic swallowing manoeuvre: to close the vocal cords when swallowing
  - ○ Subjects hold their breath while swallowing and then exhale forcefully afterwards

Other measures to support eating and swallowing

- ☐ Avoid background noise and distraction when eating
- ☐ Breathing and relaxation exercises: to optimize respiration when eating
- ☐ Facilitation techniques, e.g. vibration
- ☐ Ice application: to improve articulation
- ☐ Heimlich manoeuvre if choking

Communication aids

- ☐ Pencil and paper
- ☐ Alphabet board
- ☐ Word or picture boards
- ☐ Laser pointers on glasses or headband
- ☐ Electronic communication devices: with head or eye movement control

Dietary modifications

- ☐ Serve meals in small portions if there is easy fatigue
- ☐ Serve cool drinks to make swallowing easier
- ☐ Use special eating or drinking aids
- ☐ Use fine-bore nasogastric tubes for short term feeding
- ☐ Use enteral feeding for long-term nutrition
- ☐ Keep well-hydrated to avoid thick saliva
- ☐ Serve fruits and vegetables: these improve function possibly due to an antioxidant effect

Interventional care for secretions

- ☐ Mechanical cough assist (insufflators): if secretions are thick and cough is weak
- ☐ Tracheostomy: to reduce the risk of aspirating secretions

Nutritional management

- ☐ Monitor oral intake
- ☐ Weigh at each visit
- ☐ Provide mobile arm supports for independent eating
- ☐ Use modified cutlery
- ☐ Monitor for causes of anorexia, e.g. depression
- ☐ Serve thickened fluids
- ☐ Augment dietary calories
- ☐ Perform a gastrostomy if there is weight loss of 10–15%

Spinal muscular atrophy

SPINAL MUSCULAR ATROPHY (SMA): CLASSIFICATION

Classical SMA types

- ☐ SMA I: Infantile: Werdnig-Hoffman
- ☐ SMA II: Intermediate
- ☐ SMA III: Juvenile: Kugelberg-Welander
- ☐ SMA IV: Adult

Major SMA variants

- ☐ X linked spinal and bulbar muscular atrophy (SBMA, Kennedy disease)
- ☐ Juvenile segmental SMA: Hirayama disease

Riboflavin transporter deficiencies (RTDs)

- ☐ Brown-Vialetto-van Leare (BVVL) syndrome
- ☐ Fazio Londe syndrome

Other SMA variants

- ☐ Scapuloperoneal SMA (Davidenkow disease)
- ☐ Distal SMA
- ☐ Monomelic muscular atrophy
- ☐ Hexosaminidase A deficiency
- ☐ Infantile cerebellar atrophy with SMA
- ☐ SMA with brain atrophy
- ☐ SMA with congenital fractures of bone
- ☐ Pontocerebellar hypoplasia with SMA
- ☐ X-linked infantile SMA with arthrogryposis
- ☐ SMA with respiratory distress type 1
- ☐ SMA lower extremity dominant (SMALED)
- ☐ Dominant congenital (DSMA, SMALED2)

SPINAL MUSCULAR ATROPHY (SMA): TYPES I-IV

SMA type I (Werdnig-Hoffman syndrome)

- ☐ The onset is in infancy: the onset age is 0–6 months
- ☐ The child never learns to sit
- ☐ There is poor head control
- ☐ The tongue is atrophic with fasciculations
- ☐ The limbs are weak and hypotonic
- ☐ The chest is bell-shaped: there is abdominal protrusion and chest collapse
- ☐ The breathing is abdominal and paradoxical
  - ○ The intercostal muscles are degenerated but the diaphragm is spared
- ☐ Distal digital necrosis occasionally occurs
- ☐ The renal structure and function are impaired
- ☐ There is no electrocardiographic or clinical hand tremor

SMA type II

- ☐ The onset age is between 7–18 months: intermediate onset age
- ☐ The patients are unable to stand or walk
- ☐ They are able to sit unsupported
- ☐ They have difficulty coughing and swallowing
- ☐ There is a fine tremor
- ☐ There is mandibular dysfunction
- ☐ Joint contractures occur
- ☐ Kyphoscoliosis is present
- ☐ There is an associated electrocardiographic and clinical hand tremor

SMA type III (Kugelberg-Welander syndrome)

- ☐ This is late or juvenile onset SMA
- ☐ The onset age is after 18 months
- ☐ The phenotype is mild
- ☐ Patients achieve independent walking but they may lose it subsequently
- ☐ There is mandibular dysfunction
- ☐ Swallowing impairment occurs rarely
- ☐ Coughing difficulties may occasionally develop
- ☐ There is scoliosis
- ☐ There is associated electrocardiographic and clinical hand tremor

SMA type IV

- ☐ This is adult onset SMA
- ☐ The onset age is in the 2nd or 3rd decade
- ☐ The phenotype is mild
- ☐ There is calf hypertrophy
- ☐ There are no respiratory or gastrointestinal features

DOI: 10.1201/9781003221258-67

SPINAL MUSCULAR ATROPHY (SMA): GENERAL TREATMENTS

Respiratory treatment

- ☐ Cough assist devices
- ☐ Airway clearance: for impaired cough
- ☐ Non-invasive ventilation (NIV): with bilevel positive airway pressure (BiPAP)
- ☐ Routine vaccinations to prevent chest infections

Nutritional management

- ☐ Semisolid foods
- ☐ Thickened fluids
- ☐ Elemental formula
- ☐ Reduced fat diet
- ☐ Protein supplementation

Measures to improve swallowing

- ☐ Positioning and seating
- ☐ Orthotic devices

Measures to improve intestinal function

- ☐ Antacids
- ☐ Prokinetics
- ☐ Anti-reflux surgery

Orthopaedic care

- ☐ Monitor growth chart
- ☐ Monitor for scoliosis
- ☐ Consider thoraco-lumbo-sacral-orthosis (TLSO) bracing
- ☐ Consider spinal fusion for scoliosis

Prevention of contractures

- ☐ Physiotherapy
- ☐ Occupational therapy
- ☐ Serial casting

Other treatment considerations

- ☐ Salbutamol
- ☐ Monitor coagulation profile: impairments have been reported

SPINAL MUSCULAR ATROPHY (SMA): GENE THERAPY

Nusinersen

- ☐ This is an antisense oligonucleotide (ASO)
- ☐ It alters SMN2 splicing
- ☐ It increases the amount of functional survival motor neuron (SMN) protein
- ☐ It is mainly indicated in infants and children
- ☐ Benefit is also reported in adults and subjects with later-onset SMA
- ☐ Best outcomes correlate with early treatment
- ☐ It is administered intrathecally
- ☐ There is a risk of post lumbar puncture headache and meningitis
- ☐ Other side effects are recurrent pneumonia and proteinuria

Onasemnogene abeparvovec

- ☐ This is adeno-associated viral vector gene therapy
- ☐ It is beneficial for bi-allelic SMN1 gene mutations
- ☐ It is indicated in subjects <2 years
- ☐ It is administered as a single infusion
- ☐ Subjects may achieve independent sitting, standing, and ability to walk
- ☐ It also improves survival

Other anterior horn cell disorders

MONOMELIC AMYOTROPHY: PATHOLOGY AND EPIDEMIOLOGY

Pathogenesis

- ☐ This is a cervical flexion myelopathy
- ☐ It possibly results from repeated or sustained neck flexion

Pathology

- ☐ Anterior horn cell necrosis and gliosis C5-T1
- ☐ Chronic microcirculatory changes in the lower cervical spinal cord
- ☐ Tight dural canal

Epidemiology

- ☐ It is sporadic
- ☐ There is no preceding trauma or infection
- ☐ The onset is in adolescence or young adult age
- ☐ The median onset age is 20 years
- ☐ The onset age is wider in Europe: range is 18 to 65 years
- ☐ Males are more frequently affected: the gender ratio is 10:1
- ☐ An increased risk has been reported in basketball players

Synonyms

- ☐ Hirayama disease
- ☐ Juvenile muscular atrophy
- ☐ Juvenile non-progressive amyotrophy of the upper limb

MONOMELIC AMYOTROPHY: CLINICAL FEATURES

Weakness and wasting

- ☐ This typically affects the distal limb muscles: the C7-T1 innervated muscles
- ☐ Weakness may demonstrate cold paresis: transient worsening in the cold
- ☐ Reflexes may be normal, reduced, or increased

Patterns of weakness and wasting

- ☐ Oblique amyotrophy: this is the typical pattern of forearm muscle wasting
  - ○ This results from brachioradialis sparing (C5,6 roots)
- ☐ Contralateral upper limb involvement: this occurs in about 18% of cases
- ☐ Bilaterally symmetrical upper limb involvement: this develops in severe cases

Other features

- ☐ Finger minipolymyoclonus: irregular coarse tremors
- ☐ Causalgia
- ☐ Hyperhidrosis
- ☐ Fasciculations: these are uncommon
- ☐ Hand tremor on neck flexion

Preserved functions

- ☐ Sensation
- ☐ Cranial nerves
- ☐ Lower limb pyramidal tract
- ☐ Sphincters
- ☐ Cerebellar system

Differential diagnosis: major types

- ☐ Motor neurone disease (MND): especially brachial amyotrophic diplegia (BAD)
- ☐ Multifocal motor neuropathy (MMN)
- ☐ Spinal muscular atrophy (SMA)
- ☐ Cervical radiculopathy
- ☐ Thoracic outlet syndrome (TOS)
- ☐ Hopkins syndrome

Progress and outcome

- ☐ Progression stabilises within 1–4 years
- ☐ Then it follows a non-progressive or slowly progressive course

Synonyms

- ☐ Hirayama disease
- ☐ Juvenile muscular atrophy
- ☐ Juvenile non-progressive amyotrophy of the upper limb

DOI: 10.1201/9781003221258-68

MONOMELIC AMYOTROPHY: MANAGEMENT

Magnetic resonance imaging (MRI) spine: features

- [ ] Flattening of the lower cervical cord
- [ ] Ischaemia of the lower cervical anterior horns
- [ ] Dilated and enhancing epidural venous plexus on flexion
- [ ] Anterior displacement of the dura
- [ ] Hyperintense anterior horn cells

Magnetic resonance imaging (MRI) spine: dynamic contrast

- [ ] Contrast MRI is performed in neck flexion
- [ ] It shows asymmetric flattening of the lower cervical spinal cord

Magnetic resonance imaging (MRI) muscles

- [ ] High signal intensity in the gastrocnemius and soleus

Electromyogram (EMG)

- [ ] Acute and chronic denervation: this is in the C7, C8, and T1 myotomes
- [ ] There may be abnormalities in unaffected limbs
- [ ] Contraction fasciculations may be present

Blood tests

- [ ] Antiganglioside antibodies may be transiently elevated

Treatments

- [ ] Cervical collar in early stages
- [ ] Duraplasty
- [ ] Anterior cervical decompression and reconstruction

Synonyms

- [ ] Hirayama disease
- [ ] Juvenile muscular atrophy
- [ ] Juvenile non-progressive amyotrophy of the upper limb

KENNEDY DISEASE (SBMA): CLINICAL FEATURES

Neuromuscular features

- [ ] Muscle pain and fatigue: these are the first features
- [ ] Weakness: this is initially distal
- [ ] Fasciculations: these are often in the lower face
- [ ] Exercise induced cramps
- [ ] Jaw drop
- [ ] Myotonia-like symptoms
- [ ] Split hand syndrome: thenar wasting with relative hypothenar sparing
- [ ] Autonomic dysfunction with impaired sweating
- [ ] Peripheral neuropathy (PN)
- [ ] Postural tremor

Central features

- [ ] Dysphagia and dysarthria
- [ ] Nasal speech
- [ ] Laryngospasm
- [ ] Sleep disturbance
- [ ] Behavioural abnormalities
- [ ] Frontal lobe dementia
- [ ] Eye movement disorders: slow saccades

Endocrine features

- [ ] Diabetes mellitus
- [ ] Androgen resistance with gynaecomastia
- [ ] Sexual dysfunction
- [ ] Testicular atrophy
- [ ] Hypospadias

Cardiac features

- [ ] ST-segment abnormalities
- [ ] Brugada syndrome
- [ ] Dilated cardiomyopathy
- [ ] Sudden cardiac death

Other features

- [ ] Lower urinary tract symptoms (LUTS)
- [ ] Bladder outlet obstruction
- [ ] Reduced bone mass
- [ ] Non-alcoholic fatty liver
- [ ] Groin hernia

Differential diagnosis

- [ ] Myasthenia gravis (MG)
- [ ] Motor neurone disease (MND)
- [ ] Limb girdle muscular dystrophy (LGMD)
- [ ] Facioscapulohumeral muscular dystrophy (FSHD)
- [ ] Hereditary neuronopathy
- [ ] Late-onset Sandhoff disease
- [ ] Polymyositis
- [ ] POEMS syndrome

Synonym

- [ ] SBMA: spinal and bulbar muscular atrophy (SBMA)
- [ ] POEMS: polyneuropathy organomegaly endocrinopathy monoclonal gammopathy and skin changes

KENNEDY DISEASE (SBMA): GENETICS AND MANAGEMENT

Genetics

- ☐ Kennedy disease is caused by an androgen receptor gene mutation
- ☐ This results in CAG repeat expansions
- ☐ There is no genetic anticipation
- ☐ The onset is in adolescence

CAG repeat expansion sizes

- ☐ Normal is 11–33 repeats
- ☐ Pathological is 40–52 repeats
- ☐ Cases have been reported with 68 repeats

Muscle enzymes elevated

- ☐ Creatinine kinase (CK)
- ☐ Aspartate aminotransferase (AST)
- ☐ Alanine aminotransferase (ALT)
- ☐ Lactate dehydrogenase (LDH)

Magnetic resonance imaging (MRI)

- ☐ There is extensive white matter atrophy
- ☐ This is worse frontally

Positron emission tomography (PET) scan

- ☐ There is reduced glucose metabolism
- ☐ This is worse frontally

Blood tests

- ☐ Fasting blood sugar: there is a risk of diabetes
- ☐ Creatinine: this is reduced
- ☐ Cholesterol and LDL: these are elevated

Investigational treatments

- ☐ Insulin-like growth factor-1 (IGF-1) mimetic

Synonym

- ☐ X-linked spinal and bulbar muscular atrophy (SBMA)

POST-POLIO SYNDROME (PPS): CLINICAL FEATURES

Potential causes

- ☐ Aging
- ☐ Persistent virus
- ☐ Stress
- ☐ Overuse
- ☐ Chronic inflammation
- ☐ Genetic predisposition

Pathology

- ☐ There is denervation which is uncompensated by re-innervation

Risk factors

- ☐ Older age
- ☐ Long duration since onset of polio
- ☐ Severity of weakness at time of polio

Clinical features

- ☐ New weakness after stability of at least 15 years
- ☐ Fatigue and functional loss
- ☐ Muscle and joint pain
- ☐ Cold intolerance
- ☐ Hypoventilation
- ☐ Cramps
- ☐ Twitching
- ☐ Restless legs
- ☐ Recurrent falls

Complications

- ☐ Osteoporosis
- ☐ Limb fractures
- ☐ Cognitive complaints
- ☐ Depression

Variant: muscular atrophy (PPMA): features

- ☐ New atrophy with fatigue
- ☐ Joint pain
- ☐ Skeletal deformities

Variant: muscular dysfunction (PPMD): features

- ☐ New muscle weakness
- ☐ Atrophy
- ☐ Pain
- ☐ Fatigue

POST-POLIO SYNDROME (PPS): DIFFERENTIALS AND MANAGEMENT

Differential diagnosis

☐ Hypothyroid myopathy
☐ Myotonic dystrophy

Investigations

☐ Creatinine kinase (CK): this is normal
☐ Electromyogram (EMG): there are chronic neurogenic changes

Fatigue treatment

☐ Amantadine
☐ Modafinil
☐ Pyridostigmine
☐ Methylphenidate

Other treatments

☐ Aerobic muscle training
☐ Monitor respiratory decline
☐ Weight control

CHAPTER 12

Root and plexus disorders

Radiculopathy

RADICULOPATHY: CAUSES

Degenerative causes

- ☐ Herniated nucleus pulposus
- ☐ Degenerative spinal stenosis
- ☐ Spondylolisthesis

Vascular causes

- ☐ Epidural spinal hematoma
- ☐ Subdural spinal hematoma
- ☐ Spinal arteriovenous malformation
- ☐ Vertebral haemangioma
- ☐ Spinal epidural cavernous haemangioma
- ☐ Vertebral dissection
- ☐ Vertebral artery tortuosity
- ☐ Haemorrhagic synovial cysts
- ☐ Ligamentum flavum hematoma
- ☐ Venous varices
- ☐ Epidural venous plexus enlargement: from inferior vena cava obstruction

Extra-spinal causes

- ☐ Occult abdominal or pelvic malignancy
- ☐ Abdominal haematoma
- ☐ Aortic aneurysms
- ☐ Iliac artery aneurysms
- ☐ Obturator artery aneurysms
- ☐ Neurilemoma of the sciatic nerve

Other causes

- ☐ Demyelination
- ☐ Infection
- ☐ Tumour infiltration
- ☐ Root avulsion
- ☐ Nerve root infarction
- ☐ Ganglion cyst of posterior longitudinal ligament
- ☐ Lumbar intervertebral disc cyst
- ☐ Spinal gout tophus
- ☐ Diabetes mellitus
- ☐ Radicular endometriosis

CERVICAL RADICULOPATHY: CLINICAL FEATURES

C2 radiculopathy

- ☐ Headache
- ☐ Pain in the eye and ear

C3-C4 radiculopathy

- ☐ Red ear syndrome
- ☐ Vague neck/trapezius pain

C5 radiculopathy

- ☐ Shoulder pain

C6 radiculopathy

- ☐ Pain in the lateral forearm and first 2 digits
- ☐ It mimics carpal tunnel syndrome (CTS)

C7 radiculopathy

- ☐ Shoulder pain
- ☐ Pain in the posterior forearm and middle digit
- ☐ Pain may also occur in the subscapular region, breast or chest
- ☐ There may be pseudomyotonia: attempt to release grip causing paradoxical finger flexion

C8-T1 radiculopathy

- ☐ Pain in the medial forearm and last 2 digits
- ☐ It may be associated with Horner's syndrome

Provocative tests

- ☐ Spurling's test
- ☐ Valsalva manoeuvre
- ☐ Shoulder abductor sign
- ☐ Upper limb tension sign
- ☐ Neck distraction

DOI: 10.1201/9781003221258-70

CERVICAL RADICULOPATHY: DIFFERENTIAL DIAGNOSIS

Orthopaedic and rheumatological differentials

- ☐ Thoracic outlet syndrome
- ☐ Fibromyalgia
- ☐ Myofascial syndrome
- ☐ Epicondylitis
- ☐ Shoulder abnormalities
- ☐ De Quervain's tenosynovitis

Neurological differentials

- ☐ Brachial plexopathy
- ☐ Syringomyelia
- ☐ Mononeuropathy
- ☐ Vertebral dissection
- ☐ Neck-tongue syndrome
- ☐ Raised intracranial pressure

LUMBOSACRAL RADICULOPATHY: CLINICAL FEATURES

Anatomy of L4-L5 disc prolapse

- ☐ Central prolapse affects the cauda equina
- ☐ Posterolateral prolapse affects the L5 nerve root
- ☐ Very lateral prolapse affects the L4 nerve root
- ☐ Very medial prolapse affects the S1 nerve root

Differentiating features

- ☐ L4 radiculopathy: there is neurogenic hypertrophy of the tibialis anterior muscle
- ☐ L5 radiculopathy: both knee and ankle jerks are spared

Red flags for sinister causes

- ☐ Pain at rest
- ☐ Pain at night
- ☐ Pain not in the L5 or S1 nerve root distribution

LUMBOSACRAL RADICULOPATHY: DIFFERENTIAL DIAGNOSIS

Femoral neuropathy

- ☐ This is a differential of L3/4 radiculopathy
- ☐ Hip adduction is affected in L3/4 radiculopathy

Common peroneal neuropathy

- ☐ This is a differential of L5 radiculopathy
- ☐ Inversion and hip abduction are affected in L5 radiculopathy
- ☐ The ankle jerk is spared in L5 radiculopathy

Hip abnormalities

- ☐ Ischial bursitis
- ☐ Iliopsoas bursitis
- ☐ Greater trochanteric bursitis

Other differential diagnoses

- ☐ Lumbosacral plexopathy
- ☐ Piriformis syndrome
- ☐ Iliopsoas band syndrome
- ☐ Pes anserine bursitis
- ☐ Plantar fasciitis
- ☐ Myofascial pain syndrome
- ☐ Abdominal aortic aneurysm
- ☐ Endometriosis (catamenial sciatica)
- ☐ Nephrolithiasis
- ☐ Raised intracranial pressure (ICP)

LUMBOSACRAL POLYRADICULOPATHY

Compressive causes

- ☐ Degenerative
- ☐ Arachnoiditis
- ☐ Ankylosing spondylitis

Infiltrative causes

- ☐ Neoplastic meningitis
- ☐ Sarcoidosis

Infective causes

- ☐ Lyme neuroborreliosis
- ☐ Herpes simplex virus 2 (HSV2)
- ☐ Cytomegalovirus (CMV) in AIDS
- ☐ Epstein Barr virus (EBV)
- ☐ Syphilis

Other causes

- ☐ Ischaemia
- ☐ Diabetes mellitus
- ☐ Radiation
- ☐ Eosinophilia-myalgia syndrome
- ☐ Raised intracranial pressure
- ☐ Systemic lupus erythematosus
- ☐ Pembrolizumab
- ☐ Ipilimumab

Clinical features

- ☐ Proximal weakness
- ☐ Radicular pain
- ☐ Weakness and denervation: these are in the paraspinal and gluteal muscles

Nerve conduction studies (NCS)

- ☐ Preserved sensory nerve action potentials (SNAPs)
- ☐ Loss of F and H late responses

CAUDA EQUINA SYNDROME (CES)

Causes

- [ ] Disc herniation
- [ ] Epidural haematoma
- [ ] Infections
- [ ] Tumours
- [ ] Metastases
- [ ] Trauma
- [ ] Postsurgical
- [ ] Ankylosing spondylitis
- [ ] Constipation
- [ ] Elsberg syndrome

Clinical features

- [ ] Low back pain
- [ ] Unilateral or bilateral sciatica
- [ ] Lower limb weakness
- [ ] Saddle sensory disturbance
- [ ] Impaired lower limb reflexes
- [ ] Impaired bowel and bladder function
- [ ] Erectile dysfunction
- [ ] Priapism on walking

Treatment

- [ ] Wide laminectomy
- [ ] Extensive decompression with foraminotomy for stenosis

ELSBERG SYNDROME

Pathology

- [ ] This is acute or subacute bilateral lumbosacral radiculitis
- [ ] It is usually associated with lower spinal cord myelitis

Causes

- [ ] Herpes simplex virus type 2 (HSV2) reactivation: this is the classical cause
- [ ] HSV2 primary infection occasionally
- [ ] Varicella zoster virus (VZV) infection
- [ ] West Nile virus
- [ ] Angiostrongylus cantonensis eosinophilic meningitis
- [ ] Human herpes virus (HHV)
- [ ] Epstein-Barr virus (EBV)
- [ ] ECHO virus

Clinical features

- [ ] Preceding sacral herpes infection
- [ ] Fever
- [ ] Headache
- [ ] Photophobia
- [ ] Malaise
- [ ] Urinary retention
- [ ] Constipation
- [ ] Saddle anaesthesia
- [ ] Lower limb weakness
- [ ] Myalgia
- [ ] Impaired lower limb sensation
- [ ] Hyper- or hypo-reflexia
- [ ] Urinary incontinence
- [ ] Diarrhoea
- [ ] Rectal ulcer

Differential diagnosis

- [ ] Spinal stenosis
- [ ] Spinal dural arteriovenous fistula (dAVF)
- [ ] Guillain–Barre syndrome (GBS)
- [ ] Chronic inflammatory demyelinating polyradiculoneuropathy (CIDP)

Magnetic resonance imaging (MRI) spine: features

- [ ] T2-hyperintense signal changes: lumbar or lower thoracic cord
- [ ] Spinal cord enhancement
- [ ] Smooth nerve root enhancement
- [ ] Nerve root thickening

Cerebrospinal fluid (CSF) analysis

- [ ] Cells: there is lymphocytic pleocytosis in about 70% of cases
  - ○ This is neutrophilic in 5%
- [ ] Protein: this is increased
- [ ] Viral polymerase chain reaction (PCR)
- [ ] Intrathecal viral IgG antibody index

Treatment

- [ ] Acyclovir
- [ ] Methylprednisolone

THORACIC OUTLET SYNDROME (TOS): CAUSES AND RISK FACTORS

Risk groups

- ☐ Women
- ☐ Age in the 3rd and 4th decades
- ☐ Violinists
- ☐ Data entry staff
- ☐ Assembly line workers
- ☐ Weightlifters
- ☐ Volleyball players
- ☐ Swimmers

Causes

- ☐ Whiplash
- ☐ Repetitive strain
- ☐ Cervical rib
- ☐ Elongated C7 transverse process
- ☐ Hypertrophic scalene muscle
- ☐ Repetitive work-related injury
- ☐ Anomalous 1st rib
- ☐ Congenital narrow interscalene triangle
- ☐ Fibrous bands

Synonym

- ☐ Gilliat–Sumner hand (neurogenic TOS)

THORACIC OUTLET SYNDROME (TOS): CLINICAL FEATURES

Sensory symptoms

- ☐ Paraesthesias and sensory loss: these involve the medial forearm and fingers
- ☐ The symptoms may be positional

Neck pain radiation territories

- ☐ Neck
- ☐ Ear
- ☐ Face
- ☐ Temple
- ☐ Mandible
- ☐ Occiput
- ☐ Trapezius
- ☐ Chest (pseudoangina)
- ☐ Shoulder
- ☐ Digits

Other features

- ☐ Weakness and fatigue: these are worse with overhead arm elevation
- ☐ Arm numbness: this is on carrying objects with the arm by the side
- ☐ Headache: this is worse on arm elevation and lifting weights
- ☐ Raynaud's phenomenon
- ☐ Tenderness: this is in the scalene, trapezius, and anterior chest muscles

Clinical signs

- ☐ Contralateral neck rotation
- ☐ Head tilt to the opposite side
- ☐ Muscle atrophy in severe cases: worst in the thenar muscles
- ☐ Scalene muscle tenderness
- ☐ Scalene pressure causing radiating symptoms
- ☐ Hand oedema
- ☐ Cold and discoloured hands: this is due to an overactive sympathetic nervous system
- ☐ Reflex sympathetic dystrophy
- ☐ Raynaud's phenomenon
- ☐ Vascular insufficiency
- ☐ Hyperhidrosis
- ☐ Hand dystonia

Differential diagnosis

- ☐ Cervical radiculopathy
- ☐ Brachial plexopathy
- ☐ Carpal tunnel syndrome (CTS)

Synonym

- ☐ Gilliat–Sumner hand (neurogenic TOS)

THORACIC OUTLET SYNDROME (TOS): PROVOCATIVE TESTS

Roos test

- ☐ This is the elevated arm stress test (EAST)
- ☐ The subject repetitively clenches and unclenches the hand for 3 minutes
- ☐ It is performed with the shoulders in 90° abduction and with the elbows flexed at 90°
- ☐ This provokes symptoms

Elvey's test

- ☐ The upper limb is held in 90° abduction and external rotation
- ☐ The wrist is held in extension
- ☐ The head is then tilted to the contralateral side

Morley's sign

- ☐ This is the supraclavicular pressure test
- ☐ It evokes pain in the supraclavicular fossa

Vascular tests

- ☐ Adson's test
- ☐ Wright's test

Other provocative tests

- ☐ Halstead maneuver: the costoclavicular maneuver or exaggerated military brace test
- ☐ Tinel's sign: pressure over the brachial plexus in the neck
- ☐ Spurling's test
- ☐ Upper limb tension test
- ☐ Cyriax release test
- ☐ Diagnostic anterior scalene block

Synonym

- ☐ Gilliat–Sumner hand (neurogenic TOS)

Plexopathy

BRACHIAL PLEXOPATHY: CAUSES

Immune-mediated

- ☐ Neuralgic amyotrophy
- ☐ Idiopathic brachial neuritis (IBN)
- ☐ Idiopathic hypertrophic brachial neuritis
- ☐ Chronic inflammatory demyelinating polyradiculoneuropathy (CIDP)
- ☐ Systemic lupus erythematosus (SLE)
- ☐ Vaccination

Surgical causes

- ☐ Surgical positioning
- ☐ Jugular vein cannulation during coronary artery bypass grafting (CABG)
- ☐ Heart valve replacement
- ☐ Open heart surgery
- ☐ Liver transplantation
- ☐ Robot-assisted trans-axillary thyroidectomy

Genetic causes

- ☐ Hereditary neuralgic amyotrophy
- ☐ Hereditary neuropathy with liability to pressure palsy (HNPP)
- ☐ Adult polyglucosan body disease

Neonatal causes

- ☐ Obstetrical brachial plexus palsy
- ☐ Familial congenital brachial plexus palsy
- ☐ Maternal uterine malformation
- ☐ Congenital varicella syndrome
- ☐ Osteomyelitis of the humerus or cervical vertebrae
- ☐ Exostosis of the first rib
- ☐ Brachial plexus region tumours
- ☐ Intrauterine maladaptation

Vasculitic causes

- ☐ Giant cell arteritis (GCA)
- ☐ Microscopic polyangiitis

Other causes

- ☐ Neurogenic thoracic outlet syndrome (TOS)
- ☐ Radiation therapy
- ☐ Traumatic brachial plexus injury
- ☐ Tumours
- ☐ Paraneoplastic
- ☐ Infective
- ☐ Intravenous heroin injection
- ☐ Bee sting
- ☐ Lightening
- ☐ Subcoracoid bursitis
- ☐ Lipomatosis

BRACHIAL NEURALGIA: RISK FACTORS

Immune diseases

- ☐ Diabetes mellitus
- ☐ Systemic lupus erythematosus (SLE)
- ☐ Polyarteritis nodosa (PAN)

Other risk factors

- ☐ Immunisation
- ☐ Viral infections
- ☐ Surgery
- ☐ Childbirth
- ☐ Hereditary
- ☐ It is usually idiopathic

Synonym

- ☐ Parsonage-Turner syndrome

DOI: 10.1201/9781003221258-71

BRACHIAL NEURALGIA: CLINICAL FEATURES

Commonest affected nerves

- [ ] Long thoracic
- [ ] Suprascapular
- [ ] Axillary
- [ ] Lateral antebrachial cutaneous (LABC)

Nerve involvement outside the plexus

- [ ] Phrenic nerve
- [ ] Recurrent laryngeal nerve
- [ ] Long thoracic nerve
- [ ] Anterior interosseous nerve
- [ ] Facial nerve
- [ ] Lower cranial nerves IX, X, XI and XII
- [ ] Abdominal nerves
- [ ] Lumbosacral plexus

Pain

- [ ] This usually awakens the patient at night or in the early morning
- [ ] It worsens over a few hours
- [ ] It is exacerbated by arm movements
- [ ] It is not aggravated by Valsalva manoeuvres or neck movement
- [ ] It radiates with arm abduction, elevation, or extension

Weakness

- [ ] This occurs in 70% of cases
- [ ] It may be patchy
- [ ] It is bilateral in a third of cases

Arm positioning

- [ ] The shoulder and arm are kept adducted
- [ ] The elbow is kept flexed
- [ ] This is the flexion-adduction sign

Diaphragmatic paralysis

- [ ] This is due to associated phrenic nerve involvement
- [ ] This occurs in about 7% of cases
- [ ] It may be bilateral
- [ ] It presents with exertional dyspnoea and orthopnoea
- [ ] It also causes disturbed sleep and fatigue

Other features

- [ ] Vocal cord paralysis

Variant presentations

- [ ] Pure pain and sensory features
- [ ] Pure motor
- [ ] Involvement of individual sensory nerves

Synonym

- [ ] Parsonage-Turner syndrome

LUMBOSACRAL PLEXOPATHY: CAUSES

Traumatic causes

- [ ] Blunt trauma
- [ ] Radiation injury: causing bilateral plexopathy

Retroperitoneal causes

- [ ] Retroperitoneal haemorrhage
- [ ] Psoas abscess
- [ ] Retroperitoneal fibrosis
- [ ] Pelvic/colonic tumours

Gynaecological and obstetric causes

- [ ] Endometrial: causing catamenial pain
- [ ] Prolonged labour
- [ ] Descending foetal head

Aortic causes

- [ ] Following aortic surgery (ischaemic)
- [ ] Aortic dissection
- [ ] Aorto-iliac bypass graft
- [ ] Common iliac artery aneurysm

Neoplastic causes

- [ ] Neurofibromas
- [ ] Plexiform neurofibroma
- [ ] Schwannomas
- [ ] Malignant peripheral nerve sheath tumours (MPNST)
- [ ] Perineurinoma
- [ ] Rectal
- [ ] Gynaecological
- [ ] Prostatic
- [ ] Bladder
- [ ] Retroperitoneal sarcoma
- [ ] Lymphoma
- [ ] Metastases

Other causes

- [ ] Idiopathic in about a third
- [ ] Diabetic lumbosacral radiculoplexus neuropathy: this is a frequent cause
- [ ] Herpes simplex virus (HSV) infection
- [ ] Heroin

LUMBOSACRAL RADICULOPLEXUS NEUROPATHY

Types

- ☐ Diabetic: Burns-Garlands syndrome
- ☐ Non-diabetic: the features and course are similar

Onset features

- ☐ There is weight loss at onset
- ☐ The onset is focal and asymmetric

Features of pain

- ☐ The onset of the pain is acute or subacute
- ☐ The pain is a severe deep aching and lancinating pain
- ☐ It may be stabbing, burning, or electric-shock like
- ☐ It is worse at night
- ☐ It is located over the anterolateral thigh
- ☐ It may however spread to the rest of the limb
- ☐ It may also spread to the contralateral limb
- ☐ There may be contact allodynia with clothes or bedsheets
- ☐ There may be associated autonomic features

Features of weakness

- ☐ The weakness evolves over weeks
- ☐ It may progress distally and contralaterally
- ☐ There is associated quadriceps muscle wasting
- ☐ The knee jerks are reduced or absent
- ☐ The upper limbs are mildly affected in about half of cases

Outcome

- ☐ The mean recovery time is 3 months
- ☐ It recurs in about 17% of non-diabetic cases

Differential diagnosis

- ☐ Chronic inflammatory demyelinating polyradiculoneuropathy (CIDP)
- ☐ Vasculitis

Electromyogram (EMG) features

- ☐ There is acute denervation
- ☐ This is in the quadriceps, iliopsoas, thigh adductors, and paraspinal muscles

Nerve biopsy features

- ☐ Ischaemia
- ☐ Microvasculitis

Treatment of pain

- ☐ Opioids
- ☐ Tricyclics
- ☐ Antiepileptic drugs (AEDs)

Other treatments

- ☐ Glycaemic control
- ☐ Intravenous (IV) Methylprednisolone 1g/week for 8–16 weeks
- ☐ Intravenous immunoglobulins (IVIg)
- ☐ Plasma exchange (PE)

CHAPTER 13

Peripheral nerve disorders

Neuropathy causes

DEMYELINATING PERIPHERAL NEUROPATHY (PN): CAUSES

Genetic causes

- ☐ Charcot–Marie–Tooth disease (CMT)
- ☐ Hereditary neuropathy with liability to pressure palsy (HNPP)
- ☐ Refsum's disease
- ☐ Metachromatic leukodystrophy (MLD)
- ☐ Cerebrotendinous xanthomatosis (CTX)
- ☐ Tangier disease

Inflammatory causes

- ☐ Guillain–Barre syndrome (GBS)
- ☐ Chronic inflammatory demyelinating polyradiculoneuropathy (CIDP)
- ☐ Multifocal motor neuropathy (MMN)
- ☐ Chronic immune sensorimotor polyradiculopathy (CISMP)

Infective causes

- ☐ Diphtheria
- ☐ Hepatitis C virus (HCV)
- ☐ HIV
- ☐ Lyme neuroborreliosis
- ☐ Leprosy
- ☐ Creutzfeldt-Jakob disease (CJD)

Drug-induced

- ☐ Amiodarone
- ☐ Ipilimumab
- ☐ Pegylated interferon alfa-2a
- ☐ Statins

Other causes

- ☐ Vasculitic neuropathy
- ☐ IgM paraproteinaemic neuropathy
- ☐ Myeloma
- ☐ Amyloidosis
- ☐ Radiculoplexus neuropathy
- ☐ Tetanus toxoid
- ☐ Paraneoplastic

HEREDITARY PERIPHERAL NEUROPATHY (PN): CAUSES

Primary hereditary neuropathies

- ☐ Charcot–Marie–Tooth disease (CMT)
- ☐ Hereditary motor neuropathy (HMN)
- ☐ Hereditary neuropathy with liability to pressure palsy (HNPP)
- ☐ Hereditary sensory and autonomic neuropathy (HSAN)

Mitochondrial neuropathies

- ☐ Mitochondrial neurogastrointestinal encephalopathy (MNGIE)
- ☐ Kearns–Sayre syndrome (KSS)
- ☐ Neuropathy, ataxia, and retinitis pigmentosa (NARP) syndrome
- ☐ Syndrome of sensory axonal neuropathy, dysarthria and ophthalmoplegia (SANDO)

Other hereditary neuropathies

- ☐ Abetalipoproteinaemia
- ☐ Adrenomyeloneuropathy (AMN)
- ☐ Ataxia telangiectasia
- ☐ Cerebrotendinous xanthomatosis (CTX)
- ☐ Cockayne syndrome
- ☐ Erythromelalgia
- ☐ Fabry disease
- ☐ Familial amyloid polyneuropathy (FAP)
- ☐ Friedreich's ataxia (FA)
- ☐ Giant axonal neuropathy
- ☐ Hereditary Vitamin E deficiency
- ☐ Infantile neuroaxonal dystrophy
- ☐ Krabbe disease (globoid cell leukodystrophy)
- ☐ Metachromatic leukodystrophy (MLD)
- ☐ Porphyria
- ☐ Peroxisomal disorders: Refsum's disease and Tangier disease

DOI: 10.1201/9781003221258-73

PERIPHERAL NEUROPATHY (PN) WITH NERVE HYPERTROPHY

Commonest causes

- [ ] Leprosy
- [ ] Charcot–Marie–Tooth disease (CMT)
- [ ] Chronic inflammatory demyelinating polyradiculoneuropathy (CIDP)

Other causes

- [ ] Neurofibromatosis (NF)
- [ ] Refsum's disease
- [ ] Amyloidosis
- [ ] Nerve tumours
- [ ] Perineuroma: this causes localised hypertrophy especially of the brachial plexus
- [ ] Diabetes mellitus
- [ ] Acromegaly
- [ ] Possibly sarcoidosis
- [ ] Chronic cutaneous trauma

Usual affected nerves

- [ ] Supraorbital
- [ ] Greater auricular
- [ ] Cervical
- [ ] Radial
- [ ] Ulnar
- [ ] Median
- [ ] Radial cutaneous
- [ ] Common peroneal
- [ ] Posterior tibial

Investigations

- [ ] Nerve conduction studies (NCS)
- [ ] Magnetic resonance imaging (MRI): this shows nerve hypertrophy and enhancement
- [ ] Genetic testing
- [ ] Cerebrospinal fluid (CSF) analysis
- [ ] Neurography
- [ ] Positron emission tomography (PET) scan: this is to identify malignant causes
- [ ] Neuropathology

PERIPHERAL NEUROPATHY (PN) WITH SPASTICITY

Nutritional causes

- [ ] Vitamin B12 deficiency myeloneuropathy
- [ ] Copper (Cu) deficiency myeloneuropathy
- [ ] Vitamin E deficiency neuropathy

Neurodegenerative causes

- [ ] Friedreich's ataxia (FA)
- [ ] Motor neurone disease (MND)
- [ ] Complicated hereditary spastic paraparesis (HSP)

Systemic causes

- [ ] Adrenomyeloneuropathy (AMN)
- [ ] HIV associated neuropathy (HAN)
- [ ] Severe liver disease

Axonal neuropathy

CHRONIC IDIOPATHIC AXONAL POLYNEUROPATHY (CIAP): DIFFERENTIAL DIAGNOSES

Metabolic

- ☐ Impaired glucose tolerance neuropathy
- ☐ Diabetic neuropathy
- ☐ Hypothyroidism
- ☐ Amyloidosis

Dysimmune

- ☐ Sensory chronic inflammatory demyelinating polyradiculoneuropathy (CIDP)
- ☐ Paraproteinaemic neuropathy

Autoimmune

- ☐ Sjogren's syndrome
- ☐ Anti-sulfatide antibody
- ☐ Vasculitic neuropathy

Nutritional

- ☐ Gluten sensitivity (Coeliac disease)
- ☐ Vitamin B12 deficiency
- ☐ Vitamin B1 deficiency
- ☐ Vitamin B6 deficiency

Miscellaneous

- ☐ Charcot–Marie–Tooth disease (CMT): axonal forms
- ☐ Lyme neuroborreliosis
- ☐ Toxins
- ☐ Alcohol
- ☐ Malignancy
- ☐ Pembrolizumab

SMALL FIBER NEUROPATHY: CAUSES

Genetic

- ☐ Sodium channel gene mutations: Nav 1.7 channelopathy
- ☐ Fabry disease
- ☐ Tangier disease

Toxic

- ☐ Alcohol
- ☐ Paraneoplastic
- ☐ Chemotherapy

Autoimmune

- ☐ Systemic vasculitis: especially Sjogren's syndrome
- ☐ Coeliac disease
- ☐ Psoriasis

Endocrine and metabolic

- ☐ Diabetes mellitus
- ☐ Thyroid disorders
- ☐ Dyslipidemia
- ☐ Obesity
- ☐ Hypertension
- ☐ Mitochondrial diseases
- ☐ Obstructive sleep apnoea (OSA)

Infectious

- ☐ Hepatitis C virus (HCV)
- ☐ HIV
- ☐ Human papilloma virus (HPV) vaccination

Other causes

- ☐ Paraproteinaemia
- ☐ Ehlers Danlos syndrome (EDS)
- ☐ Haemochromatosis
- ☐ Syndromic: with acromesomelia (small hands and feet)
- ☐ Vitamin B12 deficiency
- ☐ Idiopathic: in about a third of cases

DOI: 10.1201/9781003221258-74

DRUG-INDUCED PERIPHERAL NEUROPATHY (PN): CAUSES

Antimicrobials

- ☐ Chloroquine
- ☐ Dapsone
- ☐ Isoniazid
- ☐ Metronidazole
- ☐ Nitrofurantoin
- ☐ Fluoroquinolone

Cardiac drugs

- ☐ Amiodarone
- ☐ Hydralazine

Chemotherapy-induced PN (CIPN)

- ☐ 5 Azacytidine
- ☐ Bortezomib
- ☐ Cytarabine
- ☐ Etoposide
- ☐ Fludaribine
- ☐ Hexamethylmelamine
- ☐ Mitotane
- ☐ Platinum drugs
- ☐ Procarbazine
- ☐ Suramin
- ☐ Taxanes
- ☐ Teniposide
- ☐ Thalidomide
- ☐ VEGF receptor tyrosine kinase inhibitors (VEGFR-TKI)
- ☐ Vinka alkaloids

Anti-programmed death 1 (PD-1) monoclonal antibodies

- ☐ Nivolumab
- ☐ Pembrolizumab

Other drugs

- ☐ β Interferon
- ☐ Colchicine
- ☐ Disulfiram
- ☐ Levodopa
- ☐ Minocycline
- ☐ Perhexiline
- ☐ Phenytoin
- ☐ Propafenone
- ☐ Pyridoxine
- ☐ Statins

Acronym

- ☐ VEGF: vascular endothelial growth factor

SYSTEMIC VASCULITIC PERIPHERAL NEUROPATHY (PN): CAUSES

Primary systemic vasculitis

- ☐ Eosinophilic granulomatosis with polyangiitis (EGPA)
- ☐ Granulomatosis with polyangiitis (GPA)
- ☐ Polyarteritis nodosa (PAN)
- ☐ Microscopic polyangiitis (MPA)
- ☐ Henoch-Schonlein purpura (HSP)
- ☐ Essential cryoglobulinaemia (EC)

Connective tissue diseases

- ☐ Systemic lupus erythematosus (SLE)
- ☐ Sjogren's syndrome
- ☐ Rheumatoid arthritis (RA)

Inflammatory conditions

- ☐ Hypocomplementaemia
- ☐ Inflammatory bowel disease (IBD)
- ☐ Sarcoidosis
- ☐ Cryoglobulinaemia

Infections

- ☐ HIV
- ☐ Hepatitis C virus (HCV)
- ☐ Hepatitis B virus (HBV)
- ☐ Epstein Barr virus (EBV)
- ☐ Cytomegalovirus (CMV)
- ☐ Human T cell leukaemia virus 1 (HTLV1)
- ☐ Lyme neuroborreliosis

Drug-induced

- ☐ Sulphonamides
- ☐ Recreational drugs
- ☐ Minocycline
- ☐ Ipilumab

Other causes

- ☐ Malignancies
- ☐ Diabetic lumbosacral radiculoplexus neuropathy

SENSORY NEURONOPATHY: CAUSES

Autoimmune causes

☐ Sjogren's syndrome
☐ Systemic lupus erythematosus (SLE)
☐ Rheumatoid arthritis (RA)
☐ Autoimmune hepatitis
☐ Gluten sensitivity (Coeliac disease)
☐ Autoimmune autonomic ganglionopathy
☐ Anti-fibroblast growth factor 3 (anti FGFR3) antibodies

Platinum-based chemotherapy

☐ Cisplatin
☐ Oxaliplatin
☐ Carboplatin

Viral infections

☐ HIV
☐ HTLV-1
☐ Epstein Barr virus (EBV)
☐ Varicella zoster virus (VZV)
☐ Measles virus

Hereditary causes

☐ Charcot–Marie–Tooth disease 2B (CMT2B)
☐ Hereditary sensory and autonomic neuropathy (HSAN)

Degenerative causes

☐ Sensory ataxic neuropathy with dysarthria and ophthalmoparesis (SANDO)
☐ Facial onset sensory motor neuronopathy (FOSMN)
☐ Cerebellar ataxia neuropathy vestibular areflexia syndrome (CANVAS)

Paraneoplastic causes

☐ Anti-Hu
☐ Anti CRMP-5

Other causes

☐ Pyridoxine toxicity
☐ Heavy metals
☐ Idiopathic: this accounts for 50% of cases

Synonyms

☐ Dorsal root ganglionopathy (DRG)
☐ Sensory ganglionopathy

Acquired demyelinating neuropathy

GUILLAIN–BARRE SYNDROME (GBS): NON-INFECTIVE TRIGGERS

Vaccination

- ☐ Influenza vaccine: this has the most evidence of risk
- ☐ Rabies vaccine
- ☐ Oral polio vaccine
- ☐ Hepatitis B virus (HBV) vaccine
- ☐ Not tetanus toxoid or mumps measles and rubella (MMR) vaccine

Drug-induced and toxic

- ☐ Loperamide
- ☐ Penicillins
- ☐ Tacrolimus
- ☐ Suramin
- ☐ Streptokinase
- ☐ Thiabendazole
- ☐ Isotretinoin
- ☐ Pravastatin
- ☐ Organophosphates
- ☐ Nivolumab
- ☐ Pembrolizumab
- ☐ Pazopanib
- ☐ Ifosfamide
- ☐ Alemtuzumab

Autoimmune

- ☐ Systemic lupus erythematosus (SLE)
- ☐ Sarcoidosis
- ☐ Crohn's disease
- ☐ Ulcerative colitis
- ☐ Diabetic ketoacidotic coma
- ☐ Hashimoto's thyroiditis
- ☐ Idiopathic thrombocytopaenic purpura (ITP)

Neoplastic

- ☐ Hodgkin's lymphoma
- ☐ Non-Hodgkin's lymphoma
- ☐ Burkitt's lymphoma
- ☐ Gastric adenocarcinoma
- ☐ Chronic lymphatic leukaemia (CLL)
- ☐ Hairy cell leukaemia

Miscellaneous

- ☐ Trauma: this may predispose to immune-mediated neuro-inflammation
- ☐ Surgery: especially orthopaedic and gastrointestinal
- ☐ Heat stroke
- ☐ Severe exertion
- ☐ Snakebite
- ☐ Jellyfish stings
- ☐ Sickle cell disease
- ☐ Temporal arteritis
- ☐ Organ transplantation
- ☐ Childbirth

GUILLAIN–BARRE SYNDROME (GBS): CLINICAL FEATURES

Peripheral features

- ☐ Progressive weakness: this is predominantly proximal
- ☐ Hypotonia
- ☐ Reduced reflexes
- ☐ Facial weakness
- ☐ Ophthalmoplegia
- ☐ Severe fatigue: in about 80% of cases
- ☐ Autonomic dysfunction

Pain

- ☐ Moderate to severe pain is common early
- ☐ It is a deep ache in the back and the leg
- ☐ Pain is more frequent in children
- ☐ Dysaesthetic pain may persist after recovery

Psychiatric features

- ☐ Vivid dreams
- ☐ Delusions
- ☐ Illusions
- ☐ Hallucinations: these are usually hypnagogic (before falling asleep)

Cranial nerve features

- ☐ Loss of taste
- ☐ Bilateral vocal cord paralysis
- ☐ Exophthalmos
- ☐ Lid lag
- ☐ Bilateral hearing loss

Other features

- ☐ Headache and papilloedema
  - ○ These result from high protein impairing the flow of cerebrospinal fluid (CSF)
- ☐ Widespread fasciculations
- ☐ Tongue fasciculations
- ☐ Neck stiffness
- ☐ Spinal hyperextension
- ☐ Ballism
- ☐ Horner's syndrome
- ☐ Urinary disturbance
- ☐ Supernumerary phantom limbs (SPLs)
- ☐ Hyperreflexia: from involvement of the corticospinal tracts

Red flags against GBS

- ☐ Fever at onset
- ☐ Sharp sensory level
- ☐ Marked asymmetry
- ☐ Persistent bowel and bladder symptoms or at onset
- ☐ Severe sensory signs
- ☐ Progression beyond 4 weeks
- ☐ >50 cells or polymorphs in the cerebrospinal fluid (CSF)

DOI: 10.1201/9781003221258-75

GUILLAIN–BARRE SYNDROME (GBS): COMPLICATIONS

Neurological complications

- ☐ Posterior reversible leukoencephalopathy syndrome (PRES)
  - ○ This results from dysautonomia or IVIg
- ☐ Rhabdomyolysis
- ☐ Restless legs syndrome (RLS)
- ☐ Propriospinal myoclonus

Systemic complications

- ☐ Respiratory failure
- ☐ Dysphagia
- ☐ Labile blood pressure
- ☐ Arrhythmias
- ☐ Syndrome of inappropriate antidiuretic hormone secretion (SIADH)
- ☐ Pneumonia
- ☐ Acute heart failure: from neurogenic cardiac injury
- ☐ Post-traumatic stress disorder
- ☐ Hyper-catabolism

GUILLAIN–BARRE SYNDROME (GBS): DIFFERENTIAL DIAGNOSES

Severe neuropathies

- ☐ Chronic inflammatory demyelinating polyradiculoneuropathy (CIDP)
- ☐ Critical illness polyneuropathy
- ☐ Diphtheritic polyneuropathy
- ☐ Paraneoplastic peripheral neuropathy
- ☐ Acute Beriberi

Infective neuropathies

- ☐ West Nile virus paralysis: this presents with a GBS phenotype in 13% of cases
- ☐ Acute poliomyelitis
- ☐ Lyme neuroborreliosis
- ☐ Botulism
- ☐ HIV seroconversion
- ☐ Enterovirus D68 (EV-D68)

Drug-induced demyelinating neuropathies

- ☐ Tetanus toxoid
- ☐ Ipilimumab
- ☐ Nivolumab
- ☐ Pegylated interferon alfa-2a

Other neuromuscular disorders

- ☐ Periodic paralysis
- ☐ Myasthenia gravis (MG)
- ☐ Inflammatory myopathy

Other differentials

- ☐ Acute myelopathy
- ☐ Porphyria
- ☐ Toxic
- ☐ Lymphoma

GUILLAIN–BARRE SYNDROME (GBS): TREATMENT

Monitoring for complications
- [ ] Vital capacity
- [ ] Blood pressure
- [ ] Continuous electrocardiogram (ECG)
- [ ] Swallowing
- [ ] Autonomic function

Immune treatments
- [ ] Intravenous immunoglobulins (IVIg) and plasma exchange (PE) have similar efficacy
- [ ] IVIg after PE does not confer additional benefit
- [ ] Avoid steroids: they may slow the recovery from GBS
- [ ] IV Methylprednisolone with IVIg may quicken recovery but does not alter the outcome

Supportive treatment
- [ ] Deep vein thrombosis (DVT) prophylaxis
- [ ] Pain control: Carbamazepine or Gabapentin
- [ ] Avoid immunisations in the acute phase
- [ ] Routine future vaccinations: these do not cause GBS relapse

Cardiorespiratory support
- [ ] Cardioactive drugs
- [ ] Pacemaker
- [ ] Ventilation
- [ ] Tracheostomy: this is considered after 2 weeks

Multidisciplinary rehabilitation
- [ ] Exercise program for fatigue
- [ ] Nursing to prevent pressure sores
- [ ] Oral toileting
- [ ] Nutritional support
- [ ] Enteral or parenteral feeding
- [ ] Speech and language therapy
- [ ] Physiotherapy
- [ ] Occupational therapy
- [ ] Psychological support

CIDP: CLINICAL FEATURES

Typical clinical features
- [ ] Prominent proximal motor weakness
- [ ] Generalised sensory impairment: this is initially in the upper limbs
- [ ] Generalised areflexia
- [ ] Cranial nerve involvement
- [ ] Marked ataxia
- [ ] Pain: this may be the main presenting feature

Nerve hypertrophy
- [ ] Peripheral nerves
- [ ] Trigeminal nerve
- [ ] Oculomotor nerve

Nerve root hypertrophy
- [ ] This is usually lumbar but it may be cervical
- [ ] It may result in canal stenosis
- [ ] It may present with initial back pain
- [ ] Plexus hypertrophy may occur

Pseudotumour syndrome
- [ ] This is CIDP presenting with headache and papilloedema
- [ ] It is associated with high cerebrospinal fluid (CSF) protein
- [ ] It is responsive to steroids

Unusual CIDP presentations
- [ ] Upper limb onset of weakness: in 10% of cases
- [ ] Sensory ataxic form
- [ ] Pure motor form
- [ ] Superimposed mononeuropathies
- [ ] Presentation with phrenic nerve palsy
- [ ] Tremor
- [ ] Acute onset CIDP (A-CIDP)
- [ ] Tonic pupil
- [ ] Presentation with tumefactive demyelination
- [ ] Subclinical central nervous system presentation: this may occur in up to a third of cases
- [ ] Relapsing presentation mimicking relapsing remitting multiple sclerosis (RRMS)

Acronym
- [ ] CIDP: chronic inflammatory demyelinating polyradiculoneuropathy

CIDP: ASSOCIATED DISORDERS

Paraproteinaemia

- ☐ Monoclonal gammopathy
- ☐ Anti MAG antibody syndrome
- ☐ POEMS syndrome
- ☐ CANOMAD
- ☐ Waldenstrom's macroglobulinaemia
- ☐ Castleman's disease

Infections

- ☐ HIV
- ☐ Hepatitis B (HBV)
- ☐ Hepatitis C (HCV)

Inflammatory conditions

- ☐ Sarcoidosis
- ☐ Inflammatory bowel disease (IBD)
- ☐ Nephrotic syndrome
- ☐ Graft versus host disease (GVHD)
- ☐ Organ transplantation

Diabetes mellitus

- ☐ Consider CIDP in well-controlled diabetics with neuropathy
- ☐ The risk may be related to GFAP and S-100 acting as Schwann cell autoantigens
- ☐ Benefit of intravenous immunoglobulins (IVIG) is conflicting

Drug triggers

- ☐ Nivolumab
- ☐ Pembrolizumab
- ☐ Etanercept
- ☐ Infliximab
- ☐ Adalimumab
- ☐ Interferonα
- ☐ Procainamide

Other associations

- ☐ Systemic lupus erythematosus (SLE)
- ☐ Mercury toxicity
- ☐ Cancer
- ☐ CIDP-associated autoantibodies

Acronyms

- ☐ CIDP: chronic inflammatory demyelinating polyradiculoneuropathy
- ☐ POEMS: Polyneuropathy organomegaly endocrinopathy M-protein skin changes
- ☐ CANOMAD: Chronic ataxic neuropathy ophthalmoplegia IgM paraprotein cold agglutinins disialosyl antibodies

CIDP: INVESTIGATIONS

Nerve conduction studies (NCS): features

- ☐ Prolonged distal motor latency
- ☐ Reduced velocities
- ☐ Prolonged F wave latency
- ☐ Temporal dispersion
- ☐ Conduction block
- ☐ Slow motor nerve conduction velocity (mNCV): this is <80% of the lower limit
- ☐ Sensory NCS is not sensitive

Cerebrospinal fluid (CSF): features

- ☐ This shows albumino-cytologic dissociation: increased protein with relatively low cell count
- ☐ CSF cells >10 may be seen with HIV, Lyme neuroborreliosis, sarcoidosis, and lymphoma
- ☐ CSF sphingomyelin is an emerging marker
- ☐ The CSF is normal in 10% of cases

Nerve ultrasound

- ☐ This may show nerve, root, or plexus hypertrophy
- ☐ It may identify treatable cases even when NCS shows no inflammation

Autoantibodies

- ☐ Anti MAG antibodies
- ☐ Neurofascin 155 (NF155)
- ☐ Contactin-1 (CNTN1)
- ☐ Contactin-associated protein 1 (Caspr 1)
- ☐ LM-1 antibodies

Other investigations

- ☐ Magnetic resonance imaging (MRI)
  - ○ To assess lumbosacral and sciatic nerve hypertrophy
- ☐ Somatosensory evoked potentials (SSEPs)
  - ○ To assess nerve roots inaccessible to NCS
- ☐ Nerve biopsy
  - ○ In diagnostic doubt and to assess progression despite treatment

Emerging investigation

- ☐ Serum neurofilament (sNfL): this is increased in a third of cases

Acronym

- ☐ CIDP: chronic inflammatory demyelinating polyradiculoneuropathy

CIDP TREATMENT: IVIG

Benefits

- ☐ This is usually used as second line treatment but it is effective as first line
- ☐ It has a similar benefit as plasma exchange (PE)
- ☐ It is effective in 50% of steroid non-responders
- ☐ Reconsider the diagnosis if there is no response to both steroids and IVIg
- ☐ Plasma exchange and immunosuppression often fail if steroids and IVIg have both failed

Indications for first line use of IVIg: ahead of steroids

- ☐ Pure motor CIDP: this may deteriorate on steroids
- ☐ Acute or severe presentation
- ☐ When steroids are contraindicated
- ☐ When pregnancy is planned

Protocol

- ☐ The typical dose is 0.4g/kg/day for 5 days
- ☐ A second course is given 6 weeks after
- ☐ A maintenance dose of 1g/kg every three weeks is effective
- ☐ Longer term follow-up is 4- to 6-monthly

Response

- ☐ Maximum response is at 3 weeks
- ☐ Review treatment response at 4 weeks

Predictors of poor response

- ☐ Presence of pain
- ☐ Association with other autoimmune diseases
- ☐ Difference in severity of weakness between the upper and lower limbs
- ☐ Absent anti MAG antibodies
- ☐ Positive antibodies to neurofascin 155 (NF155)

Subcutaneous immunoglobulins (SCIG)

- ☐ SCIG is as effective as IVIg
- ☐ It is safer than IVIg
- ☐ It improves patients' quality of life

Acronym

- ☐ IVIg: intravenous immunoglobulins (IVIg)
- ☐ CIDP: chronic inflammatory demyelinating polyradiculoneuropathy

CIDP TREATMENT: IMMUNOSUPPRESSANTS

Steroids: benefits

- ☐ These are first line treatments if there are no contraindications
- ☐ They provide long term remission in a quarter of patients

Steroids: options

- ☐ Pulsed Dexamethasone: one or two courses
  - ○ This results in faster improvement, fewer relapses, and less adverse events
- ☐ Prednisolone
  - ○ This is administered daily for 8 months
- ☐ IV Methylprednisolone 500 mg daily for 4 days consecutively
  - ○ This is administered every month for 6 months

Rituximab

- ☐ Rituximab is effective in 70% of patients who fail conventional treatments
- ☐ It is beneficial in patients with paranodal antibodies
- ☐ It may however not reduce IVIg requirement in refractory cases

Treatments with poor evidence

- ☐ Azathioprine
- ☐ Mycophenolate mofetil
- ☐ Methotrexate

Investigational treatments

- ☐ Bortezomib
- ☐ Stem cell transplantation

Scoring systems

- ☐ Medical research council (MRC) sum score
- ☐ Inflammatory neuropathy cause and treatment (INCAT) sensory sum score
- ☐ INCAT overall disability sum score
- ☐ Inflammatory Neuropathy-Rasch-Built Overall Disability Scale (I-RODS)

Monitoring

- ☐ Neurophysiological follow-up may be sufficient for mild symptoms

Acronym

- ☐ CIDP: chronic inflammatory demyelinating polyradiculoneuropathy

MULTIFOCAL MOTOR NEUROPATHY (MMN): CLINICAL FEATURES

Main clinical features

- ☐ Upper limb onset weakness
- ☐ Wrist drop
- ☐ Weak grip
- ☐ Foot drop
- ☐ Frequent cramps
- ☐ Twitching
- ☐ Differential finger extension weakness
- ☐ Cold paresis: weakness is worse in the cold

Rarer clinical features

- ☐ Acute onset
- ☐ Myokymia
- ☐ Fatigue: due to activity-related conduction block
- ☐ Increased reflexes: this may occur in 8% of cases
- ☐ Minor vibration loss: this occurs in a fifth of cases
- ☐ Pseudodystonia
- ☐ Muscle hypertrophy: especially biceps and trapezius
- ☐ Hamartomas: associated with PTEN mutations
- ☐ Cranial nerve involvement
- ☐ Phrenic nerve involvement
- ☐ Bilateral long thoracic nerve involvement

Reported MMN risk factors

- ☐ The HLA-DRB1*15 haplotype: this occurs frequently
- ☐ Adalimumab
- ☐ Dengue virus infection

Monofocal motor neuropathy variant

- ☐ Weakness is restricted to one nerve
- ☐ There is partial motor conduction block
- ☐ It may be caused by Adalimumab
- ☐ It may present as cramps fasciculation syndrome
- ☐ There are no sensory features
- ☐ It is responsive to intravenous immunoglobulins (IVIg)

Differential diagnosis: motor neurone disease (MND)

- ☐ MMN is misdiagnosed as MND in 1/3 of patients
- ☐ Peripheral nerve imaging may help differentiate
- ☐ Cross sectional area (CSA) of the median and ulnar nerves are larger in MMN

Differential diagnosis: others

- ☐ Lewis Sumner syndrome (MADSAM)

Hereditary neuropathies

CHARCOT–MARIE–TOOTH DISEASE 1A (CMT1A)

Genetics

- ☐ CMT is caused by a 1.4-Mb peripheral myelin protein 22 (PMP22) gene duplication
- ☐ This is on chromosome 17
- ☐ PMP22 point mutation is also causative
- ☐ Gene dosage correlates with phenotype
- ☐ Onset is in the first or second decade
- ☐ Early onset forms are severe

Main neurological features

- ☐ Muscle weakness: this is slowly progressive and symmetrical
- ☐ Muscle atrophy: this starts in the peroneal and distal leg muscles
- ☐ Pes cavus
- ☐ Hammer toes
- ☐ Hyporeflexia
- ☐ Calf pseudohypertrophy: this is asymmetric
- ☐ Nerve hypertrophy: this occurs in some cases
- ☐ Knee bob sign: the knees bob up and down on standing
  - ○ It is a sign of ankle plantar flexion weakness

Other neurological features

- ☐ Hearing loss
- ☐ Phrenic nerve palsy
- ☐ Oculomotor nerve palsy: this may be unilateral
- ☐ Cord compression: this is due to nerve root hypertrophy
- ☐ Cauda equina syndrome (CES): this is due to nerve root hypertrophy
- ☐ Essential tremor (Roussy-Levy syndrome)
- ☐ Cognitive impairment: this occurs in 70% of cases
  - ○ It is associated with reduced brain white matter volume
- ☐ Restless legs syndrome (RLS): this is present in about 40% of cases
- ☐ Periodic limb movements of sleep (PLMS): this occurs in about 40% of cases
- ☐ Obstructive sleep apnoea: this develops in about a third of cases

Abnormal gait patterns

- ☐ Pseudo-normal pattern
- ☐ Foot drop only
- ☐ Foot drop and push-off deficit
- ☐ Steppage: there is augmented hip and knee flexion
- ☐ Vaulting: ankle plantar flexion occurs mid-stance

Overlap features

- ☐ Hereditary motor neuropathy (HMN)
- ☐ Hereditary sensory and autonomic neuropathy (HSAN)
- ☐ Hereditary spastic paraparesis (HSP)

CHARCOT–MARIE–TOOTH DISEASE 2A (CMT2A)

Genetics and epidemiology

- ☐ This is mainly caused by mitofusin 2 (MFN2) gene mutations
- ☐ The gene is on chromosome 1p
- ☐ It may also be caused by MPZ mutations

Onset phenotypes

- ☐ Early onset phenotype: this starts before the age of 5 years
  - ○ It is a severe phenotype with distal weakness
- ☐ Later onset phenotype: this starts in adolescence
  - ○ It is a milder phenotype

Clinical features

- ☐ Optic atrophy: this may partially recover with time
- ☐ Scoliosis
- ☐ Vocal cord paralysis
- ☐ Macrocephaly
- ☐ Hyperreflexia
- ☐ Contractures
- ☐ Leg pain
- ☐ Cerebral involvement: this is especially in mild phenotypes
- ☐ Argyll Robertson pupil
- ☐ Deafness
- ☐ Dysphagia

Occasional features

- ☐ Asymmetry
- ☐ Brisk reflexes
- ☐ Extensor planter response
- ☐ Calf hypertrophy
- ☐ Hand tremor: this develops in about 30% of cases

Magnetic resonance imaging (MRI)

- ☐ The brain MRI is abnormal in about 40% of early-onset cases
- ☐ It shows periventricular and subcortical white matter high signal changes
- ☐ These are confluent and involve large areas
- ☐ They may also involve the grey matter
- ☐ They may manifest as cavitating leukodystrophy
- ☐ Magnetic resonance spectroscopy (MRS) is also abnormal

DOI: 10.1201/9781003221258-76

FAMILIAL TTR AMYLOID POLYNEUROPATHY (FAP TTR): CLINICAL FEATURES

Genetics

- ☐ TTR is the commonest cause of familial amyloid polyneuropathy
- ☐ Transmission is autosomal dominant with possible anticipation
- ☐ There are more than 100 TTR mutations
- ☐ The Val30Met mutation is the commonest mutation
- ☐ 30% have a non-familial presentation

Peripheral neuropathy (PN) patterns

- ☐ Length-dependent sensorimotor neuropathy (PN)
  - ○ This is the most frequent pattern
  - ○ There is near-simultaneous upper and lower limb involvement
- ☐ Predominantly motor neuropathy
  - ○ This mimics motor neuron disease (MND)
- ☐ Autonomic neuropathy
- ☐ Carpal tunnel syndrome (CTS)
- ☐ Sensory neuropathy
- ☐ Pure dysautonomia
- ☐ Demyelinating peripheral neuropathy

Cardiomyopathy

- ☐ Conduction block
- ☐ Thick ventricles
- ☐ Heart failure

Ophthalmic features

- ☐ Vitreous opacity
- ☐ Dry eyes
- ☐ Glaucoma
- ☐ Pupillary changes
- ☐ Scalloped pupils (dyscoria)
- ☐ Conjunctival lymphangiectasia

Other features

- ☐ Anaemia
- ☐ Hoarseness
- ☐ Reduced skin temperature
- ☐ Gastrointestinal impairment
- ☐ Nephropathy
- ☐ Leptomeningeal amyloidosis in advanced stages

Red flag indicators of FAP

- ☐ Family history of neuropathy
- ☐ Autonomic dysfunction
- ☐ Cardiac hypertrophy
- ☐ Gastrointestinal symptoms
- ☐ Unexplained weight loss
- ☐ Carpal tunnel syndrome (CTS)
- ☐ Renal impairment
- ☐ Ocular involvement

Mean duration to death

- ☐ This is about 7 years in adult onset forms
- ☐ It is 10–12 years in the classic forms

FAMILIAL TTR AMYLOID POLYNEUROPATHY (FAP TTR): TREATMENT

Liver transplantation: options

- ☐ Combined kidney-liver transplant
- ☐ Combined heart-liver transplant
- ☐ Domino liver transplant

Tafamidis

- ☐ Tafamidis stabilizes TTR
- ☐ It slows the progression of peripheral neuropathy
- ☐ Outcomes are better when it is started early

Diflunisal

- ☐ Diflunisal stabilises the TTR tetramer
- ☐ It increases TTR levels
- ☐ It inhibits progression of peripheral neuropathy
- ☐ It may cause renal impairment and thrombocytopaenia

Inotersen

- ☐ Inotersen is an antisense oligonucleotide inhibitor of TTR
- ☐ It prevents TTR synthesis in the liver
- ☐ It improves neuropathy
- ☐ It may cause glomerulonephritis and thrombocytopenia

Patisiran

- ☐ Patisiran is an RNA interference therapeutic agent
- ☐ It reduces TTR levels
- ☐ It improves peripheral neuropathy
- ☐ It increases the risk of respiratory tract infections

Neuropathic treatments

- ☐ Gabapentin
- ☐ Pregabalin
- ☐ Duloxetine
- ☐ Tricyclics

Other symptomatic treatments

- ☐ Orthostatic hypotension: Midodrine
- ☐ Gastroparesis: Domperidone
- ☐ Arrhythmias: pacemaker
- ☐ Cardiac failure: diuretics
- ☐ Ocular amyloidosis: vitrectomy
- ☐ Glaucoma: trabeculectomy

Pre-symptomatic management

- ☐ Genetic testing of at-risk individuals
- ☐ Clinical follow up of genetic carriers
- ☐ Early treatment at symptom onset

Investigational treatments

- ☐ Anti-SAP monoclonal antibody
- ☐ Doxycycline-ursodeoxycholic acid
- ☐ Antisense oligonucleotides

HNPP: CLINICAL FEATURES

Genetics

- [ ] HNPP is caused by PMP22 gene deletions on chromosome 17p
- [ ] The transmission is autosomal dominant
- [ ] The onset is in the 2nd to 3rd decades

Clinical features

- [ ] HNPP causes recurrent mononeuropathies
- [ ] There are episodes of painless weakness
- [ ] The symptoms are triggered by minor nerve compression
- [ ] Full recovery occurs in 50% of episodes

Frequently affected peripheral nerves

- [ ] Peroneal
- [ ] Ulnar
- [ ] Brachial plexus
- [ ] Radial
- [ ] Median

Occasionally affected cranial nerves

- [ ] Facial
- [ ] Trigeminal
- [ ] Hypoglossal
- [ ] Vagus: recurrent laryngeal branch

HNPP phenotypes

- [ ] Asymptomatic
- [ ] Recurrent short term positional sensory symptoms
- [ ] Progressive mononeuropathy
- [ ] Chronic sensory neuropathy
- [ ] Chronic sensorimotor neuropathy
- [ ] Chronic inflammatory demyelinating polyneuropathy-like
- [ ] Recurrent subacute polyneuropathy
- [ ] Subacute quadriparesis
- [ ] Scapuloperoneal phenotype
- [ ] Charcot–Marie–Tooth (CMT) disease phenotype
  - ○ Pes cavus develops in about half of HNPP cases

Unusual HNPP presentations

- [ ] Executive dysfunction
- [ ] Fulminant cases: provoked by physical training
- [ ] Recurrent dysphagia
- [ ] Prominent respiratory failure
- [ ] Subclinical central nervous system (CNS) involvement

Acronym

- [ ] HNPP: hereditary neuropathy with liability to pressure palsies

Paraproteinaemic neuropathy

IGG AND IGA MGUS PARAPROTEINAEMIC NEUROPATHY

Criteria for MGUS

- [ ] Monoclonal component ≤30g/L
- [ ] Bence Jones protein (BJP) ≤1g/24 hours
- [ ] <10% bone marrow infiltration
- [ ] No lytic bone lesions
- [ ] No evolution to myeloma or other lymphoproliferative disease within 12 months
- [ ] No anaemia
- [ ] No hypercalcaemia
- [ ] No chronic renal failure

MGUS neuropathy types

- [ ] Demyelinating MGUS neuropathy type: this is treated as CIDP
- [ ] Pure or predominantly axonal neuropathy type: this is typically mild and slowly progressive
- [ ] Distal acquired demyelinating sensory (DADS) phenotype

Treatment: limited evidence

- [ ] Plasma exchange (PE)
- [ ] Cyclophosphamide
- [ ] Prednisolone
- [ ] Intravenous immunoglobulins (IVIg)

Acronyms

- [ ] CIDP: Chronic inflammatory demyelinating polyradiculoneuropathy
- [ ] MGUS: Monoclonal gammopathy of uncertain significance

IGM ANTI-MAG PARAPROTEINAEMIC NEUROPATHY: CLINICAL FEATURES

Epidemiology

- [ ] Anti MAG antibodies are present in 50% of IgM neuropathy
- [ ] About 70% of these have MGUS
- [ ] The mean onset age is just over 60 years: the range is about 25–90 years
- [ ] It usually affects men with no other associated diseases
- [ ] There is no M protein in about 6% of cases
- [ ] There may be associated anti SGPG and anti-ganglioside antibodies

Risk factors

- [ ] Myeloma
- [ ] Plasmacytoma
- [ ] Waldenstrom's macroglobulinaemia
- [ ] Monoclonal gammopathy of uncertain significance (MGUS)
- [ ] Amyloidosis: associated with free light chains
- [ ] Myeloid differentiation factor 88 (MYD88) gene mutation:
  - ○ This is present in about 50% of IgM MGUS cases

Clinical presentation

- [ ] It usually presents as distal acquired demyelinating sensory (DADS)
- [ ] This is a large fiber sensory demyelinating neuropathy
- [ ] It may also be mixed axonal and demyelinating

Typical clinical features

- [ ] Tremor
- [ ] Sensory ataxia
- [ ] Paraesthesias
- [ ] Mild or absent distal weakness
- [ ] Cerebellar ataxia

Atypical clinical features

- [ ] Acute or chronic sensorimotor polyradiculoneuropathies
- [ ] Asymmetric neuropathy
- [ ] Multifocal neuropathy

Differential diagnosis of IgM without anti MAG antibody

- [ ] Cryoglobulinaemia
- [ ] Waldenstrom's macroglobulinaemia
- [ ] Amyloidosis
- [ ] Lymphoma

Nerve conduction studies (NCS)

- [ ] Conduction block (CB) is less frequent than in typical CIDP
- [ ] There is distal accentuation of slowing

DOI: 10.1201/9781003221258-77

Outcome

- ☐ It follows a chronic indolent course
- ☐ About a fifth of cases are severely disabled

Acronyms

- ☐ CIDP: chronic inflammatory demyelinating polyradiculoneuropathy
- ☐ MAG: myelin associated glycoprotein
- ☐ MGUS: monoclonal gammopathy of undetermined significance (MGUS)

CANOMAD PARAPROTEINAEMIC NEUROPATHY

Demographics

- ☐ This usually affects men in their mid-50's

Clinical features

- ☐ Severe sensory ataxic neuropathy
- ☐ Pseudoathetosis
- ☐ Areflexia
- ☐ Normal limb power
- ☐ Oculomotor and bulbar weakness
- ☐ Acral and perioral paraesthesia
- ☐ Bilateral abducens nerve palsy

Blood tests

- ☐ IgM
- ☐ Anti GD1b
- ☐ Anti GD3
- ☐ Anti GT1b
- ☐ Anti GQ1b

Magnetic resonance imaging (MRI)

- ☐ Brain: ischaemia, demyelination, or atrophy
- ☐ Spine: nerve root hypertrophy

Nerve conduction studies (NCS)

- ☐ Mixed demyelinating and axonal pattern
- ☐ Reduced or absent sensory responses

Nerve biopsy

- ☐ There is near complete loss of myelinated axons
- ☐ Smaller axons are preserved

Differential diagnosis

- ☐ Miller Fisher syndrome (MFS)
- ☐ Brainstem vascular pathology
- ☐ Brainstem demyelination

Treatment

- ☐ Intravenous immunoglobulin (IVIg)
- ☐ Plasma exchange (PE)
- ☐ Rituximab: this is the most effective treatment

Acronym

- ☐ CANOMAD: Chronic ataxic neuropathy ophthalmoplegia IgM paraprotein cold agglutinins disialosyl antibodies

PARAPROTEINAEMIC NEUROPATHY: MANAGEMENT

General investigations

- ☐ Routine bloods
- ☐ Immunoglobulin concentrations: IgG, IgA, IgM
- ☐ Serum protein immunofixation (IF)
- ☐ Serum plasma electrophoresis (SPEP)
- ☐ Bence Jones protein
- ☐ Cryoglobulins
- ☐ C reactive protein (CRP)
- ☐ Lactic dehydrogenase (LDH)
- ☐ Bone marrow aspiration

Conditional general investigations

- ☐ Free light chains: if IF and SPEP are normal
- ☐ Anti MAG antibodies: if IgM is raised
- ☐ Hepatitis C virus (HCV): if cryoglobulinaemia is present
- ☐ TTR gene mutation: if amyloid is present

Neurological investigations

- ☐ Nerve conduction studies (NCS)
- ☐ Cerebrospinal fluid (CSF)
- ☐ Nerve biopsy

Radiological investigations

- ☐ Computed tomography (CT): chest, abdomen, and pelvis
- ☐ X-ray skeletal survey
- ☐ Magnetic resonance imaging (MRI) skeletal survey

Treatment

- ☐ Local irradiation of isolated plasmacytoma
- ☐ Resection of isolated plasmacytoma
- ☐ Melphalan ± steroids for POEMS syndrome

Acronym

- ☐ CIDP: chronic inflammatory demyelinating polyradiculoneuropathy

Mononeuropathies

CARPAL TUNNEL SYNDROME (CTS): CAUSES AND RISK FACTORS

Causes

- ☐ Arthritis
- ☐ Flexor tenosynovitis
- ☐ Sarcoidosis
- ☐ Amyloidosis
- ☐ Hereditary neuropathy with liability to pressure palsy (HNPP)
- ☐ Trauma
- ☐ Cysts
- ☐ Lipomas
- ☐ Diabetes mellitus
- ☐ Hypothyroidism
- ☐ Connective tissue diseases

Individual risk factors

- ☐ Genetic predisposition
- ☐ Obesity: in young people
- ☐ Pregnancy
- ☐ Menopause
- ☐ Fluid retention states
- ☐ Thenar atrophy
- ☐ Smoking
- ☐ Square shaped wrist

Occupational risk factors

- ☐ Typing
- ☐ Hand-help powered vibratory tools
- ☐ Factory assembly work
- ☐ Food processing and packaging
- ☐ Forestry workers
- ☐ Quarry drillers
- ☐ Rock drillers
- ☐ Chainsaw workers
- ☐ Electricity assembly workers
- ☐ Grocery cashiers
- ☐ Textile and garment workers
- ☐ Dental hygienists

CARPAL TUNNEL SYNDROME (CTS): CLINICAL FEATURES

Pain and paraesthesias

- ☐ These involve the lateral 3 and a half fingers
- ☐ They may involve the whole hand
- ☐ They may radiate up to shoulder
- ☐ They often wake the patient up from sleep
- ☐ They are worse with the arms raised
- ☐ They exacerbate with hand use
- ☐ They are relieved by flicking the hand: the flick sign

Other symptoms

- ☐ Sensation of a swollen hand
- ☐ Clumsiness
- ☐ Cold sensitivity
- ☐ Isolated third digit numbness

Clinical signs

- ☐ Weakness: especially of the abductor pollicis brevis (APB)
- ☐ Sensory impairment: in the median nerve distribution
- ☐ Thenar muscle atrophy
- ☐ Volar wrist swelling: hot dog shaped

Provocative manoeuvres

- ☐ Hand elevation
- ☐ Tinel's test: wrist percussion
- ☐ Phalen's test: wrist flexion
- ☐ Closed fist
- ☐ Pressure provocation
- ☐ Carpal compression test

Differential diagnosis

- ☐ Ulnar neuropathy: the signs of CTS are on the ulnar side in 37% of cases
- ☐ Tendonitis
- ☐ Generalised peripheral neuropathy (PN)
- ☐ Motor neurone disease (MND)
- ☐ Syringomyelia
- ☐ Thumb metacarpophalangeal (MCP) joint arthritis
- ☐ Pronator teres syndrome
- ☐ Anterior interosseous nerve (AIN) syndrome
- ☐ Cervical radiculopathy
- ☐ Brachial plexopathy
- ☐ Thoracic outlet syndrome
- ☐ Multiple sclerosis (MS)
- ☐ Stroke

DOI: 10.1201/9781003221258-78

CUBITAL TUNNEL SYNDROME: CAUSES AND RISK FACTORS

Occupational risks

- ☐ Truck drivers
- ☐ Baseball pitchers
- ☐ Repetitive elbow flexion and extension
- ☐ Constant tool-holding position
- ☐ Vibrating tool use

Habitual risk factors

- ☐ Sleeping in foetal position
- ☐ Sleeping prone with hands under the pillow
- ☐ Prolonged elbow flexion
- ☐ Habitual telephone use
- ☐ Prolonged mobile phone use (cell phone elbow)
- ☐ Possibly smoking

Medical causes

- ☐ Diabetes mellitus
- ☐ Obesity
- ☐ Medial epicondylitis (Golfer's elbow)
- ☐ Wheelchair use
- ☐ Tumours
- ☐ Rheumatoid arthritis
- ☐ Gout
- ☐ Haematoma
- ☐ Other entrapment syndromes

Orthopaedic causes

- ☐ Trauma and compression of the cubital tunnel
- ☐ Elbow fracture (tardy ulnar nerve palsy)
- ☐ Elbow deformity: valgus or varus
- ☐ Repeated elbow dislocation
- ☐ Ganglions
- ☐ Bony spurs
- ☐ Hypertrophic callus
- ☐ Previous medial epicondyle fracture with non-union

CUBITAL TUNNEL SYNDROME: CLINICAL FEATURES

Sensory features

- ☐ These present as paraesthesias and numbness
- ☐ They affect the medial 1½ fingers
- ☐ The dorsum of the hand is affected: this is spared in Guyon's canal syndrome
- ☐ There may be elbow pain

Weakness

- ☐ Clumsiness
- ☐ Poor grip
- ☐ Difficulty doing buttons
- ☐ Difficulty typing
- ☐ Problems with opening jars and bottles
- ☐ Muscle wasting occurs in severe cases
- ☐ Clawing of little and ring fingers develop
- ☐ The little finger may be trapped when the hand is put in trouser pockets

Froment's sign

- ☐ This is the inability to pinch with the thumb and forefinger
- ☐ It results from weakness of the adductor pollicis
- ☐ Subjects compensates by gripping with the fingertips

Ulnar paradox

- ☐ There is less clawing than in Guyon's canal lesions
- ☐ This is because the flexor digitorum profundus (FDP) is spared

Elbow flexion sign

- ☐ This is the provocation of symptoms by elbow flexion/supination and wrist extension
- ☐ This occurs with nerve compression proximal to the cubital tunnel

Other clinical signs

- ☐ Tinel's sign: a radiating sensation triggered by tapping over the cubital tunnel
- ☐ Wartenberg's sign: the little finger abducts when the digits are extended
- ☐ Papal benediction sign: the little and ring fingers do not extend when undoing a fist

Differential diagnosis: C8 radiculopathy

- ☐ C8 radiculopathy involves the abductor pollicis brevis (APB)
  - ○ It is innervated by the median nerve
- ☐ C8 radiculopathy involves the extensor carpi ulnaris (ECU)
  - ○ It is innervated by the radial nerve

Differential diagnosis: others

- ☐ Thoracic outlet syndrome (TOS)
- ☐ Motor neurone diseases (MND)
- ☐ Peripheral neuropathy (PN)

ULNAR NEUROPATHY: ANOMALOUS ANASTOMOSES

Martin-Gruber anastomosis (MGA)

- ☐ This is a median-to-ulnar nerve communication
- ☐ The anastomosis is with the median nerve trunk or its anterior interosseous branch
- ☐ A distal type occurs in the forearm and is commoner
- ☐ A proximal type occurs at or above the elbow

The Riche-Cannieu anastomosis (RCA)

- ☐ This is an ulnar-to-median nerve communication
- ☐ The anastomosis occurs in the palmar hand
- ☐ It may be inherited with autosomal dominant transmission
- ☐ It may be bilateral
- ☐ The deep branch of the ulnar nerve innervates the normally median nerve innervated thenar muscles
- ☐ Carpal tunnel syndrome (CTS) developing in this situation will spare the thenar muscles
- ☐ The whole hand may be innervated by the ulnar nerve: this is the all-ulnar hand

Marinacci communication

- ☐ This is a reversed Martin-Gruber anastomosis
- ☐ There is an ulnar-to-median nerve communication in the forearm

Berretini anastomosis

- ☐ This is a communication between the common digital nerves of the ulnar and median nerves
- ☐ This is a very common variation
- ☐ There is impaired sensation in the interdigital regions

SCIATIC NEUROPATHY: CAUSES

Iatrogenic

- ☐ Gluteal injections
- ☐ Total hip arthroplasty
- ☐ Hysterectomy
- ☐ Vascular surgery
- ☐ Radiotherapy
- ☐ Sciatic nerve stump hypertrophy post amputation
- ☐ Popliteal fossa nerve block

Posture-related

- ☐ Sitting lotus position: legs flexed and abducted
- ☐ Lying flat on a hard surface
- ☐ Exercise bicycle
- ☐ Unicyclists
- ☐ Pregnancy/late labour

Extrinsic compression

- ☐ Disc prolapse
- ☐ Piriformis syndrome
- ☐ Osteochondroma
- ☐ Ectopic endometriosis: this causes cyclical sciatica
- ☐ Ovarian cysts
- ☐ Fibroids

Abscesses

- ☐ Pelvic
- ☐ Psoas
- ☐ Tubo-ovarian

Trauma

- ☐ Fractures
- ☐ Traction
- ☐ Hamstring injuries
- ☐ Gunshot wounds
- ☐ Hip fracture/dislocation

Vascular lesions

- ☐ Arteriovenous malformations (AVM)
- ☐ Deep vein thrombosis (DVT)
- ☐ Ischaemia

Other causes

- ☐ Inflammatory
- ☐ Cryoglobulinaemia
- ☐ Sacroiliatis
- ☐ Radiotherapy
- ☐ Hereditary neuropathy with liability to pressure palsies (HNPP)
- ☐ Idiopathic: this accounts for about 15% of cases

SCIATIC NEUROPATHY: CLINICAL FEATURES

Sensory features

- [ ] These present as radicular pain and numbness
- [ ] They are in the posterolateral leg and in the foot

Motor features

- [ ] Knee flexion weakness
- [ ] Ankle plantar flexion (foot drop)
- [ ] Foot inversion weakness
- [ ] Reduced ankle jerk

Features of severe cases

- [ ] Ankle dorsiflexion weakness
- [ ] Hamstrings weakness
- [ ] Toe extension/flexion weakness

Investigations

- [ ] Nerve conduction studies (NCS)
- [ ] Electromyogram (EMG)
- [ ] Magnetic resonance imaging (MRI)
- [ ] Computed tomography (CT): for bony and vascular causes

Predictors of good outcome

- [ ] Preserved ankle plantar and dorsiflexion
- [ ] Recordable compound muscle action potential (CMAP)
  - ○ In the extensor digitorum brevis (EDB) muscle

COMMON PERONEAL NEUROPATHY: CAUSES

Traumatic causes

- [ ] Fractures: hip, knee, acetabulum
- [ ] Nerve traction or stretch
- [ ] Laceration
- [ ] Ligament injury: especially anterior cruciate
- [ ] Ankle injury and sprain
- [ ] Knee dislocation
- [ ] Hip rotation: with gynaecological and abdominal surgery

Orthopaedic surgery

- [ ] Hip osteotomy or traction
- [ ] Knee arthrodesis, arthroscopy, or replacement
- [ ] Prolonged positioning

Extrinsic compression

- [ ] Ankle splint/cast
- [ ] Knee osteoarthritis
- [ ] Knee varus deformity
- [ ] Post-partum
- [ ] Plaster casts
- [ ] Tight knee-high boots
- [ ] Squatting in 'skinny jeans'

Posture-related

- [ ] Prolonged bed rest or being bedridden
- [ ] Prolonged squatting
- [ ] Habitual leg crossing
- [ ] Kneeling
- [ ] Jogging

Nerve lesions

- [ ] Intraneural ganglion cyst
- [ ] Schwannoma
- [ ] Neurofibroma
- [ ] Osteochondroma
- [ ] Neurogenic sarcoma
- [ ] Glomus tumour
- [ ] Desmoid tumour
- [ ] Focal hypertrophic neuropathy
- [ ] Nerve sheath haematoma

Other causes

- [ ] Underlying neuropathy
- [ ] Diabetes mellitus
- [ ] Leprosy
- [ ] Hereditary neuropathy with liability to pressure palsy (HNPP)
- [ ] Entrapment in fibular tunnel
- [ ] Fabellas: sesamoid bones in the gastrocnemius tendon
- [ ] Anterior tibial compartment syndrome

Synonym

- [ ] Common fibular neuropathy

COMMON PERONEAL NEUROPATHY: CLINICAL FEATURES

Weakness

- ☐ Foot drop: this is due to foot dorsiflexion and eversion weakness
- ☐ Toe extension weakness

Sensory loss: distribution

- ☐ Lateral cutaneous nerve of the calf
- ☐ Deep peroneal nerve
- ☐ Superficial peroneal nerve
- ☐ Sensory loss is variable and may be absent

Preserved functions

- ☐ Foot inversion: this is affected in L5 radiculopathy
- ☐ Biceps femoris: this arises from the peroneal division of the sciatic nerve
- ☐ Knee and ankle jerks

Differential: L4/L5 radiculopathy

- ☐ This involves the tibialis posterior (foot inversion)

Synonym

- ☐ Common fibular neuropathy

LONG THORACIC NERVE PALSY: CAUSES

Traumatic

- ☐ Sudden shoulder girdle depression
- ☐ Neck and shoulder twisting motions
- ☐ Road traffic accidents (RTA)
- ☐ Fall from a height
- ☐ Prolonged lying with abducted arms propping the head up
- ☐ Sport collisions
- ☐ Chiropractic manoeuvres
- ☐ Use of axillary crutches

Surgical

- ☐ Anterior cervical decompression
- ☐ Mastectomy
- ☐ First rib resection
- ☐ Axillary dissection
- ☐ Thoracostomy tube insertion
- ☐ Scalenotomy
- ☐ Surgery for spontaneous pneumothorax
- ☐ General anaesthesia positioning: shoulder strapping

Neuromuscular

- ☐ Facioscapulohumeral muscular dystrophy (FSHD)
- ☐ C7 radiculopathy
- ☐ Brachial neuritis
- ☐ Guillain–Barre syndrome (GBS)

Infections

- ☐ Poliomyelitis
- ☐ Lyme neuroborreliosis

Drugs and toxins

- ☐ Drugs overdose
- ☐ Drug allergic reaction
- ☐ Tetanus toxin
- ☐ Herbicides

Other causes

- ☐ Arnold–Chiari malformation
- ☐ Coarctation of aorta
- ☐ Subscapular bursa inflammation
- ☐ Electric shock
- ☐ Systemic lupus erythematosus (SLE)

LONG THORACIC NERVE PALSY: OCCUPATIONAL RISKS

Sporting risks

- ☐ Archery
- ☐ Ballet
- ☐ Baseball
- ☐ Basketball
- ☐ Bowling
- ☐ Football
- ☐ Golf
- ☐ Hockey
- ☐ Tennis
- ☐ Weight lifting
- ☐ Gymnastics
- ☐ Wrestling

Work related risks

- ☐ Car washing
- ☐ Carpenters
- ☐ Digging
- ☐ Hedge clipping
- ☐ Labourers
- ☐ Meat packers
- ☐ Mechanics
- ☐ Scaffolders
- ☐ Welders

Military risks

- ☐ Navy
- ☐ Airmen

SCAPULA WINGING: CAUSES

Mononeuropathies

- ☐ Long thoracic nerve
- ☐ Spinal accessory nerve
- ☐ Dorsal scapular nerve
- ☐ Thoracodorsal nerve

Other neurological causes

- ☐ Facioscapulohumeral muscular dystrophy (FSHD)
- ☐ Cervical syringomyelia: this causes bilateral scapula winging
- ☐ Psychogenic

Soft tissue and orthopaedic causes

- ☐ Shoulder joint contracture
- ☐ Deltoid fibrosis
- ☐ Scapulothoracic bursitis
- ☐ Subacromial bursitis
- ☐ Adhesive capsulitis
- ☐ Rotator cuff tears
- ☐ Osteochondromas
- ☐ Fracture malunion

SCAPULA WINGING: CLINICAL FEATURES

Spinal accessory nerve winging

- ☐ This is usually caused by damage to the nerve in the posterior cervical triangle
- ☐ It is iatrogenic in many cases
- ☐ It usually results from cervical lymph node biopsy or excision
- ☐ It results in trapezius muscle weakness
- ☐ It manifests as lateral winging
- ☐ The whole medial border of the scapula is elevated
- ☐ Winging is accentuated by shoulder abduction to 90°

Long thoracic nerve winging

- ☐ This is the most frequent cause of unilateral scapula winging
- ☐ It is usually related to neuralgic amyotrophy
- ☐ It results in serratus anterior muscle weakness
- ☐ It causes medial scapula winging
- ☐ The inferior tip of the scapula rotates medially
- ☐ The scapula lifts off the rib cage
- ☐ Winging is accentuated by pushing forward (shoulder flexion)

Dorsal scapular nerve winging

- ☐ This results from weakness of the rhomboids muscles
- ☐ It is caused by nerve entrapment in the scalenus medius muscle
- ☐ It may also be caused by trauma and anterior shoulder dislocation
- ☐ It manifests as lateral winging
- ☐ The inferior angle of the scapula rotates laterally
- ☐ Winging is accentuated by elevating the arm above the head

Thoracodorsal nerve winging

- ☐ This results from weakness of the latissimus dorsi muscle
- ☐ Winging is mild
- ☐ It is tested by pressing the dorsum of the hand against the ipsilateral buttock

Differential diagnosis (mimics) of scapula winging

- ☐ Brachial plexopathy
- ☐ Radial neuropathy

FOOT DROP: CAUSES

Cranial causes

- ☐ Parasagittal meningioma
- ☐ Anterior cerebral artery (ACA) stroke
- ☐ Lesions affecting the pyramidal tract

Spinal causes

- ☐ Cervical spinal stenosis
- ☐ Spinal cord tumours
- ☐ Spinal dural arteriovenous fistula (dAVF)
- ☐ Cauda equina/conus lesions: these cause bilateral foot drop

Root and plexus causes

- ☐ L5 radiculopathy
- ☐ Lumbar plexopathy

Anterior horn cell disorders

- ☐ Motor neurone disease (MND)
- ☐ Poliomyelitis

Neuropathic causes

- ☐ Sciatic neuropathy
- ☐ Peroneal neuropathy
- ☐ Hereditary neuropathy with liability to pressure palsy (HNPP)
- ☐ Multifocal motor neuropathy (MMN)

Neuromuscular junction (NMJ) disorders

- ☐ Myasthenia gravis (MG)

Muscle causes

- ☐ Distal myopathies
- ☐ Facioscapulohumeral muscular dystrophy (FSHD)
- ☐ Scapuloperoneal muscular dystrophy

FOOT DROP: LOCALISATION

L5 root lesions

- ☐ Weak inversion
- ☐ Weak eversion

Sciatic nerve lesions (L4–5, S1–3)

- ☐ Weak inversion
- ☐ Weak plantar flexion
- ☐ Weak short head of biceps femoris: assessed at EMG
- ☐ Absent ankle jerk

Common peroneal nerve lesions

- ☐ Weak eversion
- ☐ Spares inversion
- ☐ Spares ankle and knee reflexes

Superficial peroneal nerve lesions

- ☐ Weak eversion
- ☐ Spares dorsiflexion

Lesions causing inversion weakness

- ☐ L4 radiculopathy
- ☐ Tibial neuropathy
- ☐ Peroneal neuropathy

Lesions causing dorsiflexion weakness

- ☐ L4/5 radiculopathy
- ☐ Peroneal neuropathy

Lesions causing eversion weakness

- ☐ S1 radiculopathy
- ☐ Peroneal neuropathy

Lesions causing planar flexion weakness

- ☐ S1/2 radiculopathy
- ☐ Tibial nerve lesions

DIAPHRAGMATIC PARALYSIS: NEUROLOGICAL CAUSES

Radiculopathies

- ☐ C1-C2 root lesions: these cause complete diaphragmatic paralysis
- ☐ C3-C5 root lesions: these cause partial diaphragmatic paralysis

Spinal cord disorders

- ☐ Spinal cord infarction
- ☐ Chiari malformation
- ☐ Syringomyelia
- ☐ Chiropractic cervical manipulation
- ☐ Endotracheal intubation
- ☐ Severe cervical spondylosis
- ☐ Multiple sclerosis (MS)

Anterior horn cell (AHC) disorders

- ☐ Poliomyelitis
- ☐ Motor neurone disease (MND)
- ☐ Spinal muscular atrophy (SMA)
- ☐ IGHMBP2-related neuropathy

Neuropathic causes

- ☐ Charcot–Marie–Tooth disease (CMT)
- ☐ Chronic inflammatory demyelinating polyradiculoneuropathy (CIDP)
- ☐ Guillain–Barre syndrome (GBS)
- ☐ Neuralgic amyotrophy
- ☐ Critical illness neuropathy
- ☐ Paraneoplastic motor neuropathies
- ☐ Diabetic phrenic neuropathy

Neuromuscular junction (NMJ) disorders

- ☐ Myasthenia gravis (MG)
- ☐ Lambert–Eaton myasthenic syndrome (LEMS)

Muscle causes

- ☐ Limb girdle muscular dystrophy (LGMD)
- ☐ Acid maltase (Pompe) disease
- ☐ Dermatomyositis

DIAPHRAGMATIC PARALYSIS: SYSTEMIC CAUSES

Medical causes

- ☐ Idiopathic: this may respond to Valaciclovir
- ☐ Phrenic nerve trauma: from cardiac or neck surgery
- ☐ Hypothyroidism
- ☐ Malignant invasion
- ☐ Trauma
- ☐ Amyloidosis
- ☐ Giant cell arteritis
- ☐ IgG kappa monoclonal gammopathy
- ☐ Lung hyperinflation
- ☐ Prolonged vomiting

Infective causes

- ☐ Lyme neuroborreliosis
- ☐ Thoracic herpes zoster
- ☐ Botulism

Autoimmune causes

- ☐ Systemic lupus erythematosus (SLE)
- ☐ Systemic sclerosis
- ☐ Mixed connective tissue disease (MCTD)

Drug-induced and toxic causes

- ☐ Carbon monoxide poisoning
- ☐ Organophosphates
- ☐ Steroids
- ☐ Aminoglycosides
- ☐ Adalimumab
- ☐ Tetanus toxin

DIAPHRAGMATIC PARALYSIS: CLINICAL FEATURES

Respiratory features

- ☐ Diaphragmatic dyspnoea: this is shortness of breath when immersed in water above the waist level
- ☐ Decreased exercise tolerance
- ☐ Excessive use of the accessory muscles of respiration
- ☐ Paradoxical abdominal wall movements: the abdomen moves inwards on inspiration
- ☐ Atelectasis
- ☐ Respiratory failure

Sleep-related features

- ☐ Sleep disordered breathing
- ☐ Fragmented sleep
- ☐ Hypersomnia
- ☐ Subjects sleep in a reclined position

Systemic features

- ☐ Morning headaches
- ☐ Fatigue

PHRENIC NERVE PALSY

Neurological causes

- ☐ Idiopathic
- ☐ Neuralgic amyotrophy (brachial neuritis)
- ☐ Bilateral isolated phrenic neuropathy
- ☐ Motor neurone disease (MND)
- ☐ Guillain–Barre syndrome (GBS)
- ☐ Chronic inflammatory demyelinating polyneuropathy (CIDP)
- ☐ Critical illness neuropathy

Cardiothoracic causes

- ☐ Coronary artery bypass graft (CABG)
- ☐ Thoracic aortic aneurysm
- ☐ Open heart surgery
- ☐ Intrathoracic masses
- ☐ Jugular or subclavian vein catheterisation
- ☐ Mediastinal radiation

Infective causes

- ☐ Tuberculosis (TB)
- ☐ Lyme neuroborreliosis: this may be bilateral
- ☐ Herpes zoster

Syndromic causes

- ☐ The Red Cross syndrome
  - ○ This is compression of the phrenic nerve by the transverse cervical artery
- ☐ Rowland Payne syndrome
  - ○ This is phrenic nerve palsy with Horner's syndrome and recurrent laryngeal nerve palsy

Other causes

- ☐ Diabetes mellitus
- ☐ Sarcoidosis
- ☐ Liver transplantation

MONONEUROPATHY MULTIPLEX: CAUSES

Vasculitic causes

- ☐ Polyarteritis nodosa (PAN)
- ☐ Eosinophilic granulomatosis with polyangiitis (EGPA)
- ☐ Granulomatosis with polyangiitis (GPA)
- ☐ Cryoglobulinaemia
- ☐ Microscopic polyangiitis
- ☐ Henoch-Schonlein purpura
- ☐ Sjogren's syndrome
- ☐ Giant cell arteritis (GCA)
- ☐ Behcet's disease
- ☐ Systemic lupus erythematosus (SLE)

Infective and inflammatory causes

- ☐ Lyme disease
- ☐ Leprosy
- ☐ Sarcoidosis

Malignant causes

- ☐ Tumour infiltration
- ☐ Lymphoid granulomatosis
- ☐ Paraneoplastic

Drug-induced

- ☐ Simvastatin
- ☐ Adalimumab
- ☐ Minocycline

Other causes

- ☐ Diabetes
- ☐ Paraproteinaemia
- ☐ Hereditary neuropathy with liability to pressure palsy (HNPP)
- ☐ Non-vasculitic steroid responsive mononeuropathy multiplex
- ☐ Lividoid vasculopathy

Synonym

- ☐ Mononeuritis multiplex

CHAPTER 14

Neuromuscular junction disorders

Myasthenia gravis: general features

MYASTHENIA GRAVIS (MG): CLASSIFICATION

Early-onset MG with acetylcholine receptor antibodies

- ☐ This usually occurs in females
- ☐ The age at onset is <50 years
- ☐ It is associated with thymic hyperplasia

Late-onset MG with acetylcholine receptor antibodies

- ☐ This is mainly in males
- ☐ Age at onset is >50 years
- ☐ There is associated thymic atrophy

MUSK associated MG

- ☐ This accounts for 1–4% of cases
- ☐ It is rare in children or the very old
- ☐ There is no thymic involvement
- ☐ Also see topic: Anti MUSK myasthenia gravis

LRP4 associated MG

- ☐ This accounts for 2–27% of double seronegative cases
- ☐ There is a female predominance
- ☐ 20% are strictly ocular for up to 2 years
- ☐ Also see topic: Anti LRP4 myasthenia gravis

Antibody negative (seronegative) MG

- ☐ There are no detectable antibodies to AChR, MUSK, or LRP4
- ☐ Low affinity antibodies account for 20–50% of AChR negative cases
- ☐ Low antibody levels account for other cases

Thymoma associated MG

- ☐ Also see topic: Myasthenia gravis (MG) with thymoma

Ocular MG

- ☐ This accounts for 20–50% of MG
- ☐ AChR antibodies are detected in 50% of cases
- ☐ 50–60% generalise: usually in the first 2 years
- ☐ Generalisation is not prevented by any treatment
- ☐ Also see topic: Ocular myasthenia gravis

Other MG types

- ☐ Bulbopharyngeal MG: see related topic
- ☐ Generalised MG: see related topic

Acronyms

- ☐ AChR: acetylcholine receptor
- ☐ MUSK: muscle-specific receptor tyrosine kinase
- ☐ LRP4: low density lipoprotein receptor-related protein 4

MYASTHENIA GRAVIS (MG): DRUG TRIGGERS

Antibiotics

- ☐ Aminoglycosides
- ☐ Ampicillin
- ☐ Clindamycin
- ☐ Colistin
- ☐ Levofloxacin
- ☐ Macrolides
- ☐ Erythromycin
- ☐ Fluoroquinolones
- ☐ Oxytetracycline
- ☐ Quinolones
- ☐ Polymyxin B

Cardiac drugs

- ☐ Verapamil
- ☐ Nifedipine
- ☐ Felodipine
- ☐ Beta blockers
- ☐ Procainamide
- ☐ Quinidine

Anaesthetic drugs

- ☐ Ketamine
- ☐ Lidocaine
- ☐ Trimethaphan

Antiepileptic drugs (AEDs)

- ☐ Diazepam
- ☐ Gabapentin
- ☐ Phenytoin

Anti-inflammatory drugs

- ☐ D-Penicillamine
- ☐ Prednisolone
- ☐ Interferon

Anti-malarial drugs

- ☐ Chloroquine
- ☐ Quinine

Other drugs

- ☐ Anti PD-1 monoclonal antibodies
- ☐ Alendronate
- ☐ Carnitine
- ☐ Contrast media: meglumine
- ☐ Lithium
- ☐ Magnesium
- ☐ Methimazole
- ☐ Oxytocin
- ☐ Permethrin cream
- ☐ Pyrantel pamoate
- ☐ Trimethadone

DOI: 10.1201/9781003221258-80

MYASTHENIA GRAVIS (MG): NON-DRUG TRIGGERS

Environmental

- ☐ Physical exertion
- ☐ Hot temperature

Physiological

- ☐ Emotional upsets
- ☐ Menses
- ☐ Pregnancy
- ☐ Post-partum

Medical

- ☐ Infections
- ☐ Hyperthyroidism
- ☐ Hypokalaemia
- ☐ Surgery
- ☐ In-vitro fertilisation procedure
- ☐ Orbital marginal zone lymphoma: case report

Vaccinations

- ☐ Human papilloma virus (HPV) vaccination
- ☐ Hepatitis B virus (HBV) vaccination
- ☐ Intravesical BCG

MYASTHENIA GRAVIS (MG): DIFFERENTIAL DIAGNOSIS

Lambert–Eaton myasthenic syndrome (LEMS)

- ☐ LEMS does not present with initial ocular weakness or isolated upper limb weakness as in MG
- ☐ LEMS does not progress caudally as in MG

Congenital myasthenic syndromes (CMS)

- ☐ CMS may mimic late-onset seronegative myasthenia gravis
- ☐ RAPSN CMS is most likely to present like this
- ☐ It usually presents in adolescence or early adulthood

Ophthalmic differentials

- ☐ Oculopharyngeal muscular dystrophy (OPMD)
- ☐ Progressive external ophthalmoplegia (PEO)
- ☐ Thyroid ophthalmopathy

Neuromuscular differentials

- ☐ Guillain–Barre syndrome (GBS)
- ☐ Inflammatory myopathies
- ☐ Metabolic and toxic myopathies
- ☐ Acquired neuromyotonia
- ☐ Motor neurone disease (MND): this is especially a differential of anti-MUSK MG

Other differentials

- ☐ Botulism
- ☐ Cranial nerve palsies
- ☐ Brainstem disorders
- ☐ Intracranial space occupying lesions

Monoclonal antibody-induced MG

- ☐ Nivolumab
- ☐ Ipilimumab
- ☐ Pembrolizumab

Other drugs

- ☐ D-Penicillamine
- ☐ Interferon (IFN) alpha
- ☐ Statins

Myasthenia gravis types

OCULAR MYASTHENIA GRAVIS (MG)

Ptosis

- [ ] This is often partial
- [ ] It is unilateral or bilateral
- [ ] Eyelids fatigue with sustained up-gaze for ≥ 30 seconds
- [ ] It improves after sleep: the sleep test
- [ ] It improves with the ice pack test

Enhanced ptosis

- [ ] Ptosis worsens in one eye when the other eyelid is manually held up
- [ ] This occurs in patients with asymmetric ptosis

Ophthalmoplegia

- [ ] The medial rectus is the most frequently affected muscle
- [ ] It is pupil sparing
- [ ] Diplopia may be elicited by 20–30 seconds of sustained lateral gaze

Cogan's lid twitch

- [ ] This is elicited by downward eye deviation for 10–20 seconds
- [ ] The upper eyelid elevates and then drops or twitches on return to the primary position
- [ ] It may also be seen with brainstem and ocular disorders

Other signs

- [ ] Lid hopping sign: lid twitching develops with horizontal eye movements
- [ ] Hypometric saccades with intra-saccadic fatigue

Treatment options

- [ ] Anticholinesterase: this is the first line treatment
- [ ] Prednisolone: this is indicated if symptoms persist on anticholinesterases
- [ ] Methylprednisolone intravenously 1000 mg daily given 1–3 times within 6 months
  - ○ This may be more rapidly acting than Prednisolone
- [ ] Immunosuppression: this is indicated if symptoms recur on Prednisolone withdrawal
- [ ] Thymectomy: for thymoma and for AchR antibody positive subjects <45 years of age

BULBOPHARYNGEAL MYASTHENIA GRAVIS (MG)

Bulbar weakness

- [ ] Dysarthria
- [ ] Dysphagia: this may be the only feature
- [ ] Difficulty chewing

Facial and neck weakness

- [ ] Expressionless face
- [ ] Weak eye closure: the eyelashes are visible when the eyes are shut (Barre sign)
- [ ] Hanging jaw
- [ ] Jaw support with hand or finger
- [ ] Snarling on attempted smiling
- [ ] Head drop: this is frequent in late-onset MG
- [ ] Trissulcated tongue

Pharyngeal weakness

- [ ] Nasal voice
- [ ] Nasal regurgitation
- [ ] Dysphonia
- [ ] The curtain sign: this is deviation of the uvula

DOI: 10.1201/9781003221258-81

GENERALISED MYASTHENIA GRAVIS (MG)

Limb girdle weakness
- ☐ This is worse in the evening
- ☐ It demonstrates a craniocaudal progression

Respiratory muscle weakness
- ☐ Dyspnoea on exertion or at rest
- ☐ Orthopnoea
- ☐ Diaphragmatic paradox

Chronic fatigue
- ☐ This usually correlates with severity of MG
- ☐ It may develop during remission
- ☐ It may be associated with impaired thermoregulation
- ☐ It may also be related to sleep disturbance and depression

JUVENILE MYASTHENIA GRAVIS (MG)

Classification
- ☐ Very early onset group: the onset age is <8 years
  - ○ This has a genetic predisposition
- ☐ Puberty onset group: the onset age is between 8–18 years

Clinical presentation
- ☐ This usually manifests as generalised MG
- ☐ Ocular MG is more frequent with very early onset cases

Thymic abnormalities
- ☐ The thymus is abnormal in a third of cases
- ☐ This is usually hyperplasia
- ☐ Hyperplasia is more frequent in early onset cases

Antibody profile
- ☐ 50% have anti acetylcholine receptor (AChR) antibodies
- ☐ 8% have anti-MUSK antibodies
- ☐ 40% are seronegative

Prognosis
- ☐ There is a high morbidity
- ☐ 30% require intensive care on follow up
- ☐ Spontaneous remission occurs in 18% of cases

Treatment
- ☐ Consider early introduction of Rituximab

ANTI-MUSK MYASTHENIA GRAVIS (MG): CLINICAL FEATURES

Pathology

- ☐ Anti-MUSK antibodies are present in 30–50% of antibody-negative MG
- ☐ They cause pre-synaptic and post-synaptic dysfunction
- ☐ There is no loss of junctional folds
- ☐ There is no loss of acetylcholine receptor (AChR) density

Aetiology

- ☐ Anti-MUSK antibodies may be induced by D-Penicillamine
- ☐ Anti-MUSK MG may be an IgG4 related disease

Genetics

- ☐ There is a possible HLA gene susceptibility
- ☐ There is increased risk with HLA DQB1*05, DRB1*14 and DRB1*16
- ☐ There is reduced risk with HLA DQB*03

Facial and bulbar features

- ☐ Oropharyngeal weakness
- ☐ Tongue atrophy: this may be reversible
- ☐ Facial and bulbar muscle weakness
- ☐ Facial and bulbar muscle atrophy with fatty replacement
  - ○ This is possibly due to long-term steroid use

Ocular features

- ☐ Ocular features may be the first presentation
- ☐ There is symmetrical ophthalmoplegia with conjugate gaze restriction
- ☐ Some may progress to chronic ophthalmoplegia

Generalised features

- ☐ Neck weakness
- ☐ Respiratory muscle weakness
- ☐ Myasthenic crisis: this is more frequent than with anti-AChR MG

Anti-MUSK MG and pregnancy

- ☐ Pregnancy has no effect on the course of anti-MUSK MG
- ☐ Anti-MUSK MG does not affect pregnancy

Variant presentations

- ☐ Purely ocular symptoms
- ☐ Vocal cord paresis

Features distinguishing anti-MUSK from anti-AChR MG

- ☐ The onset age is earlier in anti-MUSK MG: it is usually in the third or fourth decade
- ☐ The onset is more acute in anti-MUSK MG
- ☐ Cranial and bulbar involvement are more frequent in anti-MUSK
- ☐ The clinical phenotype is worse with anti-MUSK

ANTI-LRP4 MYASTHENIA GRAVIS (MG)

Pathology

- ☐ This is caused by antibodies against the low-density lipoprotein receptor protein 4 (LRP4)
- ☐ LRP4 is the agrin receptor needed to activate MUSK
- ☐ It is present in 9–90% of double-seronegative patients
- ☐ It may co-exist with anti AChR and MUSK antibody MG

Clinical features

- ☐ It usually affects middle-aged women
- ☐ The onset age is earlier than in anti-AChR MG
- ☐ The phenotype is also milder
- ☐ It is frequently ocular

Electromyogram (EMG)

- ☐ This is usually normal

Treatment

- ☐ Steroids
- ☐ Pyridostigmine
- ☐ Treatment response is good

MYASTHENIA GRAVIS (MG) WITH THYMOMA

Thymic thymoma

- ☐ Thymomas are present in 15% of MG
- ☐ They are microscopic in 4% of cases: with diameter <1mm
- ☐ They are often invasive and cause severe myasthenia
- ☐ They are medullary, mixed, cortical, or well-differentiated carcinomas

Extra-thymic thymoma

- ☐ These are especially in the lungs, breast, gastrointestinal tract, thyroid, kidney, and liver
- ☐ They are associated with older age and longer disease duration of MG

Other thymic pathologies

- ☐ Thymus hyperplasia: this occurs in 60% of MG: it is usually in younger females
- ☐ Thymic malignancies: these are extra-thymic in 20% of cases

Myasthenia gravis with thymoma

- ☐ MG with thymoma is associated with acetylcholine, titin, or ryanodine receptor antibodies
- ☐ It may be antibody negative
- ☐ MG may first manifest after thymectomy

Other thymoma neurological manifestations

- ☐ Thymoma associated paraneoplastic encephalitis (TAPE)
  - ○ One case report was associated with anti-NMDAR antibodies
- ☐ Thymoma associated multi-organ autoimmunity (TAMA)

Myasthenia gravis: complicated types

REFRACTORY MYASTHENIA GRAVIS (MG)

Defining features

- [ ] 10% of people with MG develop refractory features
- [ ] This is inadequate response to conventional MG treatment for ≥12 months
- [ ] Subjects relapse when the dose of immunosuppressing drugs is lowered
- [ ] It typically develops in females and those with young onset age MG
- [ ] It is more frequent with anti-MUSK MG, thymoma, or thymectomy
- [ ] There may be associated diabetes and hyperlipidemia

Treatment: plasma exchange (PE)

- [ ] This is a conventional treatment for refractory MG
- [ ] It is also used to achieve remission pre-surgery

Treatment: intravenous immunoglobulins (IVIg)

- [ ] This is also a conventional treatment for refractory MG
- [ ] The dose is 1–2g/kg body weight
- [ ] It is also safe and effective subcutaneously

Treatment: Rituximab

- [ ] This is indicated if standard treatments fail
- [ ] It is especially effective in MUSK positive MG
- [ ] Low doses may be sufficient and effective long-term
- [ ] It gives a durable and sustained beneficial effect
- [ ] The response is best in younger patients with less severe disease
- [ ] Repeat treatments may be required: this is because of the resurgence of memory B cells
- [ ] The use of Rituximab reduces the annual cost of MG treatment

Treatment: Eculizumab

- [ ] This improves weakness and perceived fatigue
- [ ] The benefit is sustained
- [ ] It is well-tolerated

Emerging treatments

- [ ] Leflunomide
- [ ] Ruxolitinib
- [ ] Etanercept
- [ ] Bortezomib
- [ ] Belimumab
- [ ] Tacrolimus
- [ ] Autologous hematopoietic stem cell transplantation
- [ ] Granulocyte–macrophage colony-stimulating factor (GMCSF)

MYASTHENIC CRISIS: RISK FACTORS

Disease-related risk factors

- [ ] Disease duration >6 years
- [ ] Previous myasthenic crisis
- [ ] Bulbar symptoms
- [ ] Acetylcholine receptor (AChR) antibody level >100nmol/L
- [ ] Vital capacity (VC) <2.9L

MG drugs-related risk factors

- [ ] Altered medication regimen
- [ ] Steroid therapy: this worsens MG in 50% of cases
  - ○ It results in crises in 10–20% of these
- [ ] Pyridostigmine dose >750 mg daily
- [ ] Tapering of immune-modulators

Other drug related risk factors

- [ ] Contrast agents
- [ ] Muscle relaxants
- [ ] Benzodiazepines
- [ ] Beta blockers
- [ ] Iodinated contrast agents

Medical risk factors

- [ ] Co-existing lung disease
- [ ] Previous respiratory problems
- [ ] Chest infection
- [ ] Cardiac disease
- [ ] Aspiration
- [ ] Hypokalaemia
- [ ] Hypophosphataemia
- [ ] Systemic infections
- [ ] Hyperthyroidism

Others risk factors

- [ ] Emotional stress
- [ ] Surgery
- [ ] Temperature extremes
- [ ] Sudden body temperature increase
- [ ] Trauma
- [ ] Menses
- [ ] Pregnancy
- [ ] Sleep deprivation
- [ ] Environmental stressors
- [ ] Pain

DOI: 10.1201/9781003221258-82

MYASTHENIC CRISIS: DIFFERENTIAL DIAGNOSIS

Infections and toxins

- [ ] Botulism
- [ ] Diphtheritic polyneuropathy
- [ ] West Nile virus
- [ ] Rabies
- [ ] Tetanus
- [ ] Spider bite
- [ ] Snake venom
- [ ] Organophosphate overdose

Peripheral nerve disorders

- [ ] Guillain–Barre syndrome (GBS)
- [ ] Motor neuronopathy
- [ ] Acute intermittent porphyria (AIP)
- [ ] Vasculitic neuropathy
- [ ] Critical illness myoneuropathy

Anterior horn cell (AHC) disorders

- [ ] Motor neurone disease (MND)
- [ ] Spinal muscular atrophy (SMA)
- [ ] Brown-Vialetto-von Leare (BVVL) syndrome
- [ ] Spinal and bulbar muscular atrophy (SBMA, Kennedy disease)
- [ ] Poliomyelitis

Neuromuscular junction (NMJ) disorders

- [ ] Lambert–Eaton myasthenic syndrome (LEMS)
- [ ] Cholinergic crisis

Myopathies

- [ ] Polymyositis
- [ ] Hypothyroid myopathy
- [ ] Hyphophosphataemic myopathy
- [ ] Rhabdomyolysis
- [ ] Acid maltase deficiency
- [ ] Distal myopathy with vocal cord palsy

Muscular dystrophies

- [ ] Duchenne muscular dystrophy (DMD)
- [ ] Myotonic dystrophy type 1
- [ ] Oculopharyngeal muscle dystrophy (OPMD)

Drugs

- [ ] Alcohol
- [ ] Barbiturates
- [ ] Recreational drugs
- [ ] Sedatives

Central differentials

- [ ] Spinal cord injury
- [ ] Cervical spinal cord transection
- [ ] Brainstem lesions

MYASTHENIA GRAVIS (MG): CHOLINERGIC CRISIS

Triggers

- [ ] Anticholinergic drugs
- [ ] Rodenticide poisoning with aldicarb: a carbamate insecticide
- [ ] Organophosphate poisoning: the effect may be delayed
- [ ] Methomyl-alphamethrin poisoning: the effect may be delayed
- [ ] Distigmine bromide
- [ ] Echothiophate iodide

Neurological features

- [ ] Muscle weakness
- [ ] Nausea and vomiting
- [ ] Diarrhoea
- [ ] Bradycardia
- [ ] Cardiac arrhythmias
- [ ] Myocardial infarction
- [ ] Fasciculations

Systemic features

- [ ] Increased sweating
- [ ] Fast respiration
- [ ] Increased tearing
- [ ] Excessive salivation
- [ ] Increased pulmonary secretions
- [ ] Respiratory failure

Edrophonium test: benefit

- [ ] This differentiates cholinergic from myasthenic crisis
- [ ] Edrophonium worsens cholinergic crisis
- [ ] It improves myasthenic crisis

Edrophonium test: causes of false positive worsening

- [ ] Anti-MUSK MG
- [ ] Motor neuron disease (MND)
- [ ] Brainstem tumours

Treatment

- [ ] Reduce or stop acetylcholinesterase inhibitors

Myasthenia gravis treatment

MYASTHENIA GRAVIS (MG) TREATMENT: PYRIDOSTIGMINE

Dosing regime

- ☐ The dose is 30 mg three to four times daily for 2–4 days
- ☐ It is then increased to 60 mg three to four times daily for 5 days
- ☐ It may be increased to 90 mg four times daily over one week if required

Precautions

- ☐ It must be used with caution in people with anti-MUSK MG
- ☐ They are hypersensitive to Pyridostigmine

Side effects

- ☐ Cramps
- ☐ Diarrhoea
- ☐ Sweating
- ☐ Excessive secretions: respiratory and gastrointestinal
- ☐ Bradycardia
- ☐ Fasciculations

Treatment of side effects

- ☐ Propantheline
- ☐ Mebeverine

MYASTHENIA GRAVIS (MG) TREATMENT: STEROIDS

Indications

- ☐ This is the first choice if immunosuppression is necessary

Regime for ocular MG

- ☐ The starting dose is Prednisolone 5 mg alternate daily for three doses
- ☐ It is then increased by 5 mg every three doses until symptom control
- ☐ The maximum dose is 50 mg alternate daily or 0.75 mg/kg body weight for ocular MG

Regime for generalised MG

- ☐ The starting dose is Prednisolone 10–25 mg alternate daily for three doses
- ☐ It is then increased by 10 mg every three doses until symptom control
- ☐ The maximum dose is 100 mg alternate daily or 1.5 mg/kg body weight

Steroid withdrawal

- ☐ Prednisolone is withdrawn after 2–3 months of achieving remission
- ☐ It is reduced by 10 mg alternate daily per month until the dose is 40 mg alternate daily
- ☐ It is then reduced by 5 mg alternate daily per month until a dose of 20 mg alternate daily
- ☐ Subsequent dose reduction is by 2.5 mg alternate daily per month until 10 mg alternate daily
- ☐ The dose is then reduced by 1 mg per month

Long-term steroid therapy

- ☐ Steroids may be continued long-term at a low dose
- ☐ Consider other immunosuppression if the requirement is >15–20 mg alternate daily

Predictors of response to steroids

- ☐ Age <40 years
- ☐ Age >60 years

Steroid dip

- ☐ This is worsening of weakness 4–10 days after starting steroids
- ☐ This usually occurs with high dose steroids
- ☐ The highest risk is with Cortisone followed by Prednisolone and then Methylprednisolone
- ☐ It is more frequent in generalised and severe myasthenia gravis with bulbar symptoms
- ☐ It is more likely to occur in older patients
- ☐ Thymoma and thymectomy also increase the risk

Precautions on steroids

- ☐ Monitor for diabetes
- ☐ Use with gut and bone protection

DOI: 10.1201/9781003221258-83

MYASTHENIA GRAVIS (MG): NON-STEROID IMMUNOSUPPRESSION

Indications for the sole use of non-steroid immunosuppressants

- ☐ When steroids are contraindicated
- ☐ When steroid side effects develop
- ☐ When there is pre-existing osteoporosis
- ☐ When there is pre-existing ischaemic heart disease
- ☐ When there are significant bulbar or respiratory symptoms

Indications for combining steroids with non-steroid immunosuppressants

- ☐ To reduce the high risk of steroid side effects
- ☐ To improve an inadequate response to steroids
- ☐ When the steroid requirement is exceeding 15–20 mg alternate daily of Prednisolone

Azathioprine

- ☐ This is the first line non-steroid option
- ☐ It is administered if MPTP level is sufficient: this is the enzyme that metabolizes Azathioprine
- ☐ The dose is built up over one month to 2.5 mg/kg body weight daily
- ☐ Weekly blood tests are required during dose titration

Methotrexate

- ☐ This is indicated if Azathioprine is not tolerated
- ☐ It may be as effective as Azathioprine
- ☐ One report however suggests it is not effective in MG

Other conventional options

- ☐ Cyclosporine
- ☐ Mycophenolate
- ☐ Cyclophosphamide
- ☐ Rituximab

Tacrolimus

- ☐ This is especially effective if anti RyR antibodies are positive
- ☐ Adequate concentrations are essential for treatment response

Lambert–Eaton myasthenic syndrome (LEMS)

LAMBERT–EATON MYASTHENIC SYNDROME (LEMS): CLINICAL FEATURES

Limb weakness

- [ ] This especially involves the proximal lower limb muscles but it may also be distal
- [ ] Lambert's sign may be positive: the grip strengthens over seconds
- [ ] The reflexes are reduced in >90% of cases
- [ ] Post-tetanic potentiation of reflexes occurs in almost 80% of cases

Ptosis

- [ ] This may improve with up-gaze
- [ ] There may be enhanced ptosis

Other neuromuscular features

- [ ] Bulbar weakness
- [ ] Dropped head syndrome
- [ ] Reversible tongue atrophy

Autonomic features

- [ ] Dry mucosa
- [ ] Erectile dysfunction
- [ ] Reduced sweating
- [ ] Constipation
- [ ] Sluggish pupillary reflexes
- [ ] Metallic taste

Associated autoimmune disorders

- [ ] Myasthenia gravis (MG)
- [ ] Thyroid disorders
- [ ] Systemic lupus erythematosus (SLE)
- [ ] Insulin dependent diabetes mellitus (IDDM)
- [ ] Pernicious anaemia
- [ ] Vitiligo

Differential diagnosis: myasthenia gravis (MG)

- [ ] Ocular onset is more likely with MG
- [ ] Isolated upper limb weakness is more likely with MG
- [ ] External ophthalmoplegia supports MG over LEMS
- [ ] Caudal progression favours MG

Differential diagnoses: others

- [ ] Myositis: there is muscle tenderness
- [ ] Myopathy: creatinine kinase (CK) is raised
- [ ] Guillain–Barre syndrome (GBS): the CSF is abnormal

Acronym

- [ ] CSF: cerebrospinal fluid

LAMBERT–EATON MYASTHENIC SYNDROME (LEMS): PARANEOPLASTIC

Epidemiology

- [ ] LEMS is associated with cancer in 50–60% of cases
- [ ] The risk of cancer reduces after 2 years of the diagnosis

Small cell cancer (SCLC)

- [ ] This is more frequent in older patients
- [ ] It accounts for most cases of LEMS
- [ ] It is predicted by the absence of the HLA-B8 haplotype
- [ ] SOX1 antibody is a marker of SCLC in LEMS
- [ ] SOX1 can be used in cancer surveillance of LEMS

Other associated cancers

- [ ] Prostate
- [ ] Non-small cell lung cancer (non-SCLC)

DELTA-P paraneoplastic score: benefit

- [ ] This determines the risk of underlying cancer
- [ ] High scores should trigger an intensive and frequent search for cancer
- [ ] Low scores reassure of low risk

DELTA-P paraneoplastic score: scoring items

- [ ] Age ≥ 50 years
- [ ] Smoking at diagnosis
- [ ] ≥ 5% weight loss
- [ ] Bulbar involvement (especially dysarthria)
- [ ] Erectile dysfunction
- [ ] Karnofsky performance status score <70
- [ ] 1 point is given for each within 3 months of diagnosis

Investigations for cancer

- [ ] Computed tomography (CT) scan
- [ ] Positron emission tomography (PET) scan: if CT is negative
- [ ] Monitor for malignancy for 5 years: repeat CT at 3 months and then 6-monthly

DOI: 10.1201/9781003221258-84

LAMBERT–EATON MYASTHENIC SYNDROME (LEMS): ANTIBODIES

P/Q type VGCC antibody

- ☐ This is the most important antibody for the diagnosis of LEMS
- ☐ It is present in 75–100% of paraneoplastic LEMS
- ☐ It is present in >90% of non-paraneoplastic LEMS
- ☐ It however has a low specificity with a high false positive rate

N type VGCC antibodies

- ☐ This is present in about 50–60% of LEMS
- ☐ It may cause a myasthenia gravis-LEMS overlap syndrome (MLOS)
- ☐ It correlates with dysautonomia in LEMS

Anti SOX1 antibody

- ☐ This is frequently positive in small cell lung cancer (SCLC) LEMS
- ☐ It is useful in monitoring tumour-negative cases
- ☐ It is also present in Anti-Hu neurological syndromes

Anti GRP78 antibody

- ☐ This is anti-glucose related protein 78
- ☐ It is present in LEMS associated with paraneoplastic cerebellar degeneration (PCD-LEMS)
- ☐ It also plays a role in neuromyelitis optica (NMO)

Acronym

- ☐ VGCC: voltage gated calcium channel

LAMBERT–EATON MYASTHENIC SYNDROME (LEMS): TREATMENT

3,4 diaminopyridine (3,4 DAP)

- ☐ This is the treatment of choice
- ☐ The dose is 5–10 mg 3–4 times daily
- ☐ It blocks pre-synaptic potassium channels
- ☐ It prevents deterioration in strength
- ☐ It may cause paraesthesias and seizures

Complementary treatments to 3,4 DAP

- ☐ Pyridostigmine
- ☐ Guanidine: this carries a risk of bone marrow suppression and renal failure

Second line treatments

- ☐ Steroids ± Azathioprine: if LEMS is mild and chronic
- ☐ Intravenous immunoglobulin (IVIg)
- ☐ Plasma exchange
- ☐ Rituximab

Other immunosuppressants

- ☐ Cyclosporine
- ☐ Mycophenolate
- ☐ Cyclophosphamide

Drugs to avoid

- ☐ D-tubocurarine (DTC)
- ☐ Pancuronium
- ☐ Aminoglycosides
- ☐ Antiarrhythmics
- ☐ Beta blockers
- ☐ Calcium channel blockers
- ☐ Magnesium
- ☐ Iodinated contrast agents

Annual surveillance

- ☐ Neurophysiology
- ☐ VGCC antibody titre
- ☐ Neurological examination
- ☐ Electrocardiogram (ECG)
- ☐ Spirometry
- ☐ Quantitative myasthenia gravis (QMG) score

Congenital myasthenic syndromes (CMS)

CONGENITAL MYASTHENIC SYNDROME (CMS): CLASSIFICATION BY PATHWAY

Presynaptic defects

- [ ] CHAT: choline acetyl transferase mutations (CMS 6)
- [ ] Synaptotagmin 2: synaptic vesicle-associated calcium sensor (CMS 7)
- [ ] SNAP25B: synaptic vesicle exocytosis (CMS 18)
- [ ] VAChT: vesicular acetylcholine transporter SLC5A7 (CMS 20)
- [ ] VAChT: vesicular acetylcholine transporter SLC18A3 (CMS 21)
- [ ] SLC25A1 (CMS 23)
- [ ] VAMP1: vesicle associated membrane protein 1 (CMS 25)

Synaptic defects

- [ ] COLQ: collagen-like tail subunit (CMS type 5)
- [ ] LAMB2: laminin-β2

Endplate development and maintenance defects

- [ ] AGRN: agrin (CMS 8)
- [ ] MUSK: muscle specific receptor tyrosine kinase (CMS 9)
- [ ] DOK7 (CMS 10)
- [ ] RAPSN: rapsyn (CMS 11)
- [ ] LRP4 (CMS 17)

Postsynaptic (acetylcholine receptor) defects

- [ ] ACHRN: nicotinic acetylcholine receptor deficiency (CMS types 1–4)
  - ○ CHRNA1 (α), CHRNB1 (β), CHRND (δ), CHRNE (ϵ), CHRNG (γ)
  - ○ With fast and slow channel syndromes
- [ ] AChE: endplate acetylcholine esterase
- [ ] AChR: acetylcholine receptor deficiency
- [ ] COL13A1 (CMS 19)
- [ ] MYO9A: unconventional myosin (CMS 24)

Glycosylation pathway defects

- [ ] GFPT1 (CMS 12)
- [ ] DPAGT1 (CMS 13)
- [ ] ALG2 (CMS 14)
- [ ] ALG14 (CMS 15)
- [ ] GMPPB

Myasthenia associated with centronuclear myopathies

- [ ] BIN1: amphiphysin
- [ ] MTM1: myotubularin
- [ ] DNM2: dynamin 2

Other myasthenic syndromes

- [ ] SCN4A: sodium channel 4A (CMS type 16)
- [ ] PREPL (CMS type 22)
- [ ] Plectin
- [ ] Myasthenic symptoms with mitochondrial citrate carrier defects

CONGENITAL MYASTHENIC SYNDROME (CMS): GENERAL FEATURES

Demographic features

- [ ] There is usually a positive family history but this may be absent
- [ ] It has an early onset age but this may be delayed until adulthood
- [ ] Conventional myasthenic antibodies are negative: AChR, MUSK, P/Q type VGCC

Electromyogram (EMG) features

- [ ] Repetitive nerve stimulation at 2–3Hz shows a decremental response
- [ ] Single fiber EMG shows abnormal jitter or blocking
- [ ] Abnormalities may be absent or episodic

Differential diagnosis

- [ ] Congenital myopathies
- [ ] Congenital muscular dystrophies
- [ ] Limb girdle muscular dystrophy (LGMD)
- [ ] Facioscapulohumeral muscular dystrophy (FSHD)
- [ ] Infantile myotonic dystrophy
- [ ] Mitochondrial myopathy
- [ ] Congenital fibrosis of the external ocular muscles (CFEOM)
- [ ] Infantile botulism
- [ ] Autoimmune myasthenia gravis (MG): seropositive and seronegative
- [ ] Chronic fatigue syndrome (CFS)
- [ ] Hypermobility syndromes

DOI: 10.1201/9781003221258-85

CONGENITAL MYASTHENIC SYNDROME (CMS): DOK7

Pathology

- [ ] DOK7 interacts with MUSK
- [ ] There are no tubular aggregates on muscle biopsy
- [ ] Acetylcholine receptor (AChR) antibodies are negative
- [ ] The onset age is from birth to the third decade

Ophthalmic features

- [ ] Ptosis
- [ ] Ophthalmoplegia: this may develop later
- [ ] Transient diplopia: this develops in some cases

Facial and bulbar features

- [ ] Facial weakness
- [ ] Bulbar weakness
- [ ] Mild tongue atrophy occasionally

Limb weakness

- [ ] Limb girdle weakness
- [ ] Waddling gait
- [ ] Frequent falls
- [ ] Exercise-induced weakness

Skeletal features

- [ ] Scoliosis
- [ ] Lordosis

Respiratory features

- [ ] Frequent respiratory problems
- [ ] Stridor

Treatment

- [ ] Ephedrine
- [ ] Salbutamol
- [ ] Avoid cholinesterase inhibitors: they may worsen the symptoms

CONGENITAL MYASTHENIC SYNDROME (CMS): RAPSN

Genetics and pathology

- [ ] This results from Rapsyn deficiency
- [ ] The causative mutations are on chromosome 11p
- [ ] It is a post-synaptic disorder
- [ ] It causes acetylcholine receptor deficiency

Onset

- [ ] The onset is typically at birth
- [ ] Late-onset phenotypes occur in adolescence or early adulthood
- [ ] Late-onset cases usually present as seronegative myasthenia gravis (MG)

Clinical features

- [ ] Dysmorphic appearance
- [ ] Episodic severe sudden apnoeic attacks
- [ ] Upper respiratory tract infections
- [ ] Mild joint contractures
- [ ] Fluoxetine may worsen the symptoms: case report

Treatment

- [ ] Pyridostigmine
- [ ] 3,4 diaminopyridine (3,4 DAP)

CONGENITAL MYASTHENIC SYNDROME (CMS): FAST CHANNEL

Pathology

- ☐ This causes impaired synaptic transmission
- ☐ It results from brief channel opening events
- ☐ It is the most severe form of CMS

Bulbar symptoms

- ☐ Poor sucking
- ☐ Choking
- ☐ Poor cry
- ☐ Stridor

Weakness

- ☐ Limb
- ☐ Trunk
- ☐ Bulbar
- ☐ Facial
- ☐ Jaw
- ☐ Neck
- ☐ Generalised hypotonia

Ophthalmic features

- ☐ Ptosis: often at birth
- ☐ Ophthalmoplegia with abnormal eye movements

Foetal features

- ☐ Reduced foetal movements
- ☐ Arthrogryposis
- ☐ Joint contractures
- ☐ Respiratory crises

Electromyogram (EMG)

- ☐ Decremental response on repetitive nerve stimulation

Treatment

- ☐ Acetylcholinesterase inhibitors
- ☐ 3,4 diaminopyridine (3,4 DAP)

CONGENITAL MYASTHENIC SYNDROME (CMS) PRESENTING IN ADULTHOOD

Frequent adult forms

- ☐ DOK7
- ☐ RAPSN
- ☐ LRP4
- ☐ COLQ
- ☐ Slow-channel syndrome

Rare adult forms

- ☐ Primary acetylcholine receptor deficiency
- ☐ AGRN
- ☐ GFPT1
- ☐ SCN4A
- ☐ CHRNA1

Demographic features

- ☐ The onset age is from birth to about 40 years
- ☐ The median onset age is 5 years
- ☐ There is frequently a positive family history
- ☐ Pregnancy is often a trigger for adult onset cases

Clinical features

- ☐ Mild ophthalmoparesis
- ☐ Isolated ptosis
- ☐ Limb-girdle weakness
- ☐ Fatigable weakness
- ☐ Prominent finger extension weakness: with slow channel syndrome
- ☐ Creatine kinase (CK) may be elevated

Differential diagnosis

- ☐ Seronegative myasthenia gravis (MG)
- ☐ Myopathy
- ☐ Motor neuron disease (MND)
- ☐ Peripheral neuropathy (PN)
- ☐ Limb girdle muscular dystrophy (LGMD)
- ☐ Facioscapulohumeral muscular dystrophy (FSHD)
- ☐ Mitochondrial myopathy

Treatment

- ☐ Intravenous immunoglobulins (IVIg)
- ☐ Plasma exchange
- ☐ Ephedrine or Salbutamol for DOK7
- ☐ Fluoxetine for slow channel syndrome
- ☐ Pyridostigmine: this may worsen symptoms in DOK7

CONGENITAL MYASTHENIC SYNDROME (CMS): DRUG TREATMENT

Pyridostigmine: indications

- ☐ ChAT
- ☐ Sodium channel
- ☐ Fast channel
- ☐ Rapsyn

Pyridostigmine: contraindications

- ☐ DOK7
- ☐ COLQ
- ☐ Slow channel

3,4 diaminopyridine (3,4 DAP): indications

- ☐ Fast channel
- ☐ Rapsyn

3,4 diaminopyridine (3,4 DAP): contraindications

- ☐ DOK7
- ☐ COLQ
- ☐ Slow channel

Treatment of slow channel

- ☐ Fluoxetine
- ☐ Quinidine

Treatment of DOK7

- ☐ Ephedrine
- ☐ Salbutamol

CHAPTER 15

Muscle disorders

Muscle symptoms and signs

DROPPED HEAD SYNDROME (DHS): NEUROMUSCULAR CAUSES

Inflammatory myopathies

- ☐ Polymyositis
- ☐ Inclusion body myositis (IBM)

Metabolic myopathies

- ☐ Carnitine deficiency
- ☐ Multiple Acyl CoA dehydrogenase deficiency (MADD)
- ☐ Adult onset acid maltase deficiency (Pompe disease)
- ☐ Mitochondrial myopathy

Endocrine myopathies

- ☐ Cushing syndrome
- ☐ Hypothyroid myopathy
- ☐ Hypokalaemic myopathy
- ☐ Hyperparathyroidism

Other myopathies

- ☐ Isolated paraspinal myopathy (with bent spine)
- ☐ Isolated neck extensor myopathy (INEM)
- ☐ Nemaline myopathy
- ☐ Anti-SRP myopathy
- ☐ Anti-GAD myopathy

Muscular dystrophies

- ☐ Facioscapulohumeral muscular dystrophy (FSHD)
- ☐ Proximal myotonic myopathy
- ☐ Congenital muscular dystrophy with Lamin A/C (LMNA) gene mutations
- ☐ Selenoprotein deficiency

Anterior horn cell (AHC) disorders

- ☐ Motor neurone disease (MND)
- ☐ Post-polio syndrome (PPS)
- ☐ Spinal muscular atrophy (SMA)

Neuromuscular junction disorders and neuropathies

- ☐ Myasthenia gravis (MG)
- ☐ Chronic inflammatory demyelinating polyradiculoneuropathy (CIDP)

DROPPED HEAD SYNDROME (DHS): NON-NEUROMUSCULAR CAUSES

Cervical diseases

- ☐ Syringomyelia
- ☐ Cervical spondylosis
- ☐ Ankylosing spondylitis
- ☐ Forced cervical hyperflexion
- ☐ Cervical dystonia (spasmodic torticollis)

Neurodegenerative causes

- ☐ Chorea acanthocytosis
- ☐ Multiple system atrophy (MSA)
- ☐ Huntington's disease (HD)

Miscellaneous causes

- ☐ Idiopathic
- ☐ Botulinum toxin treatment
- ☐ High dose irradiation
- ☐ Primary amyloidosis
- ☐ Anticonvulsant-induced carnitine deficiency

Causes of intermittent head drop

- ☐ Epilepsy
- ☐ Tic disorders
- ☐ Stereotypies
- ☐ Paroxysmal dyskinesia
- ☐ Narcolepsy
- ☐ Nodding syndrome
- ☐ Sandifer syndrome

DOI: 10.1201/9781003221258-87

MYOPATHY WITH RESPIRATORY FAILURE: CAUSES

Metabolic myopathies

- ☐ Acid maltase deficiency (Pompe disease)
- ☐ Carnitine deficiency

Congenital myopathies

- ☐ Centronuclear myopathy
- ☐ Nemaline myopathy
- ☐ Myofibrillar myopathy due to BAG3 mutation
- ☐ Multiminicore disease
- ☐ Hereditary myopathy with early respiratory failure (HMERF)

EMARDD: features

- ☐ Early onset myopathy
- ☐ Areflexia
- ☐ Respiratory distress
- ☐ Dysphagia
- ☐ Associated with MEGF10 gene mutations

SMARD1

- ☐ This is a spinal muscular atrophy
- ☐ It is caused by IGHMBP2 gene mutations
- ☐ It causes respiratory distress

Other muscle diseases

- ☐ Myotonic dystrophy type 1
- ☐ MELAS
- ☐ Polymyositis
- ☐ Amyloid myopathy
- ☐ Cytoplasmic body myopathy
- ☐ FHL1-related myopathy
- ☐ Laminopathy

Acronym

- ☐ MELAS: mitochondrial encephalomyopathy lactic acidosis and stroke-like events

RAPIDLY PROGRESSIVE WEAKNESS: CAUSES

Neuropathic causes

- ☐ Guillain–Barre syndrome (GBS)
- ☐ Chronic inflammatory demyelinating polyradiculoneuropathy (CIDP)
- ☐ Miller Fisher syndrome (MFS)
- ☐ Charcot–Marie–Tooth disease type 4J (CMT 4J)
- ☐ Lead neuropathy

Myopathic causes

- ☐ Periodic paralysis
- ☐ Steroid myopathy
- ☐ Polymyositis

Other neurological causes

- ☐ Myasthenia gravis (MG)
- ☐ Myelopathy

Infective causes

- ☐ Botulism
- ☐ Diphtheria
- ☐ Tic paralysis
- ☐ Lyme neuroborreliosis
- ☐ HIV
- ☐ West Nile virus
- ☐ Poliomyelitis

Systemic causes

- ☐ Porphyria
- ☐ Vasculitis
- ☐ Sarcoidosis
- ☐ Paraneoplastic
- ☐ Thyrotoxicosis
- ☐ Diabetes mellitus

MUSCLE HYPERTROPHY: CAUSES

Myopathic causes

- ☐ Childhood acid maltase deficiency
- ☐ Hypokalaemic periodic paralysis
- ☐ Congenital hypothyroidism myopathy (Kocher-Debre-Semelaigne)
- ☐ Myositis

Muscular dystrophies

- ☐ Duchenne (DMD)
- ☐ Becker (BMD)
- ☐ Limb girdle (LGMD)

Other muscle disorders

- ☐ Myotonia congenital: this confers a Herculean appearance
- ☐ Lipodystrophy syndromes
- ☐ Myostatin (MSTN) gene mutation

Anterior horn cell (AHC) and root disorders

- ☐ Spinal muscular atrophy (SMA)
- ☐ L4 and L5 lumbar radiculopathy: these cause tibialis muscle hypertrophy

Neuropathic disorders

- ☐ Chronic inflammatory demyelinating polyradiculoneuropathy (CIDP)
- ☐ Peripheral nerve partial denervation
- ☐ Accessory nerve mononeuropathy: this causes trapezius muscle hypertrophy

Other causes

- ☐ Neuromyotonia
- ☐ Stiff person syndrome (SPS)
- ☐ Amyloidosis
- ☐ Sarcoidosis
- ☐ Acromegaly
- ☐ Fliers syndrome (insulin resistance)
- ☐ Cysticercosis
- ☐ Tethered cord syndrome

FASCICULATIONS: CAUSES

Physiological causes

- ☐ Benign fasciculations
- ☐ Coffee
- ☐ Physical activity

Anterior horn cell (AHC) disorders

- ☐ Motor neurone disease (MND)
- ☐ Spinal muscular atrophy (SMA)
- ☐ X-linked spinal and bulbar muscular atrophy (SBMA, Kennedy disease)
- ☐ Monomelic amyotrophy
- ☐ Post-polio syndrome

Nerve disorders

- ☐ Multifocal motor neuropathy (MMN)
- ☐ Charcot–Marie–Tooth disease 4C (CMT4C)
- ☐ Radiculopathy

Cerebral causes

- ☐ Creutzfeldt Jakob disease (CJD)
- ☐ Spinocerebellar ataxia type 3 (SCA3)
- ☐ Spinocerebellar ataxia type 36 (SCA36)
- ☐ Multiple system atrophy (MSA)

Hereditary spastic paraplegia (HSP)

- ☐ HSP10 (SPG10)
- ☐ HSP55 (SPG55)
- ☐ HSP79 (SPG79)

Systemic causes

- ☐ Debrancher enzyme deficiency
- ☐ Acute viral infections
- ☐ Syndrome of inappropriate ADH secretion (SIADH)
- ☐ Hyperthyroidism
- ☐ Hyperparathyroidism
- ☐ Hypophosphataemia
- ☐ Organophosphate poisoning
- ☐ Mercury

Drug-induced fasciculations

- ☐ Neostigmine
- ☐ Succinylcholine
- ☐ Steroids
- ☐ Isoniazid
- ☐ Flunarizine
- ☐ Lithium
- ☐ Nortriptyline

Causes of tongue fasciculations

- ☐ Charcot–Marie–Tooth disease 4C (CMT4C)
- ☐ Spinocerebellar ataxia type 36 (SCA36)
- ☐ Organophosphate poisoning
- ☐ Myasthenia gravis (MG): case report
- ☐ Osmotic demyelination disorder (ODD)
- ☐ TTR familial amyloid neuropathy (FAP)

CAMPTOCORMIA: CAUSES

Idiopathic camptocormia

- ☐ This is a late-onset idiopathic axial myopathy
- ☐ There is a female preponderance
- ☐ There may be a family history
- ☐ It is limited to the spinal muscles
- ☐ It causes forward spinal flexion
- ☐ It resolves in the horizontal position
- ☐ There is back pain in some cases
- ☐ There is associated spondyloarthrosis in almost all cases
- ☐ Creatinine kinase (CK) may be elevated
- ☐ Imaging shows fatty infiltration of paravertebral muscles

Parkinsonian causes

- ☐ Idiopathic Parkinson's disease (PD) with axial dystonia
- ☐ Parkin PD
- ☐ Multiple system atrophy (MSA)
- ☐ Post-encephalitic parkinsonism

Other neurodegenerative causes

- ☐ Alzheimer's disease (AD)
- ☐ Dopa-responsive dystonia (DRD)

Neuromuscular causes

- ☐ Focal paraspinal myopathy
- ☐ Inclusion body myositis (IBM)
- ☐ Nemaline myopathy
- ☐ Facioscapulohumeral muscular dystrophy (FSHD)
- ☐ Duchenne muscular dystrophy (DMD) carriers
- ☐ Motor neurone disease (MND)
- ☐ Myotonic dystrophy
- ☐ Tetanus
- ☐ Mitochondrial diseases

Drug-induced

- ☐ Valproate
- ☐ Olanzapine
- ☐ Donepezil
- ☐ Systemic steroids
- ☐ Dopamine agonist

Miscellaneous causes

- ☐ Spinal deformities
- ☐ Stroke
- ☐ Psychogenic
- ☐ Thyrotoxicosis
- ☐ Paraneoplastic
- ☐ Tourette syndrome

Synonym

- ☐ Spinal flexion

Inflammatory myopathies

INFLAMMATORY MYOPATHY: CLASSIFICATION

Primary inflammatory myopathies

- [ ] Dermatomyositis (DM)
- [ ] Juvenile dermatomyositis
- [ ] Amyopathic dermatomyositis
- [ ] Dermatomyositis with vascular pathology (DM-VP)
- [ ] Polymyositis (PM)
- [ ] Juvenile myositis other than dermatomyositis
- [ ] Inclusion body myositis (IBM): sporadic
- [ ] Immune-mediated necrotising myopathy (IMNM)
- [ ] Overlap myositis
- [ ] Anti-synthetase syndrome
- [ ] Immune myopathies with perimysial pathology (IMPP)
- [ ] Brachiocervical inflammatory myopathy
- [ ] Macrophagic myofasciitis

Secondary inflammatory myopathies

- [ ] Myositis associated with cancer
- [ ] Myositis associated with other connective tissue diseases
- [ ] Drug-induced inflammatory myopathies

Acronyms

- [ ] HMGCoA: 3-hydroxy-3-methylglutaryl-CoA
- [ ] SRP: signal recognition particle

DERMATOMYOSITIS: CLINICAL FEATURES

Possible risk factors

- [ ] Exposure to ultraviolet light
- [ ] TIF1 gene mutations
- [ ] Some class 2 HLA alleles

Major dermatological features

- [ ] Heliotrope rash: this is a violaceous oedematous periorbital rash
- [ ] Gottron's papules: this is an erythematous rash on the extensor surface of joints
- [ ] Mechanics hands: these are cracked fingers
- [ ] Shawl or V sign (poikiloderma): this is an erythematous rash over the face, neck, and chest
- [ ] Red rash: this is over the knees, elbows, and malleoli
- [ ] Calcinosis: this is especially associated with NXP2 dermatomyositis

Other dermatological features

- [ ] Periungual telangiectasias
- [ ] Cuticular hypertrophy
- [ ] Holster sign: on the hips
- [ ] Leukokeratosis
- [ ] Hiker's feet: plantar hyperkeratosis
- [ ] Pruritus
- [ ] Ulcers: these are usually on flexor surfaces of the digits and the palm
  - ○ They are most frequently seen in MDA5 positive cases
- [ ] Suntan sign: these are hyperchromic and erythematous patches on the face and nose

Neurological features

- [ ] Myopathy
- [ ] Dysphagia
- [ ] Ophthalmoplegia: case reports

Oral features

- [ ] Erythema
- [ ] Haemorrhages
- [ ] Ulcers
- [ ] Vesicles
- [ ] Gingival telangiectasias

Anti-MDA5 features

- [ ] Rapidly progressive interstitial lung disease (ILD)
- [ ] Severe skin vasculopathy and frequent myositis
- [ ] Palmar papules: inverse Gottron
- [ ] Diffuse hair loss
- [ ] Digital and oral ulcers
- [ ] Panniculitis
- [ ] Polyarthritis

DOI: 10.1201/9781003221258-88

Associated disorders

- ☐ Malignancy: especially ovarian
- ☐ Interstitial lung disease: this is severe with anti MDA5 cases
- ☐ Heart failure
- ☐ Arrhythmias
- ☐ Arthralgia
- ☐ Gastrointestinal bleeding

DERMATOMYOSITIS: MANAGEMENT

Autoantibody tests

- ☐ Anti MDA5
- ☐ Anti mi2
- ☐ Anti NXP2
- ☐ Anti SAE
- ☐ Anti TIF1

Muscle enzymes

- ☐ Creatinine kinase (CK): this is usually elevated but it may be normal
  - ○ A normal CK may predict a poor prognosis
- ☐ Aldolase: this may be elevated when the CK is normal

Electromyogram (EMG): features

- ☐ Myopathic motor units
- ☐ Fibrillations
- ☐ Spontaneous sharp waves

Muscle biopsy: features

- ☐ Perifascicular atrophy: this has >90% specificity but <50% sensitivity
- ☐ Perifascicular human myxovirus resistance protein: this has >70% sensitivity
- ☐ Perifascicular retinoic acid-inducible gene 1: this has 50% sensitivity
- ☐ Cellular infiltrates: plasmacytoid dendritic cells, B cells, CD4 T cells, and macrophages
- ☐ Microtubular inclusions: these are on intramuscular capillaries
- ☐ Class-1 major histocompatibility complex upregulation
- ☐ Necrosis: this may predominate

Magnetic resonance imaging (MRI): muscle

- ☐ This shows high signal intensities on contrast T1 sequences
  - ○ These are subcutaneous and fascial
- ☐ They have a honeycomb pattern
- ☐ The distribution is peripheral

POLYMYOSITIS

Demographic features

☐ The onset is typically after the of age 16 years
☐ The onset may be triggered by TNF-α blocking agents

Neurological features

☐ It spares the face and eyes
☐ It may present with muscle hypertrophy
☐ It may present with prominent neck extension weakness

Cardiac features

☐ These are more frequent in polymyositis than in dermatomyositis
☐ They are usually subclinical
☐ Heart failure is the commonest clinical presentation
☐ Anti-Ro is a marker for cardiac injury

Neoplastic features

☐ There is a malignancy risk
☐ This is especially ovarian

Differential diagnosis

☐ Inclusion body myositis (IBM)
☐ Limb girdle muscular dystrophy 2B (LGMD 2B)
☐ Myositis associated with a connective tissue disease
☐ Muscular dystrophies with inflammation
☐ Diabetes mellitus

IMMUNE MEDIATED NECROTISING MYOPATHY (IMNM): CAUSES

Idiopathic

☐ Idiopathic accounts for about half of cases

Autoimmune

☐ Anti HMGCoA reductase: this is found in about a third of cases
☐ Anti SRP: this is present in about a quarter of cases

Statins

☐ This causes statin induced necrotising autoimmune myopathy (SINAM)
☐ Statins cause up-regulation of HMGCR
☐ Symptoms may persist even on stopping the drug

Paraneoplastic

☐ Malignancies occur in 20% of seronegative cases
☐ They are present in about 10% of anti HMGCR positive cases
☐ They are not associated with anti SRP positive cases

Other causes

☐ Viral infections
☐ Overlap syndromes

Synonym

☐ Necrotising autoimmune myopathy (NAM)

Acronyms

☐ HMGCoA: 3-hydroxy-3-methylglutaryl-CoA
☐ SRP: signal recognition particle

IMMUNE MEDIATED NECROTISING MYOPATHY (IMNM): CLINICAL FEATURES

Antibody profile

- ☐ Anti SRP: this frequently involves the lungs
- ☐ Anti HMGCR: this is seen in statin exposed subjects
- ☐ Antibody negative (seronegative): this has a strong association with cancer

Clinical features

- ☐ Subacute lower limb predominant proximal weakness: this is worse in anti-SRP cases
- ☐ Dysphagia
- ☐ Dyspnoea
- ☐ Facial weakness: especially with anti SRP positive cases
- ☐ Risk of malignancy: but not with anti SRP cases
- ☐ Cardiac involvement: especially with anti SRP cases

Features of seronegative IMNM

- ☐ There is a female predominance
- ☐ It is more frequently associated with connective tissue diseases
- ☐ There is a higher risk of malignancy
- ☐ There are more frequent extra-muscular features

Muscle biopsy

- ☐ This shows necrosis with minimal lymphocytes
- ☐ The necrosis is worse with anti SRP cases
- ☐ There is no perifascicular atrophy

Other investigations

- ☐ Creatine kinase (CK): the level is very high
- ☐ Electromyogram (EMG): this is myopathic
- ☐ Endomyocardial biopsy: this is indicated in selected cases

Differential diagnosis

- ☐ Limb girdle muscular dystrophy (LGMD)

Prognostic features

- ☐ Anti HMGCR is a marker of treatment response
- ☐ Anti-SRP is an indicator of severe disease
- ☐ Younger subjects have a worse outcome

Synonym

- ☐ Necrotising autoimmune myopathy (NAM)

INCLUSION BODY MYOSITIS (IBM): RISK FACTORS

Infections

- ☐ Hepatitis C virus (HCV)

Anti-cytosolic 5'-nucleotidase 1A (anti NT5c1A)

- ☐ This is present in about 35% of cases
- ☐ It is associated with less frequent proximal upper limb weakness
- ☐ It confers a higher mortality risk
- ☐ Muscle biopsy shows more cytochrome oxidase deficient fibers
- ☐ The type 2 muscle fibers are smaller

VCP-related multisystem proteinopathy (MSP): components

- ☐ Frontotemporal dementia and Paget's disease of the bone (IBMPFD)
- ☐ Amyotrophic lateral sclerosis (ALS)
- ☐ Charcot–Marie–Tooth disease type 2 (CMT2)
- ☐ Hereditary spastic paraplegia (HSP)
- ☐ Early onset Parkinson's disease (PD)

Possible IBM risk associations

- ☐ Chronic lymphocytic leukemia (CLL)
- ☐ Sjogren's syndrome
- ☐ FYCO1 missense variants
- ☐ Spinocerebellar ataxia types 3 and 6 (SCA3 and SCA6)

INCLUSION BODY MYOSITIS (IBM): CLINICAL FEATURES

Quadriceps weakness

- ☐ This manifests as knee extension weakness
- ☐ This is usually asymmetric: unlike polymyositis (PM) or dermatomyositis (DM)
- ☐ It typically presents with recurrent falls

Long finger flexion weakness: difficulties

- ☐ Buttons
- ☐ Zippers
- ☐ Jars
- ☐ Turning keys
- ☐ Tying knots
- ☐ Holding golf clubs

Other weakness features

- ☐ Foot drop: this results from weakness of the foot dorsiflexors
- ☐ Facial weakness: this occurs an a third of cases
- ☐ Neck weakness: this is due to weakness of the neck flexors and extensors
- ☐ Head drop
- ☐ Camptocormia
- ☐ Dysphagia: this occurs in 60% of cases
- ☐ Positive Beevor's sign

Peripheral neuropathy (PN)

- ☐ This is common
- ☐ It is frequently asymptomatic

Spared muscles and organs

- ☐ Extraocular muscles
- ☐ Small hand muscles (unlike MND)
- ☐ Cardiac disease
- ☐ Interstitial lung disease (ILD)
- ☐ Malignancy

Differential diagnosis: motor neurone disease (MND)

- ☐ Dysphagia occurs without dysarthria in 40% of IBM cases: this is unusual in MND
- ☐ Cramps are unusual in IBM unlike in MND
- ☐ Visible fasciculations are unusual in IBM
- ☐ Definite upper motor neurone signs are unusual in IBM

INFLAMMATORY MYOPATHY: INVESTIGATIONS

Electromyogram (EMG): features

- ☐ Spontaneous fibrillations: at rest and with needle insertion
- ☐ Short-duration, small-amplitude polyphasic motor unit potentials
- ☐ Spontaneous high-frequency discharges

Magnetic resonance imaging (MRI) muscle: features

- ☐ Active inflammation and oedema: these enhance on T2-weighted images
- ☐ Late stage lipomatosis: these enhance on T1- and T2-weighted images
- ☐ STIR sequences can differentiate oedema from fatty infiltration

Muscle biopsy: features

- ☐ The inflammation may be patchy with skip areas
- ☐ The inflammatory infiltrate is predominantly lymphocytic
- ☐ The infiltrates are intra-fascicular in polymyositis and inclusion body myositis
- ☐ The infiltrates are perivascular and perifascicular in dermatomyositis
- ☐ Perifascicular atrophy is seen in dermatomyositis
- ☐ There may be myophagocytosis by macrophages
- ☐ Centralisation of myofibril nuclei may be seen
- ☐ Fibrosis may be present

Muscle ultrasound

- ☐ Muscle atrophy
  - ○ This is symmetrical and proximal in polymyositis
  - ○ It is severe in inclusion body myositis (IBM)
  - ○ It is rare in dermatomyositis
- ☐ Increased echointensity
  - ○ This is worse in lower limb muscles in polymyositis
  - ○ It is worse in forearm muscles in dermatomyositis
- ☐ Inflammation and oedema
  - ○ These are seen in polymyositis

High resolution chest CT: features

- ☐ Diffuse ground glass attenuation: especially in the lung bases
- ☐ Interlobular septal thickening
- ☐ Bronchiectasis
- ☐ Reticular opacities
- ☐ Honeycombing
- ☐ Air space consolidation

Other tests

- ☐ Pulmonary function tests (PFTs)
- ☐ Electrocardiogram (ECG)
- ☐ Echocardiogram: if there are features of heart failure
- ☐ Cardiac MRI
- ☐ Video fluoroscopy: for dysphagia

INFLAMMATORY MYOPATHY: TREATMENT

Acute treatment

- ☐ Prednisolone
- ☐ Intravenous immunoglobulins (IVIg) if steroid resistant

Long-term treatment

- ☐ Azathioprine
- ☐ Methotrexate
- ☐ Mycophenolate
- ☐ Ciclosporin
- ☐ Tacrolimus

Treatment of refractory cases

- ☐ Rituximab
- ☐ Cyclophosphamide
- ☐ Tacrolimus
- ☐ Rapamycin: a TNF alpha inhibitor
- ☐ Abatacept
- ☐ Tocilizumab

JAK inhibitors: indications

- ☐ Refractory juvenile dermatomyositis
- ☐ Refractory interstitial lung disease in MDA5 associated dermatomyositis

JAK inhibitors: types

- ☐ Tofacitinib
- ☐ Ruxolitinib
- ☐ Baricitinib

Glycogen storage diseases

POMPE DISEASE (GSD TYPE II): CLINICAL FEATURES

Neuromuscular features

- [ ] Weakness: proximal lower limbs, paraspinal, diaphragm, and respiratory muscles
- [ ] Exercise intolerance
- [ ] Fatigue
- [ ] Ptosis: this occurs in a third of cases
- [ ] Positive Beevor's sign
- [ ] Bent spine syndrome
- [ ] Macroglossia

Intracranial features

- [ ] Vertebrobasilar dolichoectasia (VBD)
- [ ] Intracranial aneurysms
- [ ] Basilar artery fenestration
- [ ] Microbleeds
- [ ] Hearing impairment

Skeletal features

- [ ] Back pain
- [ ] Kyphoscoliosis
- [ ] Hyperlordosis
- [ ] Rigid spine
- [ ] Bent spine syndrome
- [ ] Vertebral fractures

Gastrointestinal features

- [ ] Dysphagia
- [ ] Early satiety
- [ ] Chronic diarrhoea
- [ ] Urinary and bowel incontinence
- [ ] Hepatomegaly

Cardiorespiratory features

- [ ] Chest infections
- [ ] Respiratory failure
- [ ] Exertional dyspnoea
- [ ] Hypertrophic cardiomyopathy
- [ ] Aortic aneurysms
- [ ] Arrhythmias

Differential diagnosis

- [ ] Limb girdle muscular dystrophy (LGMD)
- [ ] Becker muscular dystrophy
- [ ] Inclusion body myositis (IBM)
- [ ] Scapuloperoneal syndromes
- [ ] Rigid spine syndrome
- [ ] Myasthenia gravis
- [ ] Spinal muscular atrophy (SMA)
- [ ] Polymyositis
- [ ] Glycogen storage diseases
- [ ] Danon disease
- [ ] Rheumatoid arthritis
- [ ] Mitochondrial myopathies
- [ ] Hydroxychloroquine induced toxic myopathy
- [ ] Fibromyalgia

DOI: 10.1201/9781003221258-89

POMPE DISEASE (GSD TYPE II): INVESTIGATIONS

Dried blood spot (DBS) test

☐ This is positive in 2.5% of people with raised CK and limb girdle weakness
☐ Consider screening in this circumstance

Tissue GAA activity

☐ Skin fibroblast (gold standard)
☐ Muscle

Mutational analysis

☐ This is especially indicated for family carriers
☐ The commonest mutation is the c.-32–13T_>G splice site mutation

Prenatal diagnosis: techniques

☐ Uncultured chorionic villus sample
☐ Amniocentesis
☐ Pre-implantation genetic diagnosis

Cardiorespiratory assessments

☐ 24-hour electrocardiogram (ECG): for conduction defects
☐ Echocardiogram: for cardiomyopathy
☐ Pulmonary function test
☐ Supine vital capacity
☐ Sleep respiratory function: for disordered breathing
☐ Polysomnography: at diagnosis

Other tests

☐ Creatinine kinase (CK): this is raised in 95% of cases
☐ Urine glucose tetrasaccharide (Glc4): this is raised
☐ Muscle biopsy: this shows glycogen positive vacuoles
  ○ It may mimic hydroxychloroquine myopathy
☐ Video-fluoroscopy: for risk of aspiration
☐ Chest X ray
☐ DEXA bone screening
☐ Hearing assessment

POMPE DISEASE (GSD TYPE II): ENZYME REPLACEMENT THERAPY (ERT)

Benefits

☐ The agent is alglucosidase alpha
☐ It is beneficial in adult-onset Pompe disease
☐ It improves muscle strength
☐ It stabilises or improves pulmonary function
☐ It improves quality of life
☐ It improves survival

Indications

☐ It is recommended only for symptomatic adult-onset subjects
☐ It may benefit subjects with advanced disease
☐ The benefit should be re-evaluated after one year of use

Use in pregnancy

☐ It has been used successfully through pregnancy
☐ It increases the frequency of interventional deliveries
☐ Symptoms worsen if the treatment is stopped in early pregnancy
☐ Recommencing treatment results in adverse reactions

Limitations

☐ ERT does not prevent slowly progressive white matter abnormalities
☐ Its efficacy is impaired by Propranolol
☐ Adjunctive Salbutamol gives little additional benefit

MCARDLE'S DISEASE (GSD TYPE V): CLINICAL FEATURES

Exercise-induced symptoms

- ☐ Proximal weakness: this is permanent in a third of cases
- ☐ Fatigue: this is chronic in 40% of cases
- ☐ Muscle stiffness
- ☐ Myalgia
- ☐ Weakness
- ☐ Cramps: in the limbs, chest, jaw, and paraspinal muscles
- ☐ Contractures
- ☐ Myoglobinuria

Second wind phenomenon

- ☐ Strength improves after 6–8 minutes of weakness
- ☐ This is absent in a fifth of cases

Muscle wasting

- ☐ Paraspinal
- ☐ Periscapular
- ☐ Proximal upper limbs

Other features

- ☐ Muscle hypertrophy is present in a quarter of patients

Differential diagnosis

- ☐ Becker muscular dystrophy (BMD)

Complications

- ☐ Rhabdomyolysis
- ☐ Renal failure
- ☐ Risk of gout: urate levels should be monitored
- ☐ Weight gain

MCARDLE'S DISEASE (GSD TYPE V): MANAGEMENT

Non-ischaemic forearm test

- ☐ This has a high risk of false positive results
- ☐ It however has a lesser risk of compartment syndrome than the ischaemic test

Function tests

- ☐ Functional cycle test
- ☐ 12-minute walk challenge

Muscle biopsy

- ☐ This is falsely positive in critical illness
- ☐ It is falsely negative soon after rhabdomyolysis

Other neurological tests

- ☐ Creatinine kinase (CK)
- ☐ Electromyogram (EMG): this is normal in 50% of cases

Genetics

- ☐ Myophosphorylase gene (PYGM) mutations
- ☐ These are on chromosome X 11q13
- ☐ The p.Arg 50X mutation is the commonest form in the UK and North America
- ☐ Heterozygotes are asymptomatic

Treatment

- ☐ Pre-exercise sucrose
- ☐ High carbohydrate diet
- ☐ Teach second wind strategy
- ☐ Aerobic exercise: this increases work capacity
- ☐ Creatine

Lipid storage myopathies

CARNITINE PALMITOYL TRANSFERASE (CPT II) DEFICIENCY: CLINICAL FEATURES

Epidemiology and pathology
- ☐ This is the commonest familial cause of myoglobinuria

Onset types
- ☐ Infantile
- ☐ Neonatal
- ☐ Late onset

Clinical features
- ☐ Attacks of myalgia: from childhood
- ☐ Attacks of myoglobinuria: from adolescence
- ☐ Exercise induced muscle pain and weakness: after prolonged exertion
- ☐ Isolated myalgia: this is an atypical feature
- ☐ Rhabdomyolysis
- ☐ Renal failure

Common triggers for attacks
- ☐ Exercise
- ☐ Infection
- ☐ Fasting
- ☐ Cold

Uncommon triggers for attacks
- ☐ Mild exercise
- ☐ Emotional stress
- ☐ Anaesthesia
- ☐ Diazepam
- ☐ Valproate
- ☐ Ibuprofen

Differential diagnosis: McArdle's disease
- ☐ There is weakness between attacks in a quarter of people with McArdle's disease
  - ○ This is not seen in CPT II deficiency
- ☐ There are associated cramps in McArdle's disease
  - ○ These are not present in CPT II deficiency

Synonym
- ☐ Di Mauro's disease

CARNITINE PALMITOYL TRANSFERASE (CPT II) DEFICIENCY: MANAGEMENT

Blood tests
- ☐ Long chain acylcarnitines: the levels are increased
- ☐ Creatinine kinase (CK): this is normal between attacks

Mutations in blood cells
- ☐ S113: this is present in up to 95% of cases
- ☐ P50H
- ☐ Q413fs-F448L

Muscle biopsy
- ☐ There is no pathological hallmark unlike in carnitine deficiency

Treatment
- ☐ Frequent meals
- ☐ Carbohydrates before exercise
- ☐ Restrict long chain fatty acids
- ☐ Avoid fasting
- ☐ Bezafibrate
- ☐ Medium chain fatty acid supplementation

Synonym
- ☐ Di Mauro's disease

DOI: 10.1201/9781003221258-90

MULTIPLE ACYL-COA DEHYDROGENASE DEFICIENCY (MADD): CLINICAL FEATURES

Genetics

- [ ] MADD is caused by mutations in the electronic transfer flavoprotein (ETF) gene
- [ ] These are ETFA, ETFB, and ETF dehydrogenase (ETFDH)
- [ ] ETFDH causes riboflavin-responsive MADD (RR-MADD)
- [ ] Transmission is autosomal recessive

Pathogenesis

- [ ] It impairs flavin transport and metabolism
- [ ] There is impaired beta oxidation by all fatty-acid acyl-CoA dehydrogenases

Types

- [ ] Type I: neonatal onset with congenital anomalies: riboflavin-unresponsive
- [ ] Type II: neonatal onset without congenital anomalies
- [ ] Type III: adult onset

Muscle features

- [ ] Late-life onset
- [ ] Proximal myopathy
- [ ] Exercise intolerance
- [ ] Dropped head syndrome (DHS): from paravertebral muscle involvement

Systemic features

- [ ] Weight loss
- [ ] Respiratory insufficiency
- [ ] Cardiomyopathy
- [ ] Pancreatitis

Features in crises

- [ ] Encephalopathy
- [ ] Lethargy
- [ ] Vomiting
- [ ] Hypoglycaemia
- [ ] Hyperammonaemia
- [ ] Rhabdomyolysis
- [ ] Renal failure

Other features

- [ ] Sensory axonal peripheral neuropathy (PN)
- [ ] Depression
- [ ] Congenital anomalies: with infantile forms

Differential diagnosis

- [ ] Primary carnitine deficiency: acyl carnitine may be decreased in MADD
- [ ] Neutral lipid storage disease with myopathy (NLSDM)
- [ ] Myasthenia gravis (MG)
- [ ] Guillain–Barre syndrome (GBS)
- [ ] Polymyositis
- [ ] Mitochondrial myopathy with MTCYB gene mutation

Synonym

- [ ] Glutaric aciduria type II (GAII)

MULTIPLE ACYL-COA DEHYDROGENASE DEFICIENCY (MADD): MANAGEMENT

Blood tests

- [ ] Serum free carnitine: this is increased
- [ ] Acyl-carnitine: this is increased
- [ ] Co-enzyme Q10: this is usually normal but it may be reduced
- [ ] Ammonia: this is increased
- [ ] Creatinine kinase (CK): this is elevated
- [ ] Lactic acidosis
- [ ] Hypoglycaemia

Urinary acid excretion

- [ ] Glutaric
- [ ] Lactic
- [ ] Ethylmalonic
- [ ] Butyric
- [ ] Isobutyric
- [ ] 2-methylbutyric
- [ ] Isovaleric
- [ ] Hexanoylglycine

Muscle biopsy

- [ ] Lipid storage
- [ ] Low muscle carnitine
- [ ] Increased coenzyme Q

Magnetic resonance imaging (MRI) muscle

- [ ] There is fatty infiltration and atrophy
- [ ] This is prominent in the posterior thigh and gluteal muscles

Magnetic resonance imaging (MRI) brain: location of high signal changes

- [ ] Periventricular white matter
- [ ] Splenium of the corpus callosum
- [ ] Basal ganglia
- [ ] Middle cerebral peduncles

Treatment

- [ ] Riboflavin 100–400 mg daily: for ETFDH
- [ ] Carnitine supplementation
- [ ] Coenzyme Q

Synonym

- [ ] Glutaric aciduria type II (GAII)

Muscle channelopathies

NEUROLOGICAL CHANNELOPATHIES: CLASSIFICATION

Muscle channelopathies: periodic paralyses

- ☐ Hyperkalaemic periodic paralysis
- ☐ Hypokalaemic periodic paralysis

Muscle channelopathies: non-dystrophic myotonias

- ☐ Myotonia congenita
- ☐ Paramyotonia congenita (PMC)
- ☐ Potassium-aggravated myotonia (PAM)
- ☐ Andersen-Tawil syndrome (ATS)

Muscle channelopathies: ryanodinopathies

- ☐ Malignant hyperthermia (MH)
- ☐ Central core disease (CCD)
- ☐ Multi-minicore disease (MmD)
- ☐ Centronuclear myopathy (CNM)

Epileptic channelopathies

- ☐ Dravet syndrome (severe myoclonic epilepsy of infancy)
- ☐ Migrating partial seizures of infancy
- ☐ Genetic epilepsy with febrile seizures + (GEFS+)
- ☐ Benign familial neonatal convulsions (BFNC)
- ☐ Generalised epilepsy with paroxysmal movement disorders
- ☐ Absence epilepsy
- ☐ Autosomal dominant nocturnal frontal lobe epilepsy (ADNFLE)

Pain syndromes

- ☐ Erythromelalgia
- ☐ Paroxysmal extreme pain disorder (PEPD)
- ☐ Congenital insensitivity to pain
- ☐ Familial episodic pain syndrome

Ataxic syndromes

- ☐ Episodic ataxia
- ☐ Spinocerebellar ataxia

Other channelopathy syndromes

- ☐ Familial hemiplegic migraine (FHM)
- ☐ Hyperekplexia
- ☐ Peripheral nerve hyperexcitability (PNH)
- ☐ Congenital myasthenic syndromes
- ☐ Acquired neuromyotonia
- ☐ Jervell–Lange–Nielsen syndrome

MUSCLE CHANNELOPATHIES: GENERAL FEATURES

Myotonia

- ☐ This is muscle stiffness due to difficulty in relaxing muscle contractions
- ☐ It is tested by percussion and handgrip
- ☐ It is relieved by exercise and repetition: this is the warm-up phenomenon

Paramyotonia

- ☐ This is muscle stiffness caused by difficulty in relaxing muscle contractions
- ☐ It is induced by cold and exercise
- ☐ It worsens with repetition

Episodic weakness: triggers

- ☐ Waking
- ☐ Rest after exercise
- ☐ Stress
- ☐ Fasting
- ☐ Carbohydrate meal (hypokalaemic)
- ☐ Cold (especially paramyotonia)

Other features

- ☐ Hyporeflexia
- ☐ Muscle hypertrophy

Investigation of periodic paralysis

- ☐ McManis test

Treatment of non-dystrophic myotonia

- ☐ Lamotrigine: this is recommended as first line
- ☐ Mexiletene

DOI: 10.1201/9781003221258-91

HYPOKALAEMIC PERIODIC PARALYSIS: CLINICAL FEATURES

Genetics transmission

- [ ] This is an autosomal dominant calcium channelopathy
- [ ] It has a reduced penetrance in women

Genetic types

- [ ] Type 1: with CACNA1AS mutations: this accounts for 70% of cases
- [ ] Type 2: with SCN4A mutation
- [ ] MCM3AP mutation has also been reported

Prodrome

- [ ] Fatigue
- [ ] Paraesthesias
- [ ] Cognitive changes
- [ ] Behavioural changes

Clinical features

- [ ] The onset is in the second decade of life
- [ ] The attacks last hours to days
- [ ] Weakness is often on waking or at night
- [ ] Weakness is focal or generalised
- [ ] It usually spares the facial and respiratory muscles
- [ ] Fixed weakness develops with repeated attacks
- [ ] Fixed weakness may be the only presentation
- [ ] Reflexes are reduced in attacks
- [ ] There is no myotonia
- [ ] The attacks improve with age

Differential diagnosis: hyperkalaemic periodic paralysis

- [ ] The attacks are less severe in hyperkalaemic periodic paralysis
- [ ] They are also more frequent

HYPOKALAEMIC PERIODIC PARALYSIS: TREATMENT

Oral potassium

- [ ] Potassium chloride is preferred
- [ ] The dose is 0.2–0.4mEq/kg every 30 minutes: the maximum dose is 200–250mEq/day
- [ ] It is taken with plenty of water
- [ ] Avoid slow release preparations

Intravenous potassium

- [ ] This is infused in Mannitol and not Dextrose
- [ ] The dose is 40 mEq/L in 5% Mannitol
- [ ] The maximum infusion rate is 20 mEq/hour
- [ ] The maximum dose is 200 mEq daily
- [ ] It must be infused under electrocardiogram (ECG) monitoring

Potassium sparing diuretics

- [ ] Triamterene 50–150 mg daily
- [ ] Spironolactone 25–100 mg daily
- [ ] Eplerenone 50–100 mg daily

Other diuretics

- [ ] Acetazolamide: 125–1,000 mg daily: some cases may worsen on this
- [ ] Dichlorphenamide
- [ ] Thiazides

Other treatments of attacks

- [ ] Lithium if diuretics fail
- [ ] Insulin/glucose in severe cases

Triggers to avoid

- [ ] High carbohydrate meals
- [ ] High salt intake
- [ ] Alcohol
- [ ] Stress
- [ ] Heavy meals
- [ ] Exercise

Preventative diet

- [ ] Low sodium
- [ ] Low carbohydrate
- [ ] High potassium
- [ ] Take frequent small meals

Preventative potassium intake

- [ ] Liquid or aqueous potassium: taken before triggering activities
- [ ] Sustained release potassium at bedtime: if attack frequency is high
  - ○ Use with proton pump inhibitor (PPI)

Perioperative measures

- [ ] Avoid volatile anaesthetics
- [ ] Avoid depolarising muscle relaxants

HYPERKALAEMIC PERIODIC PARALYSIS: CLINICAL FEATURES

Clinical features

- ☐ The onset is in the first decade of life
- ☐ The attacks last 1–4 hours
- ☐ The attacks usually occur in the morning
- ☐ Weakness ascends from the lower limbs
- ☐ Bulbar and respiratory weakness develop occasionally
- ☐ Myotonia occurs in 20% of cases: this is persistent and not episodic
- ☐ Inter-ictal eyelid myotonia and lid lag may be present
- ☐ Reflexes are reduced in attacks
- ☐ The attack frequency reduces with age

Triggers

- ☐ Stress
- ☐ Fatigue
- ☐ High potassium foods
- ☐ Exercise
- ☐ Cold
- ☐ Emotional stress
- ☐ Fasting
- ☐ Pregnancy

HYPERKALAEMIC PERIODIC PARALYSIS: MANAGEMENT

Electromyogram (EMG): McManis test

- ☐ The test is done during 2–5 minutes of intermittent muscle contractions
- ☐ There is an abnormal increase in the compound muscle action potential (CMAP)
- ☐ This is followed by progressive abnormal reduction in the CMAP
- ☐ The reduction is most marked in the first 20 minutes post-exertion
- ☐ The test is also positive in other periodic paralyses

Preventative activities

- ☐ Mild exercise
- ☐ Frequent carbohydrate meals
- ☐ Early rising

Things to avoid

- ☐ Potassium-rich food: fruits and juices
- ☐ Potassium sparing diuretics
- ☐ Fasting
- ☐ Strenuous exercise
- ☐ Cold

Acute treatment

- ☐ Salbutamol: 1–2 puffs (0.1 mg)
- ☐ Calcium gluconate intravenously
- ☐ Thiazide diuretics: hydrochlorothiazide 25–75 mg daily
- ☐ Acetazolamide: 125–1,000 mg daily
- ☐ Dichlorphenamide: 50 mg twice daily and adjusted weekly: maximum is 200 mg daily

THYROTOXIC PERIODIC PARALYSIS: CLINICAL FEATURES

Genetics and pathology

- ☐ Kir2.6 gene mutations may occur
- ☐ It is associated with hyperthyroidism
- ☐ Features of thyrotoxicosis may be subtle

Demographic features

- ☐ Usual affected populations: Chinese, Japanese, Vietnamese, Filipinos, and Koreans
- ☐ Males are more frequently affected
- ☐ The male to female ratio ranges from 17:1 to 70:1
- ☐ The onset age is 20–50 years

Prodromal features

- ☐ Muscle aches
- ☐ Cramps
- ☐ Stiffness

Features of weakness

- ☐ There are recurrent sudden episodes of weakness
- ☐ The episodes may last up to 72 hours
- ☐ These usually occur at night or on waking
- ☐ They are mild to severe
- ☐ They involve all the limbs
- ☐ The weakness ascends from the lower limbs
- ☐ Proximal muscles are worse affected
- ☐ It may be asymmetrical
- ☐ It may affect respiratory, bulbar, and ocular muscles
- ☐ The reflexes are typically reduced: but they may be normal or brisk in attacks
- ☐ There are no bowel or bladder symptoms

Drug triggers

- ☐ Diuretics
- ☐ Insulin
- ☐ Steroids
- ☐ Acetazolamide
- ☐ Alcohol
- ☐ Recreational drugs, e.g. Ecstasy

Other triggers

- ☐ Heavy meals
- ☐ Sweet meals: refined carbohydrates
- ☐ Rest after rigorous exercise
- ☐ Trauma
- ☐ Hot weather
- ☐ Upper respiratory tract infections
- ☐ Emotional stress
- ☐ Menses

Differential diagnosis

- ☐ Guillain–Barre syndrome (GBS)
- ☐ Transverse myelitis (TM)
- ☐ Acute spinal cord compression
- ☐ Familial hypokalaemic periodic paralysis

THYROTOXIC PERIODIC PARALYSIS: MANAGEMENT

Urine spot test

- ☐ There is an increase in the urinary excretion ratio of calcium to phosphate

Blood tests

- ☐ Potassium: this is reduced in attacks but it may be normal
- ☐ Phosphate: this is transiently reduced
- ☐ Magnesium: this is transiently reduced
- ☐ Insulin: this is increased prior to attack
- ☐ Calcium: this is raised
- ☐ Creatinine kinase (CK): this is normal
- ☐ Thyroid function tests: these show high T4 and T3 levels
- ☐ Thyroid stimulating hormone (TSH): this is low

Electrocardiogram (ECG)

- ☐ Sinus tachycardia is prominent
- ☐ Atrial fibrillation
- ☐ Atrioventricular block
- ☐ Ventricular fibrillation
- ☐ Asystole
- ☐ Cardiac arrest

Treatment

- ☐ Avoid provoking factors
- ☐ Potassium replacement: with potassium chloride (KCl)
- ☐ Steroids if not responsive
- ☐ Propranolol
- ☐ Treatment of hyperthyroidism

MALIGNANT HYPERTHERMIA (MH): CLINICAL FEATURES

Neurological features

- ☐ Generalised muscle rigidity
- ☐ Contractures: especially of the masseter muscle
- ☐ Postoperative stiffness and myalgia
- ☐ Co-morbidity with multiminicore disease (MmD): this has been reported

Rhabdomyolysis

- ☐ The onset may be delayed
- ☐ The urine is red-coloured
- ☐ There is associated hyperkalaemia

Hyperthermia

- ☐ This is an early and rapid feature
- ☐ It may be delayed
- ☐ It is associated with excessive sweating

Cardiorespiratory features

- ☐ Inappropriate hypercapnia
- ☐ Blood pressure fluctuations
- ☐ Respiratory acidosis
- ☐ Tachyarrhythmias

Other reported associations

- ☐ Cerebellar impairment with swelling: this is due to heat-induced Purkinje cell damage
- ☐ Bleeding tendency

Complications

- ☐ Acute renal failure
- ☐ Disseminated intravascular coagulation
- ☐ Fatal cardiac arrhythmias

MALIGNANT HYPERTHERMIA (MH): MANAGEMENT

Basic investigations

- ☐ Lactic acid: this is increased
- ☐ Creatinine kinase (CK): this is frequently >10,000 iu/L
- ☐ Urinalysis: for myoglobinuria
- ☐ Renal function test: for hyperkalaemia

Magnetic resonance imaging (MRI) muscle

- ☐ The rectus femoris muscle is usually spared with RYR1-related myopathy

In-vitro contracture test (IVCT): types

- ☐ Halothane and caffeine
- ☐ Sevoflurane: this is a less sensitive alternative to Halothane

Acute treatment

- ☐ Dantrolene
- ☐ Avoid triggers of MH

Prevention of exertional rhabdomyolysis

- ☐ Avoid exercise in extreme heat
- ☐ Avoid caffeine
- ☐ Restrict alcohol consumption

Muscular dystrophies

DUCHENNE MUSCULAR DYSTROPHY (DMD): CLINICAL FEATURES

Genetics

- ☐ The dystrophin gene is on chromosome Xp21
- ☐ Out-of-frame mutations occur in 65% of cases
- ☐ These usually cause complete dystrophin deficiency
- ☐ DMD may also result from partial dystrophin deficiency: similar to Becker muscular dystrophy (BMD)
- ☐ The onset is usually between ages 2–5 years

Mobility and gait

- ☐ Delayed walking: beyond 18 months
- ☐ Waddling gait
- ☐ Toe walking
- ☐ Frequent falls
- ☐ Difficulty rising from the floor
- ☐ Wheelchair dependence by about 10 years
- ☐ Acute illness-associated weakness (AIAW)

Neuromuscular features

- ☐ Calf hypertrophy
- ☐ Positive Gower's sign
- ☐ Strong plantar flexors and everters
- ☐ Absent reflexes except the ankle jerks

Skeletal deformities

- ☐ Foot deformities
- ☐ Progressive scoliosis: this is from the early teen years

Cognitive and psychiatric features

- ☐ Global developmental delay
- ☐ Learning difficulties
- ☐ Anxiety
- ☐ Obsessive compulsive disorder
- ☐ Attention-deficit hyperactivity disorder (ADHD)
- ☐ Autism spectrum disorder

Cardiorespiratory complications

- ☐ Cardiomyopathy: this develops in 90% of cases
  - ○ It carries a risk of stroke
- ☐ Respiratory insufficiency: this develops in the late teens

Gastrointestinal complications

- ☐ Constipation
- ☐ Reflux
- ☐ Gastric distension
- ☐ Malnutrition
- ☐ Failure to thrive
- ☐ Chilaiditi syndrome: this is the interposition of the colon between the diaphragm and the liver
- ☐ Malignant hyperthermia-like reaction to suxamethonium/ halothane anaesthesia

Other complications

- ☐ Nephrolithiasis
- ☐ Adrenal crisis: from chronic steroid use
- ☐ Fat embolism: from bone fractures

DOI: 10.1201/9781003221258-92

DUCHENNE MUSCULAR DYSTROPHY (DMD): CARDIAC MANAGEMENT

Cardiac monitoring

- ☐ Routine biannual cardiac surveillance: from age 10 years
- ☐ Heightened cardiac surveillance: if the patient is on steroids
- ☐ Perform periodic Holter monitoring: if there is cardiac dysfunction
- ☐ Refer to a cardiologist with interest in DMD

Cardiac monitoring tools

- ☐ Electrocardiogram (ECG)
- ☐ Echocardiogram
- ☐ Multi-gated acquisition (MUGA) scan: if echocardiogram acoustic windows are limited
- ☐ Consider cardiac magnetic resonance imaging (MRI)

Electrocardiogram (ECG) features

- ☐ Sinus tachycardia
- ☐ Right axis deviation
- ☐ R:S ratio ≥1 in lead V1
- ☐ Deep Q waves in leads I, aVL, V5–V6
- ☐ Complete right bundle branch block

Echocardiogram features

- ☐ Left ventricular enlargement
- ☐ Systolic dysfunction
- ☐ Diastolic dysfunction

Cardiac magnetic resonance imaging (MRI) features

- ☐ This reveals early regional cardiac changes
- ☐ There is late gadolinium enhancement (LGE) with myocardial damage

Cardiac treatments

- ☐ Angiotensin converting enzyme inhibitors (ACEI)
- ☐ Beta blockers
- ☐ Diuretics
- ☐ Angiotensin II receptor antagonist (Losartan)
- ☐ Cardiac transplant

DUCHENNE MUSCULAR DYSTROPHY (DMD): GENERAL TREATMENTS

Immunisations

- ☐ Influenza: annually
- ☐ Pneumococcal: 5-yearly from the age of 2 years

Steroids

- ☐ Steroids are gold standard
- ☐ They stabilise strength and function
- ☐ They improve respiratory function
- ☐ They reduce need for scoliosis surgery
- ☐ They improve muscle mass
- ☐ A twice weekly regime may be effective

Bone health management

- ☐ Dietary advice
- ☐ Calcium and vitamin D supplementation
- ☐ Bisphosphonates after vertebral fracture: they may reduce fracture risk on steroids

Other drugs

- ☐ Dantrolene: for post-exercise pain
- ☐ Idebenone: it may slow down the loss of respiratory function
- ☐ Salbutamol

Orthopaedic treatments

- ☐ Physiotherapy
- ☐ Tendon stretching: for contractures
- ☐ Knee ankle foot orthoses (KAFOs)
- ☐ Spinal fusion for scoliosis: this is indicated if Cobb's angle is 20–40° and FVC is >30% of predicted
- ☐ Spinal brace: if spinal fusion is contraindicated

DUCHENNE MUSCULAR DYSTROPHY (DMD): GENETIC TREATMENTS

Eteplirsen (Exondys 51)
- ☐ This is an approved exon skipping gene therapy
- ☐ It restores dystrophin positive fibers
- ☐ It improves walking distance
- ☐ It reportedly slows down the rate of decline of ambulation

Ataluren (Translana)
- ☐ Ataluren has been approved by licensing authorities
- ☐ It corrects premature nonsense mutations
- ☐ It is recommended for patients older than 5 years who are ambulant
- ☐ It is most effective if the 6-minute walking distance (6MWD) is 300–400m

Drisapersen
- ☐ Drisapersen has not been approved by licensing authorities
- ☐ It is an anti-sense oligonucleotide (ASO) treatment
- ☐ It is administered subcutaneously
- ☐ It improves 6-minute walking distance (6MWD)
- ☐ It elevates Factor VIII levels
- ☐ It causes injection site erythema, hyperpigmentation, fibrosis, calcification, and ulcers

Golodirsen
- ☐ Golodirsen has been approved by licensing authorities
- ☐ It is an antisense oligonucleotide (ASO)
- ☐ It increases exon53 skipping
- ☐ It results in increased dystrophin production

Viltolersen
- ☐ Vitolersen has been approved by licensing authorities
- ☐ It is a phosphorodiamidate morpholino antisense oligonucleotide (ASO)
- ☐ It is indicated in DMD variants amenable to exon 53 skipping
- ☐ It binds to exon 53 of the dystrophin mRNA precursor
- ☐ It is administered intravenously

BECKER MUSCULAR DYSTROPHY (BMD): CLINICAL FEATURES

Genetics
- ☐ BMD is caused by X-linked in-frame mutations of the dystrophin gene
- ☐ Most mutations are in exons 45–60
- ☐ Most cases are caused by deletions
- ☐ Point-mutations and duplications also occur
- ☐ Mutations cause reduced dystrophin: this is proportional to the size of the deletions

Clinical features
- ☐ The median onset age is 8 years: the range is 3–36 years
- ☐ Patients have difficulty with sports
- ☐ They have walking difficulties and falls
- ☐ Severe myalgia and cramps often develop early
- ☐ Loss of ambulation occurs between ages 26–56 years
- ☐ Ventilatory support is rarely required
- ☐ Scoliosis surgery is occasionally needed
- ☐ Dilated cardiomyopathy occurs in 28% of cases

Atypical features
- ☐ Asymptomatic elevated creatinine kinase (CK)
- ☐ Exercise-induced cramps and myalgia
- ☐ Myalgia and cramps during normal activity
- ☐ Myoglobinuria

Severe phenotype
- ☐ This develops in those with early onset disease
- ☐ It results in earlier loss of ambulation
- ☐ Abnormal electrocardiography (ECG) features are more frequent
- ☐ Reproductive ability is reduced

Becker vs Duchenne muscular dystrophy (DMD)
- ☐ The mean onset age is about 9 years: it is about 3 years in DMD
- ☐ Gower's sign is seen in about 37%: it is in about 90% in DMD
- ☐ Calf pseudohypertrophy is present in about 60%: it is in >90% in DMD
- ☐ Contractures occur in about 20%: they are seen in >60% of DMD
- ☐ Cardiomyopathy is present in about 4%: it is in about 6% in DMD
- ☐ Scoliosis develops in about 8%: it is in about 15% in DMD
- ☐ Wheelchair use is in about 8%: it is in >35% in DMD
- ☐ Respiratory function is preserved: unlike in DMD

Treatment
- ☐ Tadalafil may improve ischaemia

FACIOSCAPULOHUMERAL MUSCULAR DYSTROPHY (FSHD): GENETIC CLASSIFICATION

FSHD type 1A (FSHD1A)

- ☐ This results from D4Z4 gene mutations on chromosome 4q35
  - ○ D4Z4 enables DUX4 protein expression
- ☐ The transmission is autosomal dominant
- ☐ There is a reduction in number of D4Z4 repeats
  - ○ The normal range is 11–1,000 D4Z4 repeats
  - ○ FSHD results if there are 1–10 repeats
- ☐ FSHD develops only if the variant distal to the D4Z4 is 4qA and not 4qB

FSHD type 1B (FSHD1B)

- ☐ This is not linked to Chromosome 4q
- ☐ The transmission is autosomal dominant

FSHD type 2

- ☐ It results from SMCHD1 and DNMT3B gene mutations on chromosome 18p
  - ○ These are D4Z4 chromatin modifiers
- ☐ FSHD2 can also be caused by LRIF1 gene mutations and monosomy 18

Acronym

- ☐ DNMT: DNA methyltransferase
- ☐ LRIF: ligand dependent nuclear receptor interacting factor
- ☐ SMCHD1: structural maintenance of chromosomes hinge domain 1

FACIOSCAPULOHUMERAL MUSCULAR DYSTROPHY (FSHD): CLINICAL FEATURES

Clinical phenotypes

- ☐ Category A: both facial and scapular girdle muscle weakness
- ☐ Category B: either facial or scapular weakness
- ☐ Category C: asymptomatic
- ☐ Category D: atypical phenotypes

Features of facial weakness

- ☐ Horizontal smile
- ☐ Protruding lips
- ☐ Sleeping with the eyes open
- ☐ Weak eye closure: with positive Bell's phenomenon
- ☐ Difficulty pursing the lips
- ☐ Difficulty whistling

Features of limb weakness

- ☐ Scapula weakness with an angel wing appearance
- ☐ Weakness and wasting of the biceps and triceps (Popeye arms)
- ☐ Sparing of the humeral muscles
- ☐ Trapezius hump
- ☐ Horizontal clavicles
- ☐ Down-sloping anterior axillary folds: this is secondary to pectoral wasting
- ☐ Congenital absence of pectorals, brachioradialis, or biceps muscles occasionally occur
- ☐ Waddling gait
- ☐ Foot drop: this is secondary to tibialis anterior weakness

Coat's disease

- ☐ Retinal capillary telangiectasias
- ☐ Microaneurysms
- ☐ Vascular occlusion and leakage
- ☐ Eventual retinal detachment

Respiratory impairment: risk factors

- ☐ Severe weakness
- ☐ Kyphoscoliosis
- ☐ Wheelchair dependence
- ☐ Co-morbid lung diseases

Cardiac features

- ☐ Cardiomegaly
- ☐ Occasional supraventricular arrhythmias
- ☐ Focal fibrosis and fat infiltration: these are seen on contrast MRI

Other features

- ☐ Trunkal weakness
- ☐ Protruding abdomen: this may be unilateral
- ☐ Positive Beevor's sign
- ☐ Chronic pain
- ☐ Hearing loss

Differential diagnosis

- ☐ Scapuloperoneal muscular dystrophy

EMERY–DREIFUSS MUSCULAR DYSTROPHY (EDMD): CLINICAL FEATURES

Genetics

- ☐ There are seven genetic forms: EDMD types 1 to 7
- ☐ Mutations are in STA, LMNA, SYNE1, SYNE2, FHL1, and TMEN genes
- ☐ The transmission may be X-linked, autosomal dominant, or autosomal recessive

Classical triad

- ☐ Contractures
- ☐ Weakness
- ☐ Cardiomyopathy

Contractures: affected joints

- ☐ Achilles
- ☐ Elbows
- ☐ Posterior cervical

Contractures: clinical features

- ☐ Toe walking
- ☐ Inability to extend the elbow
- ☐ Limited neck flexion
- ☐ Spinal rigidity

Humeroperoneal weakness and atrophy: affected muscles

- ☐ Biceps
- ☐ Triceps
- ☐ Anterior tibial
- ☐ Peroneal
- ☐ A scapulo-humero-pelvo-peroneal pattern develops later

Skeletal features

- ☐ Pes cavus: this is common

Creatinine kinase (CK)

- ☐ CK is elevated: but this is not very high

Cardiac features

- ☐ This may be the only manifestation of EDMD
- ☐ Supraventricular tachycardia (SVT)
- ☐ Atrioventricular (AV) conduction defects
- ☐ Ventricular arrhythmias
- ☐ Dilated cardiomyopathy
- ☐ Non-dilated cardiomyopathy
- ☐ Sudden death: this may occur even after pacemaker insertion
- ☐ Female carriers may develop cardiac features

Differential diagnosis

- ☐ Bethlem myopathy: COL6 mutations with collagen VI deficiency

MYOTONIC DYSTROPHY TYPE 1: NEUROLOGICAL FEATURES

Genetics

- ☐ This is caused by DMPK gene mutations on chromosome 19q
- ☐ It is a CTG repeat disorder

CTG repeats

- ☐ The normal repeat range is 5–37
- ☐ The premutation range is 38–49
- ☐ Mild disease is seen with a range between 50–100
- ☐ The classical disease phenotype is seen with a repeat range of 200–500
- ☐ Congenital/childhood onset develops with >1,000 repeats

Facial appearance

- ☐ Frontal balding
- ☐ Ptosis
- ☐ Hatchet face
- ☐ Carp mouth (tented upper lip): in congenital forms
- ☐ Malocclusion: this is due to masseter wasting

Central features

- ☐ Cognitive impairment: this correlates with CTG repeat expansion size
- ☐ Central sleep apnoea
- ☐ Hypersomnia
- ☐ Excessive daytime sleepiness (EDS)
- ☐ Ophthalmoplegia: case reports

Peripheral muscle features

- ☐ Myotonia
- ☐ Warm up phenomenon: with repeated muscle contractions
- ☐ Foot drop: this is an early feature
- ☐ Swan neck: this is from sternomastoid weakness
- ☐ Talipes

Peripheral neuropathy (PN)

- ☐ This is present in a third of cases
- ☐ It is usually demyelinating and motor
- ☐ It is often subclinical

Magnetic resonance imaging (MRI): brain

- ☐ Frontal hyperostosis
- ☐ Basal ganglia calcification
- ☐ Dilated perivascular spaces (Virchow Robin spaces)
- ☐ White matter lesions: especially in the anterior temporal pole and the external capsule: like in CADASIL
- ☐ Cortical and subcortical grey and white matter lesions: especially in the corpus callosum and limbic system

Magnetic resonance imaging (MRI): sites of fatty muscle infiltration

- ☐ Medial head of gastrocnemius
- ☐ Tibialis anterior
- ☐ Tensor fascia latae
- ☐ Other lower leg muscles: these are affected later
- ☐ Spine extensor muscles
- ☐ The rectus femoris muscle is relatively spared

Acronym

- ☐ CADASIL: cerebral autosomal dominant arteriopathy, subcortical infarcts and leukoencephalopathy

MYOTONIC DYSTROPHY TYPE 1: MAJOR SYSTEMIC FEATURES

Cardiac features

- ☐ Atrioventricular (AV) block
- ☐ Arrhythmias: supraventricular and ventricular
- ☐ Systolic and diastolic dysfunction: often subclinical
- ☐ Ischaemic heart disease
- ☐ Mitral valve prolapse (MVP)
- ☐ Hypertrophic cardiomyopathy
- ☐ Brugada syndrome

Respiratory features

- ☐ Impaired lung function: the progression is slow
- ☐ Obstructive sleep apnoea (OSA)
- ☐ Excessive daytime sleepiness
- ☐ Diaphragmatic weakness
- ☐ Alveolar hypoventilation
- ☐ Chest infections

Gastrointestinal features

- ☐ Dysphagia
- ☐ Constipation
- ☐ Gallstones
- ☐ Nausea and vomiting
- ☐ Diarrhoea with malabsorption
- ☐ Megacolon/mega-oesophagus
- ☐ Gastroesophageal reflux disease (GORD)
- ☐ Chronic liver enzyme elevation
- ☐ Chilaiditi syndrome: this is the interposition of the colon between the diaphragm and the liver

Endocrine and immune features

- ☐ Diabetes mellitus
- ☐ Testicular atrophy
- ☐ Gynaecomastia
- ☐ Impotence and reduced libido
- ☐ Fatigue
- ☐ Low immunoglobulins
- ☐ Hyperlipidemia

Cutaneous features

- ☐ Dysplastic nevi
- ☐ Alopecia
- ☐ Xerosis
- ☐ Seborrhoeic dermatitis
- ☐ Premature aging
- ☐ Basal cell carcinoma
- ☐ Possibly melanoma

MYOTONIC DYSTROPHY TYPE 1: ASSESSMENTS AND MONITORING

Baseline assessments

- ☐ Electrocardiogram (ECG): basal, 24 hour, and signal-averaged
- ☐ Echocardiogram
- ☐ Forced vital capacity (FVC)
- ☐ Liver function tests
- ☐ Thyroid function tests: TSH and free T4
- ☐ Serum lipids
- ☐ Consider baseline brain magnetic resonance imaging (MRI)

Annual clinical monitoring

- ☐ Speech and swallowing
- ☐ Mobility
- ☐ Balance
- ☐ Falls
- ☐ Activities of daily living
- ☐ Self-care
- ☐ School and social activities
- ☐ Work activities

Annual test monitoring

- ☐ Electrocardiogram (ECG)
- ☐ Fasting glucose and HbA1c
- ☐ Cataract assessment
- ☐ Slit-lamp eye examination
- ☐ Forced vital capacity (FVC)
- ☐ Liver function tests

Three-yearly test monitoring

- ☐ Serum lipids
- ☐ Thyroid function tests

Neuromuscular respiratory specialist referral: indications

- ☐ Ineffective cough: peak expiratory cough flow rate <270 L/min
- ☐ Respiratory insufficiency
- ☐ Recurrent pulmonary infections
- ☐ Prominent snoring
- ☐ Maximal inspiratory pressure of 60 cm H_2O
- ☐ Forced vital capacity (FVC) 50% less than predicted

Cardiac investigations: indications

- ☐ Palpitations
- ☐ Chest pain
- ☐ Dyspnoea
- ☐ Orthopnea
- ☐ Lightheadedness
- ☐ Syncope

Sleep studies: indications

- ☐ Excessive daytime sleepiness (EDS)
- ☐ Obstructive sleep apnoea (OSA)

CHAPTER 16

Tumours

Primary brain tumours

BRAIN TUMOURS: RISK FACTORS

Genetic risk factors

- [ ] Tuberous sclerosis
- [ ] Neurofibromatosis 1 and 2 (NF1 and NF2)
- [ ] Neavoid basal cell carcinoma syndrome
- [ ] Adenomatous polyposis
- [ ] Folate metabolism gene polymorphisms: risk of meningiomas and gliomas
- [ ] SMARCB1/INI1 gene mutations
- [ ] L-2-hydroxyglutaric aciduria (L2HGDH) gene mutations

Chemical and environmental risk factors

- [ ] Female sex hormones: these increase the risk of meningiomas
- [ ] Hormone replacement therapy (HRT)
- [ ] Dyes
- [ ] Solvents
- [ ] Pesticides
- [ ] Petroleum
- [ ] Ambient air pollution

Individual risk factors

- [ ] Higher socioeconomic status
- [ ] Allergies
- [ ] Diet
- [ ] Smoking
- [ ] Alcohol
- [ ] Head injury

Other risk factors

- [ ] Radiation therapy: risk of gliomas, glioblastomas, and meningiomas
- [ ] Viruses, e.g. measles virus
- [ ] Toxoplasmosis

Doubtful risk factors

- [ ] Mobile phone use: reports are contradictory

Factors which do not increase the risk of brain tumours

- [ ] Hair dyes (aromatic amines)

Factors which may reduce the risk of brain tumours

- [ ] Statins

BRAIN TUMOUR HEADACHES

Epidemiology

- [ ] Headaches occur in about 50% of people with brain tumours
- [ ] They occur especially with intraventricular, midline, and infratentorial tumours
- [ ] Previous headache is a risk factor

General features

- [ ] Headache is the sole symptom in only 2–3% of cases
- [ ] It is usually frontal but non-localising
- [ ] Unilateral headache is not always localising
- [ ] Most headaches are non-specific
- [ ] Severe headaches with vomiting occur in only 5% of cases
- [ ] Headaches are tension type in about 23–40% of cases
- [ ] Episodic migraine with aura occurs in about 13% of cases
- [ ] The headaches may mimic cluster headache

Migraine-type headache features

- [ ] Middle age onset
- [ ] Progressive
- [ ] Worse with Valsalva or supine position
- [ ] Nocturnal
- [ ] Unresponsive to analgesics

Cluster-type headache: causes

- [ ] Prolactinoma
- [ ] Acoustic neuroma
- [ ] Meningiomas: of cavernous sinus, sphenoid ridge, and foramen magnum

Atypical facial pain

- [ ] These occur with non-metastatic lung cancer
- [ ] They are possibly due to infiltration of the vagus nerve
- [ ] X ray or CT chest are therefore indicated in smokers with unexplained facial pain

DOI: 10.1201/9781003221258-94

BRAIN TUMOUR RELATED EPILEPSY (BTRE): CLINICAL FEATURES

Characteristics of seizure-related tumours

- [ ] Slow growth
- [ ] Cortical focus
- [ ] Temporal lobe predominance

Seizure types

- [ ] Early-onset drug-resistant epilepsy
- [ ] Focal seizures with loss of awareness
- [ ] Secondary generalised seizures: especially with low grade gliomas
- [ ] Refractory seizures: especially with low grade gliomas
- [ ] Epileptic spasms
- [ ] Tumour-associated status epilepticus (TASE): this often predicts tumour progression

Poor seizure prognostic features

- [ ] BRAF V600E genetic mutations
- [ ] Nuclear protein Ki-67 overexpression
- [ ] RINT1 expression
- [ ] Low expression of very large G-protein-coupled receptor-1 (VLGR 1)
- [ ] miR-128 dysregulation
- [ ] Low Ki-67 expression
- [ ] EGFR amplification
- [ ] High expression of cystine-glutamate exchanger (SLC7A11, xCT)

BRAIN TUMOURS: DIFFERENTIAL DIAGNOSIS

Brain abscess

- [ ] This shows the double rim sign on susceptibility weighted imaging (SWI)
- [ ] This sign is absent in necrotic glioblastomas

Other infective differentials

- [ ] Tuberculoma
- [ ] Neurocysticercosis
- [ ] Syphilitic gumma
- [ ] Aspergilloma
- [ ] Cryptococcoma
- [ ] Intracranial abscesses
- [ ] Fungal granulomas
- [ ] Whipple's disease with focal mass lesions

Congenital infections

- [ ] Toxoplasmosis
- [ ] Rubella
- [ ] Cytomegalovirus (CMV)
- [ ] Herpes simplex virus (HSV)

Vascular differentials

- [ ] Haematoma transformation
- [ ] Ischaemic stroke with mass effect
- [ ] Haemorrhagic infarction
- [ ] Arteriovenous malformations (AVM)
- [ ] Arteriovenous fistulas (AVF)
- [ ] Cavernoma
- [ ] Giant aneurysms
- [ ] Tumefactive perivascular Virchow-Robin spaces
- [ ] Systemic lupus erythematosus (SLE) vasculitis
- [ ] Primary angiitis of the central nervous system (PACNS)

Inflammatory differentials

- [ ] Progressive multifocal leukoencephalopathy (PML)
- [ ] Tumefactive demyelination
- [ ] Inflammatory pseudotumors (inflammatory myofibroblastic tumours)
- [ ] Behcet's disease
- [ ] Neurosarcoidosis

Phakomatoses and histiocytosis

- [ ] Neurofibromatosis type 1(NF1) mass-like lesions
- [ ] Tuberous sclerosis tubers
- [ ] Neuronal migration disorders
- [ ] Castleman disease: angiofollicular lymph node hyperplasia
- [ ] Erdheim-Chester disease
- [ ] Rosai-Dorfman disease: sinus histiocytosis with massive lymphadenopathy

Other differentials

- [ ] Autoimmune encephalitis: tumours may show selective limbic involvement and antibodies
- [ ] Canavan disease
- [ ] Alexander disease
- [ ] Post-operative changes
- [ ] Radiation necrosis
- [ ] Amyloidoma

LOW GRADE GLIOMAS: CLINICAL FEATURES

Types

- ☐ Astrocytoma
- ☐ Oligodendroglioma
- ☐ Oligoastrocytoma

Scoring systems

- ☐ University of California San Francisco (UCSF) 2008
- ☐ Pignatti 2002

Seizures

- ☐ Seizures occur in 80% of cases: they occur in 60% of high-grade gliomas
- ☐ They are often refractory

Poor prognostic markers

- ☐ Age >40 years
- ☐ Subtotal resection
- ☐ Astrocytic histology with >8% MIB-1 proliferation index
- ☐ Tumours larger than 4–6cm: especially if they cross the midline
- ☐ Neurologic deficits
- ☐ Poor performance status
- ☐ Location in an eloquent area
- ☐ p53 mutation
- ☐ Median survival is about 10 years

Good prognostic markers

- ☐ Seizure onset
- ☐ Chromosome 1p19q deletion (oligodendrogliomas)
- ☐ IDH1 mutation

MENINGIOMAS: RISK FACTORS

Major tumour syndromes

- ☐ Neurofibromatosis type 2 (NF2)
- ☐ Multiple endocrine neoplasia type 1 (MEN1)

Copy number alterations (CNAs)

- ☐ Loss of heterozygosity (LOH) of chromosome 22q: in 60–70% of sporadic meningiomas
- ☐ Deletion of chromosome 1p: this is associated with high grade meningiomas
- ☐ Other chromosomal CNAs: 6q, 6q, 10q, 11p, 14q, and 18q
- ☐ Gain of chromosomes 1q, 9q, 12q, 15q, and 20q
- ☐ CNAs are associated with tumour aggressiveness

Major cancer predisposition mutations

- ☐ TRAF7: tumour necrosis factor (TNF) receptor associated factor 7: chromosome 16p
- ☐ AKT1 (protein kinase B): in 10% of sporadic meningiomas
- ☐ KLF4: Kruppel-like factor 4
- ☐ PIK3CA: phosphatidylinositol 3-kinase, catalytic
- ☐ SMO: smoothened, frizzled class receptor
- ☐ TERT: telomerase reverse transcriptase promoter
- ☐ POLR2A: RNA polymerase II
- ☐ BAP1: BRCA–associated protein 1

Other cancer predisposition mutations

- ☐ NF1
- ☐ PTCH
- ☐ CREBBP
- ☐ VHL
- ☐ PTEN
- ☐ CDKN2A
- ☐ SMARCE1
- ☐ SMARCB1
- ☐ CHEK2
- ☐ CLH-22/CTCL1

Epigenomic alterations: DNA methylation

- ☐ DNA methyltransferase (DNMT) enzymes 3A and 3B
- ☐ Metalloproteinase 3 (TIMP3)
- ☐ Cyclin-dependent kinase inhibitor 2A (CDKN2A)
- ☐ Tumour protein 73 (TP73)

Epigenomic alterations: micro RNA

- ☐ miRNA-200a
- ☐ miRNA-145
- ☐ miRNA-109a
- ☐ miRNA-29c-3p
- ☐ miR-219–5p

Non-genetic risk factors

- ☐ Female hormones
- ☐ Full mouth dental X-rays
- ☐ Occupational iron exposure

MENINGIOMAS: RADIOLOGICAL DIFFERENTIALS

Neoplastic

- ☐ Dural metastasis
- ☐ Lymphoma
- ☐ Leukaemia
- ☐ Solitary fibrous tumour
- ☐ Hemangiopericytoma
- ☐ Metastases
- ☐ Melanocytic tumours
- ☐ Glioblastoma
- ☐ Epstein-Barr virus (EBV) associated smooth muscle tumours

Granulomatous

- ☐ Sarcoidosis
- ☐ Tuberculosis
- ☐ Granulomatosis with polyangiitis (GPA)
- ☐ Idiopathic hypertrophic pachymeningitis
- ☐ Extranodal sinus histiocytosis

Other differentials

- ☐ IgG4 disease
- ☐ Rosai-Dorfman disease
- ☐ Erdheim Chester disease

GERM CELL TUMOURS: CLINICAL FEATURES

Onset age

- ☐ The onset age is 0–20 years with non-germinomas
- ☐ The range is 7–30 years with germinomas

Frequent sites

- ☐ Pineal region: this is the commonest location
- ☐ Suprasellar regions
- ☐ Fourth ventricle
- ☐ Basal ganglia
- ☐ Thalamus

Features of raised intracranial pressure (ICP)

- ☐ Headache
- ☐ Impaired consciousness
- ☐ Papilloedema
- ☐ Obstructive hydrocephalus

Visual features

- ☐ Visual blurring
- ☐ Visual impairment
- ☐ Optic atrophy
- ☐ Bitemporal hemianopia

Cranial nerve palsies

- ☐ Oculomotor
- ☐ Facial

Motor features

- ☐ Weakness
- ☐ Ataxia

Endocrine features

- ☐ Diabetes insipidus
- ☐ Precocious puberty
- ☐ Delayed sexual development
- ☐ Hypopituitarism
- ☐ Isolated growth hormone deficiency

Psychiatric features

- ☐ Behavioural problems
- ☐ Depression
- ☐ Psychosis

Other features

- ☐ Parinaud's syndrome

PRIMARY CENTRAL NERVOUS SYSTEM LYMPHOMA (PCNSL): CLINICAL FEATURES

Epidemiology

☐ This is a form of non-Hodgkin's lymphoma (NHL)
☐ The mean onset age is 50 years

Risk disorders

☐ Rheumatoid arthritis (RA)
☐ Systemic lupus erythematosus (SLE)
☐ Sjogren's syndrome
☐ Sarcoidosis
☐ Immunocompromised subjects
☐ Post-organ transplant

Typical sites

☐ Periventricular
☐ Leptomeninges
☐ Optic nerve
☐ Spinal cord
☐ Intraocular
☐ Occult systemic lymphoma

Clinical features

☐ Focal neurological deficits
☐ Cognitive dysfunction
☐ Seizures: most occur at presentation: especially with cortical lesions
☐ Hypertrophic multiple cranial neuropathies

Poor prognostic markers

☐ Age >60 years
☐ Raised lactate dehydrogenase (LDH)
☐ Raised cerebrospinal fluid (CSF) protein
☐ Deep lesions

Secondary brain tumours

BRAIN METASTASES: SKULL BASE SYNDROMES

Orbital syndrome

- ☐ First division trigeminal nerve sensory loss
- ☐ Supraorbital ache
- ☐ Diplopia
- ☐ Proptosis

Parasellar syndrome

- ☐ First division trigeminal nerve sensory loss
- ☐ Frontal headache
- ☐ Ocular paresis

Gasserian ganglion syndrome

- ☐ Atypical facial pain: in the cheek, jaw, and forehead
- ☐ Facial numbness
- ☐ Abducens and facial nerve palsies

Jugular foramen syndrome

- ☐ Retro-ocular pain
- ☐ Hoarseness
- ☐ Dysphagia

Occipital condyle syndrome

- ☐ Severe unilateral occipital headache: worse with neck flexion
- ☐ Hypoglossal nerve palsy with dysarthria and dysphagia

NEOPLASTIC MENINGITIS: CLINICAL FEATURES

Epidemiology

- ☐ This occurs in 3–5% of patients with cancer
- ☐ 25% of cases are diagnosed on clinical features

Typical primary sites

- ☐ Breast adenocarcinoma
- ☐ Lung adenocarcinoma
- ☐ Melanoma
- ☐ Leukaemia
- ☐ Primary brain tumours
- ☐ Primary leptomeningeal melanocytosis

Meningeal features

- ☐ Impaired consciousness
- ☐ Headache
- ☐ Mental changes
- ☐ Seizures
- ☐ Neck stiffness: this develops in only 15% of cases
- ☐ Nausea
- ☐ Vomiting

Cranial nerve features

- ☐ Diplopia
- ☐ Hearing loss
- ☐ Visual loss
- ☐ Facial numbness

Other features

- ☐ Focal weakness
- ☐ Hemiparesis
- ☐ Gait difficulty
- ☐ Dysphasia
- ☐ Paraesthesias
- ☐ Back pain
- ☐ Testicular pain
- ☐ Bladder and bowel dysfunction

Synonyms

- ☐ Malignant meningitis
- ☐ Carcinomatous meningitis

DOI: 10.1201/9781003221258-95

NEOPLASTIC MENINGITIS: INVESTIGATIONS

Cerebrospinal fluid (CSF): routine tests

- ☐ Pleocytosis: in about 60% of cases
- ☐ Raised protein: in 80% of cases
- ☐ Reduced glucose: in 55% of cases
- ☐ High CSF opening pressure: in 57% of cases
- ☐ Cytology-negative: in about 40–50% of cases
- ☐ Flow cytometry

CSF tumour markers

- ☐ Carcinoembryonic antigen (CEA)
- ☐ Beta human chorionic gonadotrophin (β hCG)
- ☐ Alpha fetoprotein (αFP)
- ☐ Lactate dehydrogenase (LDH)

Measures to improve CSF yield

- ☐ Take the sample near to the pathological site
- ☐ Take large samples: at least 10mls
- ☐ Take more than one sample
- ☐ Process the CSF promptly
- ☐ Fix the sample in formalin within 30 minutes

Contrast magnetic resonance imaging (MRI) brain and spine: features

- ☐ Leptomeningeal enhancement
  - ○ This is focal or diffuse
  - ○ It is especially in the convexity, basal cisterns, tentorium, and ependymal surface
- ☐ Cranial nerve enhancement and enlargement
- ☐ Intradural enhancing nodules: especially in the cauda equina
- ☐ Hydrocephalus: this occurs in 8–10% of cases

Radionuclide studies

- ☐ Abnormal CSF flow dynamics: this is seen in 30–70% of cases
- ☐ Obstructions: at skull base, spinal canal, and cerebral convexities

Meningeal biopsy

- ☐ This is indicated if the CSF is inconclusive

Synonyms

- ☐ Malignant meningitis
- ☐ Carcinomatous meningitis

Paraneoplastic syndromes

PARANEOPLASTIC NEUROLOGICAL SYNDROMES: CLASSIFICATION

Cranial syndromes

- [ ] Brainstem encephalitis
- [ ] Bilateral diffuse uveal melanocytic proliferation
- [ ] Cerebellar ataxia
- [ ] Encephalomyelitis
- [ ] Limbic encephalitis
- [ ] Opsoclonus-myoclonus
- [ ] Stiff person syndrome (SPS)
- [ ] Subacute cerebellar degeneration

Spinal syndromes

- [ ] Necrotic myelopathy and bilateral optic neuritis
- [ ] Necrotising myelopathy
- [ ] Neuromyelitis optica (NMO)

Anterior horn cell and plexus syndromes

- [ ] Motor neurone disease (MND)
- [ ] Brachial neuritis

Ophthalmic syndromes

- [ ] Optic neuritis
- [ ] Retinopathy: cancer or melanoma associated

Autonomic syndromes

- [ ] Acute gastrointestinal dysautonomia
- [ ] Acute pandysautonomia
- [ ] Chronic gastrointestinal pseudoobstruction
- [ ] Guillain–Barre syndrome (GBS)

Neuromuscular junction (NMJ) syndromes

- [ ] Lambert–Eaton myasthenic syndrome (LEMS)
- [ ] Myasthenia gravis (MG)

Myopathy syndromes

- [ ] Acute necrotising myopathy
- [ ] Polymyositis
- [ ] Dermatomyositis
- [ ] Cachetic myopathy

Neuropathy syndromes

- [ ] Acquired neuromyotonia
- [ ] Paraproteinaemic neuropathy
- [ ] Peripheral neuropathy (PN)
- [ ] Pure autonomic neuropathy
- [ ] Sensorimotor neuropathy
- [ ] Subacute motor neuronopathy
- [ ] Subacute sensory neuronopathy
- [ ] Vasculitic neuropathy

PARANEOPLASTIC NEUROLOGICAL SYNDROMES: CANCER SCREENING

Small cell lung cancer (SCLC) and thymoma

- [ ] Computed tomography (CT) thorax
  - ○ At onset and after 3–6 months
  - ○ Then 6-monthly for 4 years (2 years for LEMS)
- [ ] Positron emission tomography (PET) scan
  - ○ This is indicated if the CT is negative and the lesions are difficult to biopsy

Breast cancer

- [ ] Mammography
- [ ] Magnetic resonance imaging (MRI): if mammography is negative

Ovarian teratoma and cancer

- [ ] Trans-vaginal ultrasound scan (USS)
- [ ] Computed tomography (CT) of abdomen and pelvis: if ultrasound is negative
- [ ] Magnetic resonance imaging (MRI) of abdomen and pelvis: if other imaging modalities are negative
- [ ] Exploratory surgery/oophorectomy: in deteriorating post-menopausal anti Yo positive cases

Testicular cancer

- [ ] Testicular ultrasound scan: if under the age of 50 years
- [ ] Testicular biopsy: if ultrasound shows microcalcifications

Dermatomyositis: females

- [ ] Computed tomography (CT) thorax/abdomen
- [ ] Pelvic ultrasound scan
- [ ] Mammography
- [ ] Colonoscopy: if over the age of 50 years

Dermatomyositis: males

- [ ] Computed tomography (CT) thorax/abdomen
- [ ] Testicular ultrasound: if age is <50 years
- [ ] Colonoscopy: if age is >50 years

DOI: 10.1201/9781003221258-96

Phakomatoses

NEUROFIBROMATOSIS TYPE 1 (NF1): DIAGNOSTIC AND NEUROLOGICAL FEATURES

Diagnostic criteria

- ☐ ≥6 cafe au lait spots >1.5cm
- ☐ ≥2 neurofibromas or 1 plexiform neurofibroma
- ☐ Axillary or groin freckles
- ☐ Optic pathway glioma
- ☐ Bony dysplasia
- ☐ First degree relative with NF1
- ☐ The criteria are fulfilled with any two of the above

Central neurological features

- ☐ Headache
- ☐ Epilepsy
- ☐ Sphenoid wing dysplasia
- ☐ Aqueductal stenosis
- ☐ Cognitive dysfunction
- ☐ Chiari malformation
- ☐ Macrocephaly
- ☐ Cerebrovascular disease
- ☐ Bilateral congenital ptosis
- ☐ Vertebrobasilar dolichoectasia
- ☐ Increased risk of stroke

Peripheral neuropathy (PN): types

- ☐ Facial mononeuropathy
- ☐ Poliomyelitis-like neuropathy
- ☐ Generalised peripheral neuropathy
- ☐ Small fiber neuropathy

Mosaic neurofibromatosis type 1 (MNF1)

- ☐ This was formerly referred to as segmental NF1 or NF type V
- ☐ The abnormalities are limited to one or several body segments
- ☐ Pigmentary changes and neurofibromas are the only features in most cases
- ☐ Pigmentary changes are the most frequent abnormality
- ☐ It usually manifests as café au lait spots with or without freckling
- ☐ Giant plexiform neurofibromas may occur
- ☐ There may be a risk of epilepsy, Hodgkin's lymphoma, and ganglioneuroblastoma

NEUROFIBROMATOSIS TYPE 1 (NF1): TUMOURS

Gliomas

- ☐ Optic pathway glioma (OPG)
- ☐ Brainstem gliomas
- ☐ Other brain gliomas

Glomus tumours

- ☐ These are frequently in the fingertips
- ☐ They are painful

Neurofibromas: complications

- ☐ Malignant transformation of subcutaneous neurofibromas
  - ○ Cutaneous neurofibromas do not become malignant
- ☐ Bleeding
- ☐ Growth
- ☐ Infiltration by plexiform neurofibromas
- ☐ Enlargement in pregnancy: with risk of cord compression
- ☐ Transformation to malignant peripheral nerve sheath tumours (MPNST)

Systemic tumours

- ☐ Gastrointestinal stromal tumours (GIST)
- ☐ Juvenile myelomonocytic leukaemia
- ☐ Rhabdomyosarcoma

Unidentified bright objects (UBOs)

- ☐ They are also called focal areas of signal intensity (FASI)
- ☐ They are seen on T2 MRI
- ☐ They are especially found in the thalamus
- ☐ They are also present in the basal ganglia and cerebellum
- ☐ They may occur in the spinal cord
- ☐ They result from microstructural brain damage

Emerging investigations

- ☐ Whole body magnetic resonance imaging (WB-MRI): for tumour detection

Investigational drugs for plexiform neurofibromas

- ☐ Selumetinib
- ☐ Imatinib
- ☐ Sirolimus
- ☐ Everolimus
- ☐ Pegylated interferon α-2b

DOI: 10.1201/9781003221258-97

NEUROFIBROMATOSIS TYPE 2 (NF2): CLINICAL FEATURES

Features of vestibular schwannomas

- ☐ Deafness
- ☐ Tinnitus
- ☐ Dizziness and imbalance
- ☐ Headaches
- ☐ Seizures
- ☐ Sensory disturbance
- ☐ Weakness
- ☐ Nausea
- ☐ Vomiting
- ☐ Vertigo: this is a rare and late feature

Ophthalmic features

- ☐ Reduced visual acuity
- ☐ Posterior subcapsular cataracts
- ☐ Retinal hamartoma
- ☐ Epiretinal membrane

Other features

- ☐ Skin lesions: similar to NF1
- ☐ Peripheral neuropathy (PN)
- ☐ Amyotrophy: focal and facial
- ☐ Epilepsy
- ☐ Cerebral aneurysms: these occur in 4% of cases
- ☐ Brainstem ischaemia: this develops in juvenile NF2

Differential diagnoses of unilateral vestibular schwannomas

- ☐ Mosaic NF2
- ☐ LZTR1-related schwannomatosis

NEUROFIBROMATOSIS TYPE 2 (NF2): TUMOURS

Vestibular schwannomas

- ☐ These are usually bilateral in children
- ☐ They are bilateral in 15–30% of adults
- ☐ Isolated schwannomas in subjects under the age of 18 years carry a 10% risk of NF2

Schwannomas: other locations

- ☐ Cutaneous
- ☐ Subcutaneous
- ☐ Bilateral vestibular
- ☐ Facial mononeuropathy
- ☐ Other cranial nerve except I and II
- ☐ Peripheral nerve

Meningiomas: locations

- ☐ Cranial
- ☐ Spinal
- ☐ Optic nerve

Meningiomas: implications

- ☐ Isolated meningiomas in subjects under the age of 18 years carry a 20% risk of NF2
- ☐ Multiple meningiomas predict severe disease course
- ☐ SMARCE1 mutation is a genetic risk for meningiomas

Gliomas

- ☐ Ependymomas: spinal and brainstem
- ☐ Astrocytomas: cranial and spinal

Other tumours

- ☐ Neurofibromas
- ☐ Plaque-like cutaneous skin tumours
- ☐ Nodular subcutaneous skin tumours
- ☐ Meningioangiomatosis
- ☐ Spinal cord ependymomas
- ☐ Intraneural perineuroma

SCHWANNOMATOSIS (SWN): CLINICAL FEATURES

Genetic features

- [ ] The mutations are on chromosome 22
- [ ] The transmission is autosomal dominant
- [ ] It is familial in 15–25% of cases
- [ ] Most cases are sporadic: de novo mutations

Genetic mutations

- [ ] SMARCB1 gene mutations: INI1, BAF47, or hSNF5
- [ ] LZTR1 gene mutations

Demographic features

- [ ] The peak incidence is between 30–60 years
- [ ] Some families may progress to typical NF2

Presenting features

- [ ] Pain: this is the most frequent feature
- [ ] Mass lesions
- [ ] Weakness
- [ ] Paraesthesias
- [ ] Headaches
- [ ] Depression
- [ ] Anxiety
- [ ] Polyradiculopathy

Synonym

- [ ] Neurilemommatosis

SCHWANNOMATOSIS (SWN): TUMOURS

Typical features

- [ ] These are typically multiple
- [ ] The average number of schwannomas per patient is 4.7
- [ ] They are most frequently restricted to the upper limb
- [ ] They may be restricted to a spinal segment

Usual locations

- [ ] Cranial
- [ ] Spinal
- [ ] Peripheral nerves

Unusual locations

- [ ] Bilateral maxillary sinus
- [ ] Pancreatic
- [ ] Submandibular salivary gland
- [ ] Intraosseous

Associated tumours

- [ ] Unilateral vestibular tumours: these are rare
- [ ] Intracranial meningiomas: especially falcine: these may be multiple
- [ ] Malignant peripheral nerve sheath tumors (MPNSTs)
- [ ] Cutaneous neurofibroma
- [ ] Lipomas
- [ ] Angiolipomas

Synonym

- [ ] Neurilemommatosis

TUBEROUS SCLEROSIS COMPLEX (TSC): NEUROPSYCHIATRIC FEATURES

Seizure features

- ☐ Seizures occur in >60% of cases
- ☐ They are early and severe
- ☐ They are usually focal seizures or infantile spasms
- ☐ Infantile spasms are more frequently seen with TSC1
- ☐ Diffusion tensor imaging (DTI) may identify epileptogenic tubers

TSC-associated neuropsychiatric disorder (TAND)

- ☐ Aggressive behaviour
- ☐ Autism spectrum disorders
- ☐ Cognitive impairment
- ☐ Intellectual disability
- ☐ Psychosis

Cognitive impairment: predictors

- ☐ Infantile spasms
- ☐ Polytherapy
- ☐ Corticosteroid treatment
- ☐ Older age at independent walking
- ☐ Younger age at onset of seizures
- ☐ Not using Vigabatrin as first anti-epileptic drug (AED)

Other neurological features

- ☐ Disturbed sleep pattern
- ☐ Excessive daytime sleepiness (EDS)
- ☐ Attention deficit hyperactivity disorder (ADHD)
- ☐ Possible association with cerebral aneurysms
- ☐ Spasticity

TUBEROUS SCLEROSIS COMPLEX (TSC): LESIONS

Cortical tubers: imaging features

- ☐ Broadened gyri
- ☐ Subcortical increased signal
- ☐ Blurred grey/white matter junction
- ☐ The severity of TSC is related to the tuber count

Hamartomas: locations

- ☐ Brain
- ☐ Eyes
- ☐ Heart
- ☐ Kidneys
- ☐ Skin

Other lesions

- ☐ Harmatias: non-growing lesions
- ☐ Subependymal nodules
- ☐ Subependymal giant cell astrocytoma (SEGA)
- ☐ Cerebral white matter radial migration lines
- ☐ Calcifications
- ☐ Cerebellar tubers: more frequent with TSC2 mutations
- ☐ Subtle cortical dysplasia
- ☐ Transmantle dysplasia
- ☐ Hemimegalencephaly
- ☐ Focal megalencephaly
- ☐ Cortical infoldings

Systemic lesions

- ☐ Cardiac rhabdomyoma
- ☐ Lymphangiomyomatosis
- ☐ Renal cysts
- ☐ Renal angiomyolipomas
- ☐ Hepatic angiomyolipomas
- ☐ Retinal nodular hamartomas
- ☐ Bone cysts

STURGE–WEBER SYNDROME (SWS): CLINICAL FEATURES

Genetics
- [ ] This is caused by mutations in the GNAQ gene

Central neurological features
- [ ] Intracranial haemangiomas
- [ ] Leptomeningeal angiomatosis
- [ ] Migraine
- [ ] Stroke like episodes
- [ ] Intracranial calcifications
- [ ] Seizures
- [ ] Mental retardation
- [ ] Hemianopia
- [ ] Hemiparesis
- [ ] Subarachnoid haemorrhage (SAH)
- [ ] Autism spectrum disorder (ASD)

Peripheral neurological features
- [ ] Hemiatrophy or hemihypertrophy
- [ ] Recurrent rhabdomyolysis: from lipid metabolic myopathy

Ophthalmic features
- [ ] Retinal haemangiomas
- [ ] Choroidal haemangiomas
- [ ] Episcleral haemangiomas
- [ ] Congenital glaucoma (buphthalmos)
- [ ] Bilateral exudative retinal detachment

Cutaneous haemangiomas
- [ ] Port wine stains: naevus flammeus
- [ ] Usually in the first and second trigeminal distributions
- [ ] They may be bilateral
- [ ] They may involve the lower face

Juvenile ossifying fibroma
- [ ] This is a bone hypertrophy
- [ ] It causes rapid overgrowth of the facial and jaw bones

Differential diagnosis
- [ ] Klippel Trenaunay Weber syndrome
- [ ] Rendu-Osler Weber syndrome
- [ ] Bannayan Riley Ruvalcaba syndrome
- [ ] Divry van Bogart syndrome
- [ ] Cobb syndrome
- [ ] Cerebrofacial arteriovenous metameric syndrome (CAMS)

Synonym
- [ ] Encephalofacial angiomatosis

Acronym
- [ ] GNAQ: guanine nucleotide-binding protein G(q) subunit alpha

VON HIPPEL-LINDAU DISEASE (VHL): CLINICAL FEATURES

Type 1 VHL
- [ ] VHL without pheochromocytoma

Type 2 VHL
- [ ] VHL with pheochromocytoma
- [ ] Type 2A: with other haemangioblastomas except renal cell carcinoma
- [ ] Type 2B: with other haemangioblastoma and renal cell carcinoma
- [ ] Type 2C: with only pheochromocytoma

Clinical features
- [ ] Cerebellar ataxia
- [ ] Raised intracranial pressure: from cerebellar haemangioblastoma
- [ ] Visual impairment: from retinal haemangioblastoma
- [ ] Deafness: from endolymphatic sac tumours (ELSTs)

Monitoring
- [ ] Annual ophthalmology examinations
- [ ] Brain magnetic resonance imaging (MRI): 12–36 monthly from adolescence
- [ ] Abdominal MRI or ultrasound: annually from 16 years
- [ ] Annual blood pressure monitoring
- [ ] Annual 24-hour urine catecholamines

CHAPTER 17

Metabolic and mitochodrial disorders

Lysosomal storage diseases

FABRY DISEASE: NEUROLOGICAL FEATURES

Genetic features

- ☐ This is caused by mutations in the alpha-galactosidase (GLA) gene
- ☐ This is on chromosome Xq22
- ☐ The transmission is X-linked

Demographic features

- ☐ Males are usually affected
- ☐ Female involvement may be severe
- ☐ The median age at diagnosis is around 22 years

Thrombotic stroke

- ☐ Stroke is the first presentation in many patients
- ☐ The average stroke onset age is 34 years in males and 40 years in females
- ☐ Stroke risk is predicted by increased regional cerebral blood flow

Embolic stroke: risks

- ☐ Ischaemic heart disease (IHD)
- ☐ Cardiac valve disease
- ☐ Cardiomyopathy

Other central nervous system features

- ☐ Heamorrhagic stroke
- ☐ Venous and arterial thrombosis
- ☐ High frequency sensorineural deafness
- ☐ Epilepsy
- ☐ Depression
- ☐ Peripheral vestibular abnormalities

Small fiber peripheral neuropathy (PN)

- ☐ This is present in about three-quarters of cases
- ☐ There is possible involvement of the dorsal root ganglia (DRG)
- ☐ It presents with neuropathic pain

Episodic pain (Fabry crises): triggers

- ☐ Exercise
- ☐ Temperature change
- ☐ Stress

Acroparaesthesias: differential diagnosis

- ☐ Urticaria
- ☐ C1 esterase deficiency
- ☐ Acute intermittent porphyria (AIP)
- ☐ Erythromelalgia
- ☐ Reflex sympathetic dystrophy

FABRY DISEASE: SYSTEMIC FEATURES

Cardiac features

- ☐ Left ventricular hypertrophy (LVH)
- ☐ Cardiomyopathy
- ☐ Abnormal heart valves
- ☐ Atrioventricular conduction defects

Ophthalmic features

- ☐ Corneal dystrophy
- ☐ Lens opacities
- ☐ Reduced tears and saliva
- ☐ Tortuous conjunctival and retinal blood vessels
- ☐ Central retinal artery occlusion

Angiokeratoma corporis diffusum

- ☐ This is a skin lesion
- ☐ It occurs in about 95% of cases
- ☐ It has a bathing-trunk distribution and spread
- ☐ The onset age is 14–16 years

Other dermatological features

- ☐ Thick lips
- ☐ Thick nasolabial folds
- ☐ Reduced sweating (hypohidrosis)

Other systemic features

- ☐ Renal failure
- ☐ Fever
- ☐ Nausea and vomiting
- ☐ Diarrhoea
- ☐ Fatigue
- ☐ Tinnitus
- ☐ Lymphoedema
- ☐ Jejunal diverticulosis

DOI: 10.1201/9781003221258-99

FABRY DISEASE: MANAGEMENT

Blood tests

- ☐ Alpha galactosidase: this is deficient in white cells, fibroblasts, and plasma
- ☐ DNA analysis: this is done if the alpha galactosidase level is normal or mildly reduced

Magnetic resonance imaging (MRI) brain: features

- ☐ White matter lesions
- ☐ Ischaemic stroke
- ☐ Pulvinar signal intensity: in the posterior thalamus
- ☐ Dolichoestasia: this is mainly in the vertebrobasilar arteries
- ☐ Lenticular degeneration

Magnetic resonance spectroscopy (MRS)

- ☐ There is reduced cortical and subcortical n-acetoacetate (NAA)

Slit lamp examination findings

- ☐ Lens opacities: capsular, subcapsular, or posterior
- ☐ Whorl-like corneal opacities

Other investigations

- ☐ Pathology: this shows globotriaosylceramide (Gb3) in the tissues
- ☐ Urinalysis: this shows mulberry cells and bodies

Treatment of crises

- ☐ Phenytoin
- ☐ Carbamazepine
- ☐ Gabapentin

Definitive treatments: Migalastat

- ☐ This is an oral pharmacological chaperone
- ☐ It binds and stabilizes mutant α-Gal A
- ☐ It increases glucosidase levels and improves organ function

Definitive treatments: others

- ☐ Enzyme replacement therapy (ERT): this is administered intravenously

NIEMANN–PICK C (NPC): CLINICAL FEATURES

Genetic mutations

- ☐ NPC1: this accounts for 95% of cases
- ☐ NPC2
- ☐ The mean onset age of the adult form is 25 years

Pathological features

- ☐ It results from impaired lipid transport
- ☐ There is sphingomyelinase deficiency in types A and B
- ☐ There is a possible link to copper metabolism

Neurological features

- ☐ Cognitive impairment
- ☐ Deafness
- ☐ Cerebellar ataxia
- ☐ Parkinsonian tremor
- ☐ Cataplexy
- ☐ Myoclonus
- ☐ Ataxia
- ☐ Dysarthria
- ☐ Dysphagia

Psychiatric features

- ☐ Psychosis: this may be the presenting feature
- ☐ Depression
- ☐ Agitation and hyperactivity

Vertical supranuclear gaze palsy (VSGP)

- ☐ This is also called vertical supranuclear gaze saccade palsy (VSSP)
- ☐ It occurs early and frequently in NPC
- ☐ It may be the only feature of adult NPC

Slow saccades

- ☐ This is initially vertical then horizontal
- ☐ It may be masked by blinking
- ☐ It is observed after lifting the eyelids

Systemic features

- ☐ Hepatomegaly
- ☐ Isolated splenomegaly
- ☐ Prolonged unexplained neonatal jaundice
- ☐ Acute neonatal liver failure

Differential diagnosis

- ☐ Alzheimer's disease (AD)
- ☐ Creutzfeldt Jakob disease (CJD)
- ☐ Multiple sclerosis (MS)
- ☐ Parkinson's disease (PD)
- ☐ Progressive supranuclear palsy (PSP)
- ☐ Spinocerebellar ataxia (SCA)
- ☐ Wilson's disease
- ☐ Wernicke encephalopathy

KRABBE DISEASE: CLINICAL FEATURES

Genetics and pathology

- ☐ This is caused by mutations in the glucocerebrosidase (GALC) gene
- ☐ This is on chromosome 14
- ☐ Subjects are unable to degrade galactolipids in myelin
- ☐ There are globoid cell deposits in the perivascular regions

Types

- ☐ Early infantile onset: this accounts for most cases
- ☐ Juvenile onset
- ☐ Late onset: this occurs in 10–15% of cases
  - ○ It has a milder course due to partial enzyme deficiency

Developmental features

- ☐ Poor expressive language development
- ☐ Psychomotor retardation
- ☐ Microcephaly
- ☐ Cognitive impairment
- ☐ Dementia
- ☐ Poor growth
- ☐ Abnormal motor control

Pyramidal features

- ☐ Spasticity
- ☐ Adult onset spastic paraparesis with normal MRI

Movement disorders

- ☐ Incoordination
- ☐ Ataxia
- ☐ Tremor
- ☐ Myoclonus

Other features

- ☐ Peripheral neuropathy (PN) with pes cavus
- ☐ Visual loss

Magnetic resonance imaging (MRI) features

- ☐ Tigroid appearance: these are non-contrasting symmetrical T2 hyperintensities
- ☐ T2 thalamic hypointensities
- ☐ Cerebellar hyperintensities: these are peridentate in location
- ☐ Lumbosacral root enhancement: this may precede cerebral changes

Synonym

- ☐ Globoid cells leukodystrophy

Leukodystrophies

ALEXANDER DISEASE: CLINICAL FEATURES

Genetics and pathology

- ☐ This is caused by mutations in the glial fibrillary acidic protein (GFAP) gene
- ☐ It is an astrocytopathy
- ☐ The pathology shows Rosenthal fibers: these are ubiquinated astrocytic inclusions

Types

- ☐ Infantile onset: <2 years
- ☐ Juvenile onset: 2–12 years
- ☐ Adult onset: >12 years: this has a worse brainstem involvement and a slower progression

Brainstem features

- ☐ Dysarthria
- ☐ Dysphagia
- ☐ Dysphonia
- ☐ Diplopia
- ☐ Nystagmus
- ☐ Ptosis
- ☐ Vocal cord palsy
- ☐ Palatal myoclonus (oculopalatal tremor): this is highly suggestive of Alexander disease

Other features

- ☐ Spastic quadriparesis
- ☐ Cerebellar ataxia
- ☐ Urinary symptoms
- ☐ Dysautonomia
- ☐ Sleep disorders
- ☐ Progressive microcoria: very small pupils
- ☐ Very late onset variant: it may present as late as 80 years

Rare features

- ☐ Dystonia
- ☐ Retinopathy
- ☐ Brain mass
- ☐ Functional megacolon

Features of infantile onset

- ☐ Macrocephaly
- ☐ Spasticity
- ☐ Ataxia
- ☐ Psychomotor regression
- ☐ Seizures

ADRENOLEUKODYSTROPHY (ALD): NEUROLOGICAL FEATURES

Genetics and pathology

- ☐ This is caused by mutations in the ABCD1 gene on chromosome Xq
- ☐ The gene encodes adrenoleukodystrophy protein (ADLP)
- ☐ The transmission is X-linked but autosomal recessive transmission occurs in neonatal forms
- ☐ The mutations cause impaired beta oxidation of very long chain fatty acids (VLCFAs)
  - ○ These accumulate in blood and tissues

Clinical phenotypes

- ☐ Childhood cerebral ALD: the onset age is 3–10 years
- ☐ Adolescent cerebral ALD: the onset age is 10–21 years
- ☐ Adult cerebral ALD
- ☐ Adrenomyeloneuropathy (AMN): this is usually adult onset
- ☐ Isolated adrenocortical insufficiency (Addison's disease)
- ☐ Asymptomatic and pre-symptomatic
- ☐ Symptomatic female heterozygotes: late onset
- ☐ Spinocerebellar variant

Cerebral features

- ☐ Demyelination: this may be triggered by head injury
- ☐ Seizures
- ☐ Dementia
- ☐ Ataxia
- ☐ Dysphagia
- ☐ Raised intracranial pressure (ICP)
- ☐ Multiple congenital brain development defects

Psychiatric features

- ☐ Psychosis
- ☐ Bipolar disorder
- ☐ Behavioural abnormalities, e.g. exhibitionism
- ☐ Depression
- ☐ Attention deficit hyperactivity disorder (ADHD)

Other neurological features

- ☐ Visual impairment: red-green colour blindness
- ☐ Impaired auditory discrimination
- ☐ Sensorimotor peripheral neuropathy (PN): this is axonal with multifocal demyelination
- ☐ Small fiber neuropathy

Features of adrenomyeloneuropathy (AMN)

- ☐ Myelopathy with spastic paraparesis/quadriparesis
- ☐ Peripheral neuropathy (PN)
- ☐ Hypogonadism
- ☐ Subcortical dementia: this is present in 50–60% of cases
- ☐ Urinary symptoms

DOI: 10.1201/9781003221258-100

Course and outcome

- ☐ The mean onset age is around 7 years
- ☐ It may follow a relapsing course
- ☐ A vegetative state develops within 2 years
- ☐ It is often fatal in the first decade

ADRENOLEUKODYSTROPHY (ALD): SYSTEMIC FEATURES

Addisonian features

- ☐ Bronzed skin pigmentation
- ☐ Scanty hair
- ☐ Gastrointestinal disturbance
- ☐ Fatigue
- ☐ Hypotension
- ☐ Hyponatraemia
- ☐ Impaired synacthen test
- ☐ Symptoms may develop before, with, or after neurological symptoms
- ☐ They may precede neurological features by years

Other endocrine features

- ☐ Hypogonadism with primary testicular failure
- ☐ Scanty scalp hair
- ☐ Urinary difficulty

Features of female heterozygote carriers

- ☐ Most female carriers are asymptomatic
- ☐ Symptoms develop with age
- ☐ Myelopathy occurs in about two-thirds of cases
- ☐ Peripheral neuropathy develops in more than half of cases
- ☐ Faecal incontinence is present in about a quarter of cases
- ☐ VLCFAs are normal in about a third of cases
- ☐ Sensorimotor axonal peripheral neuropathy (PN) occurs in about 60%: it is often subclinical
- ☐ Brainstem auditory evoked potentials (BAEPs) are abnormal in more 50% of cases

Acronym

- ☐ VLCFA: very long chain fatty acids

Peroxisomal disorders

REFSUM'S DISEASE: CLINICAL FEATURES

Genetic mutations

- [ ] PHYH: phytanoyl-CoA hydroxylase: this is on chromosome 10
- [ ] PEX7: peroxisomal targeting system-2 (PTS-2): this is on chromosome 6

Pathology

- [ ] It is a peroxisomal disorder
- [ ] Plasma phytanic acid levels are elevated
- [ ] There is phytanic acid accumulation in tissues: nerves, brain, and fat
- [ ] Pristanic acid levels are reduced

Tapetoretinal degeneration: features

- [ ] Bone spicule retinal pigmentation
- [ ] Retinitis pigmentosa
- [ ] Night blindness
- [ ] Visual field constriction
- [ ] Attenuated retinal vessels

Other ophthalmic features

- [ ] Miosis: from iris deposition or dysautonomia
- [ ] Optic atrophy
- [ ] Iris atrophy
- [ ] Cataracts
- [ ] Vitreous opacities
- [ ] Nystagmus

Skeletal malformations

- [ ] Epiphyseal bone dysplasia of hands and feet
- [ ] Syndactyly
- [ ] Short metacarpals giving short tubular fingers
- [ ] Short fourth metatarsal: results in a short fourth toe
- [ ] Pes cavus

Neurological features

- [ ] Demyelinating sensorimotor peripheral neuropathy (PN)
- [ ] Cranial neuropathies
- [ ] Guillain–Barre syndrome (GBS)-like presentation
- [ ] Cerebellar ataxia
- [ ] Sensorineural deafness
- [ ] Reversible vestibular neuropathy
- [ ] Anosmia
- [ ] Psychiatric disorders rarely

Systemic features

- [ ] Ichthyosis over the extremities
- [ ] Cardiomyopathy
- [ ] Arrhythmias
- [ ] Renal failure

Triggers for deterioration

- [ ] Rapid weight loss
- [ ] Acute illness
- [ ] Fasting
- [ ] Pregnancy

DOI: 10.1201/9781003221258-101

CEREBROTENDINOUS XANTHOMATOSIS (CTX): CLINICAL FEATURES

Genetics and pathology

- ☐ This is caused by mutations in the CYP27A1 gene
- ☐ This encodes sterol 27-hydroxylase
- ☐ The mutations result in cholestanol accumulation in tissues

Main features

- ☐ Intractable diarrhoea: in childhood onset forms
- ☐ Juvenile onset cataracts
- ☐ Tendon xanthomas: these develop after the second decade

Cranial features

- ☐ Cerebellar ataxia
- ☐ Epilepsy: including infantile spasms
- ☐ Distal myoclonus: this is subcortical in origin
- ☐ Dystonia
- ☐ Oromandibular myoclonus
- ☐ Parkinsonism: the most frequent movement disorder
- ☐ Corticobasal syndrome (CBS)
- ☐ Postural tremor
- ☐ Progressive ataxia and palatal tremor (PAPT)
- ☐ Progressive dementia
- ☐ Autism

Spinal features

- ☐ Spastic paraparesis
- ☐ Myelopathy

Peripheral features

- ☐ Mild peripheral neuropathy (PN)

Psychiatric features

- ☐ Personality disorder
- ☐ Learning difficulty
- ☐ Mood disorders
- ☐ Psychosis

Systemic features

- ☐ Cataracts
- ☐ Tendon xanthomas
- ☐ Premature atherosclerosis
- ☐ Osteoporosis
- ☐ Pulmonary insufficiency
- ☐ Diarrhoea
- ☐ Abdominal aortic aneurysm: case report

Differential diagnosis

- ☐ Sitosterolaemia
- ☐ Familial hypercholesterolaemia
- ☐ Langerhans cell histiocytosis
- ☐ Marinesco-Sjogren syndrome

TANGIER DISEASE

Genetics

- ☐ This is caused by mutations in the ATP-binding cassette transporter (ABCA1) gene
- ☐ This is on chromosome 9q31
- ☐ The transmission is autosomal co-dominant
- ☐ Most cases are from Tangier in Morocco

Pathology

- ☐ There are cholesterol ester deposits in macrophages and the reticulo-endothelial system
- ☐ High density lipoproteins (HDL) are almost absent
- ☐ Apo A1 is low or absent
- ☐ Total plasma cholesterol is occasionally decreased

Lymphoid-related features

- ☐ Organomegaly
- ☐ Lymphadenopathy
- ☐ Enlarged yellow tonsils

Peripheral neuropathy (PN)

- ☐ This is often the presenting feature
- ☐ It starts as a progressive mononeuropathy or polyneuropathy
- ☐ It is syringomyelia-like in adults: with dissociated sensory loss
- ☐ It may be relapsing-remitting

Ophthalmic features

- ☐ Corneal opacities
- ☐ Retinal pigmentary changes

Other features

- ☐ Premature atherosclerosis
- ☐ Thrombocytopaenia

Differential diagnosis

- ☐ Leprosy

Urea cycle disorders

UREA CYCLE DISORDERS: CLINICAL FEATURES

Types of urea cycle disorders

- ☐ Argininaemia: arginase deficiency (ARG1)
- ☐ Argininosucciniaciduria: argininosuccinase acid lyase deficiency (ASL)
- ☐ Citrullineamia type I: argininosuccinic acid synthase deficiency (ASS1)
- ☐ Citrullinemia type II
- ☐ HHH syndrome: hyperornithinemia, hyperammonemia, homocitrullinuria: it is caused by mitochondrial ornithine transporter (ORNT) deficiency
- ☐ Carbamyl phosphate synthase I (CPSI) deficiency
- ☐ Ornithine transcarbamylase (OTC) deficiency
- ☐ N-acetylglutamate synthase deficiency (NAGS)

Demographic features

- ☐ The onset is usually in the neonatal period
- ☐ Adult onset cases may occur with partial deficiencies or arginase deficiency

Clinical features

- ☐ Vomiting
- ☐ Lethargy
- ☐ Cognitive impairment
- ☐ Headaches
- ☐ Ataxia
- ☐ Protein intolerance
- ☐ Neuropsychiatric features
- ☐ Respiratory alkalosis: from hyperventilation
- ☐ Encephalopathy

Triggers for crises

- ☐ High protein intake
- ☐ Stress
- ☐ Illness
- ☐ Surgery
- ☐ Post-partum
- ☐ Valproate
- ☐ Salicylates
- ☐ Steroids
- ☐ L-asparaginase

ORNITHINE TRANSCARBAMYLASE (OTC) DEFICIENCY: CLINICAL FEATURES

Genetics and pathology

- ☐ OTC deficiency is the most frequent urea cycle disorder
- ☐ It is X-linked: other urea cycle disorders are autosomal recessive
- ☐ It usually affects males
- ☐ Female heterozygotes may be symptomatic
- ☐ The onset is usually in infancy

Clinical features

- ☐ Post prandial vomiting
- ☐ Lethargy
- ☐ Seizures
- ☐ Coma
- ☐ Hyperventilation
- ☐ Respiratory alkalosis
- ☐ Hyperammonemic crises

Triggers of hyperammonemic crises

- ☐ Pregnancy: symptoms typically present post-partum
- ☐ Febrile illness
- ☐ Fasting
- ☐ Protein loading

Outcome

- ☐ Serum ammonia level at diagnosis predicts outcome

DOI: 10.1201/9781003221258-102

ORNITHINE TRANSCARBAMYLASE (OTC) DEFICIENCY: MANAGEMENT

Serum tests

- ☐ Ammonia: high
- ☐ Glutamine: high
- ☐ Alanine: high
- ☐ Citrulline: low
- ☐ Lactate: high
- ☐ Glucose: low

Other tests

- ☐ Urinary orotic acid: high
- ☐ Arterial pH: alkalosis
- ☐ Cerebrospinal fluid (CSF): this is usually normal
- ☐ Electroencephalogram (EEG): this may show seizure activity
- ☐ Magnetic resonance imaging (MRI): this may show extensive abnormal signal changes and restricted diffusion

Nutritional supplementation

- ☐ Calories
- ☐ Essential amino acids
- ☐ Minerals
- ☐ Vitamins
- ☐ Long-chain polyunsaturated fatty acids

Treatment: sodium scavenging drugs

- ☐ Sodium phenylbutyrate 2 g qid: this is the preferred option
- ☐ Sodium benzoate 4 g qid

Treatment: others

- ☐ Arginine 500 mg qid ± Citrulline: for removal of ammonia
- ☐ Avoid triggers
- ☐ Low-protein diet

Porphyria

PORPHYRIA: CLINICAL FEATURES AND TREATMENT

Neurological features

- [ ] Anxiety
- [ ] Confusion
- [ ] Agitation
- [ ] Restlessness
- [ ] Insomnia
- [ ] Psychosis
- [ ] Seizures
- [ ] Coma
- [ ] Leukoencephalopathy
- [ ] Osmotic demyelination disorder (ODD)
- [ ] Cortical blindness: from occipital stroke
- [ ] Autonomic dysfunction: diarrhoea, vomiting, constipation
- [ ] Reversible cerebral vasoconstriction syndrome (RVCS)
- [ ] Posterior reversible encephalopathy syndrome (PRES)
- [ ] Peripheral neuropathy: see related topic

Systemic features

- [ ] Attacks of abdominal pain
- [ ] Respiratory dysfunction
- [ ] Hyponatraemia: this is due to syndrome of inappropriate ADH secretion (SIADH)
- [ ] Dark coloured urine: this is due to increased urinary δ ALA and porphobilinogen

Triggers for acute attacks

- [ ] Drugs
- [ ] Abuse substances
- [ ] Infection
- [ ] Emotional stress
- [ ] Physical exertion
- [ ] Fasting
- [ ] Smoking
- [ ] Premenstrual

Chronic features

- [ ] Skin lesions
- [ ] Anxiety states
- [ ] Epilepsy
- [ ] Neuropathy
- [ ] Myopathy

Treatment

- [ ] Intravenous haematin
- [ ] Intravenous 10% glucose: to suppress haem biosynthesis
- [ ] Betablockers: for hypertension and tachycardia
- [ ] Pyridoxine
- [ ] Opiates: for pain
- [ ] Gabapentin: for seizures

Investigational treatment

- [ ] Givosiran: this is an RNA interference therapy

PORPHYRIA: PERIPHERAL NEUROPATHY (PN)

Clinical features

- [ ] Porphyric neuropathy occurs with hepatic porphyrias
- [ ] It is predominantly an axonal motor neuropathy
- [ ] It presents with proximal rapidly ascending asymmetric weakness
- [ ] 50% have upper limb onset: it may present as severe bilateral axonal radial motor neuropathy
- [ ] There may be glove and stocking and bathing-suit sensory deficits
- [ ] There is generalised hyporeflexia but preserved ankle reflexes

Autonomic features

- [ ] Neuropathic pain
- [ ] Constipation
- [ ] Pseudo-obstruction
- [ ] Labile hypertension

Differential diagnosis

- [ ] Guillain–Barre syndrome (GBS)

Cerebrospinal fluid (CSF) analysis

- [ ] This shows dissociated protein-cell picture
- [ ] Suspect porphyria in cases of recurrent Guillain–Barre syndrome (GBS)

Nerve conduction studies (NCS)

- [ ] Axonal polyradiculopathy or neuronopathy

Prevention

- [ ] Check urinary porphyrins routinely in inflammatory neuropathy

DOI: 10.1201/9781003221258-103

PORPHYRIA: DRUG SAFETY

Unsafe drugs

- ☐ Alcohol
- ☐ Barbiturates
- ☐ Calcium channel blockers
- ☐ Carbamazepine
- ☐ Clonazepam
- ☐ Halothane
- ☐ Ketamine
- ☐ Phenytoin
- ☐ Primidone
- ☐ Progestins
- ☐ Sulphonamides
- ☐ Tranquilizers
- ☐ Valproate

Potentially unsafe drugs

- ☐ Clonidine
- ☐ Chloroquine
- ☐ Erythromycin
- ☐ Lidocaine
- ☐ Methyldopa
- ☐ Nalidixic acid
- ☐ Nortryptiline
- ☐ Oestrogens
- ☐ Pentazocine
- ☐ Rifampin
- ☐ Spironolactone

Potentially safe drugs

- ☐ Acetaminophen
- ☐ Acyclovir
- ☐ Amantadine
- ☐ Aspirin
- ☐ Beta blockers
- ☐ Cimetidine
- ☐ Chlorpromazine
- ☐ Fentanyl
- ☐ Gabapentin
- ☐ Glucocorticoids
- ☐ Haloperidol
- ☐ Insulin
- ☐ Narcotic analgesics
- ☐ Neostigmine
- ☐ Penicillin
- ☐ Phenothiazines
- ☐ Propofol
- ☐ Selective serotonin reuptake inhibitors (SSRIs)
- ☐ Streptomycin
- ☐ Tetracycline

Mitochondrial disorders: phenotypes and features

MITOCHONDRIAL DISEASES: NEUROLOGICAL FEATURES

Peripheral neuropathy (PN): common causes

- ☐ Mitochondrial neuro-gastrointestinal encephalopathy (MNGIE)
- ☐ Mitochondrial encephalopathy lactic acidosis and stroke-like episodes (MELAS)
- ☐ Myoclonic epilepsy with ragged red fibers (MERRF)

Movement disorders

- ☐ Parkinsonism
- ☐ Ataxia
- ☐ Myoclonus
- ☐ Dystonia

Ophthalmic features

- ☐ Optic atrophy
- ☐ Cataracts
- ☐ Ptosis
- ☐ Pigmentary retinopathy
- ☐ Ophthalmoplegia
- ☐ Subacute visual loss

Miscellaneous neurological features

- ☐ Encephalopathy
- ☐ Epilepsy
- ☐ Migraine
- ☐ Myopathy
- ☐ Deafness
- ☐ Stroke-like episodes (SLEs)

Psychiatric features

- ☐ Dementia
- ☐ Bipolar disorder

MITOCHONDRIAL STROKE-LIKE EPISODES (SLEs)

Pathology

- ☐ These are metabolic strokes
- ☐ They are typical of MELAS
- ☐ They arise from focal breakdown of the blood-brain barrier
- ☐ Triggers may be metabolic, epileptic, or drugs

Epidemiology

- ☐ They may be the first and only mitochondrial feature in young patients
- ☐ They are a cause of unexplained isolated strokes in subjects under the age of 50 years

Clinical features

- ☐ Headache
- ☐ Epilepsy
- ☐ Ataxia
- ☐ Visual impairment
- ☐ Vomiting
- ☐ Psychiatric features

Radiological features

- ☐ They may be focal or multifocal
- ☐ They may be cortical or subcortical
- ☐ They may be symmetrical
- ☐ They do not conform to vascular territories
- ☐ They appear as cytotoxic oedema and progress to vasogenic oedema
- ☐ They progressively expand over days to months
- ☐ They manifest as hyper-perfusion on perfusion studies
- ☐ They may resolve spontaneously: fleeting cortical lesions

Manifestations of chronic lesions

- ☐ Contrast enhancement
- ☐ Cystic change
- ☐ Laminar cortical necrosis
- ☐ Focal atrophy
- ☐ Toenail sign

Potential treatments

- ☐ L-Arginine
- ☐ L Carnitine
- ☐ L-Citrulline
- ☐ Antioxidants: Co-enzyme Q (CoQ)
- ☐ Antiepileptic drugs (AEDs)
- ☐ Ketogenic diet
- ☐ Steroids

Acronym

- ☐ MELAS: mitochondrial encephalopathy lactic acidosis and stroke-like episodes

DOI: 10.1201/9781003221258-104

MITOCHONDRIAL EPILEPSIES

Mitochondrial diseases with epilepsy

- ☐ Mitochondrial encephalomyopathy lactic acidosis and stroke-like episodes (MELAS)
- ☐ Myoclonic epilepsy with ragged red fibers (MERRF)
- ☐ Alpers syndrome
- ☐ Mitochondrial recessive ataxia syndrome (MIRAS)
- ☐ Spinocerebellar ataxia with epilepsy (SCAE)
- ☐ Myoclonus, epilepsy, myopathy, sensory ataxia (MEMSA)
- ☐ Leigh syndrome

Presentations

- ☐ Early onset epileptic encephalopathy
- ☐ Infantile spasms
- ☐ Lennox-Gastaut syndrome (LGS)

Clinical features

- ☐ Simple or complex focal seizures
- ☐ Epilepsia partialis continua (EPC)
- ☐ Bilateral convulsive seizures
- ☐ Segmental and generalised myoclonic seizures
- ☐ There is usually a combination of different focal seizures types

MITOCHONDRIAL OPTIC NEUROPATHIES AND MYOPATHIES

Causes of mitochondrial optic neuropathy

- ☐ Leber hereditary optic neuropathy (LHON)
- ☐ Dominant optic atrophy (DOA, OPA1 mutations)
- ☐ Friedreich's ataxia (FA)
- ☐ Hereditary motor sensory neuropathy 6 (HMSN 6; MFN 2)
- ☐ Hereditary spastic paraparesis 7 (SPG7; paraplegin)

Role of mitochondria in other optic neuropathies

- ☐ Charcot–Marie–Tooth disease (CMT)
- ☐ Multiple sclerosis (MS)

Causes of mitochondrial myopathy

- ☐ Mitochondrial encephalomyopathy lactic acidosis and stroke-like episodes (MELAS)
- ☐ Myoclonic Epilepsy with Ragged Red Fibers (MERRF)
- ☐ Kearns Sayre syndrome (KSS)
- ☐ Chronic progressive external ophthalmoplegia (CPEO)
- ☐ Leigh syndrome
- ☐ Long-term Zidovudine therapy

MITOCHONDRIAL DISEASES: SYSTEMIC FEATURES

Cardiorespiratory features

- ☐ Cardiomyopathy: this is usually hypertrophic but it can be dilated
- ☐ Conduction abnormalities
- ☐ Hyperventilation: from lactic acidosis
- ☐ Central hyperventilation: with encephalopathy
- ☐ Lung sepsis: this is often terminal

Renal features

- ☐ Metabolic acidosis
- ☐ Aminoaciduria
- ☐ Proximal tubulopathy
- ☐ Nephrotic syndrome
- ☐ Tubulointerstitial nephropathy

Endocrine features

- ☐ Diabetes mellitus
- ☐ Hypoparathyroidism
- ☐ Hypothyroidism

Gastrointestinal features

- ☐ Episodic nausea and vomiting
- ☐ Malabsorption
- ☐ Intestinal pseudo-obstruction
- ☐ Hepatic failure

Haematological features

- ☐ Sideroblastic anaemia
- ☐ Pancytopaenia

Other systemic features

- ☐ Short stature
- ☐ Brachydactyly: short fingers and toes
- ☐ Chronic fatigue
- ☐ Exercise intolerance
- ☐ Cervical lipomatosis

Neurological mitochondrial disorders

CHRONIC PROGRESSIVE EXTERNAL OPHTHALMOPLEGIA (CPEO)

Genetic mutations

- ☐ Polymerase gamma (POLG)
- ☐ Adenine nucleotide translocator 1 (ANT1)
- ☐ C10orf2: this encodes Twinkle
- ☐ SPG7: this is associated with a CPEO variant which manifests with spasticity
- ☐ MT-TL1: this is usually associated with MELAS

Ophthalmic features

- ☐ Bilateral ptosis: the onset is often asymmetric
- ☐ Optic atrophy
- ☐ Cataracts

Muscle features

- ☐ Mild proximal weakness
- ☐ Fatigue

Cardiac features

- ☐ Cardiac conduction defects
- ☐ Cardiomyopathy

Other features

- ☐ Ataxia
- ☐ Peripheral neuropathy (PN)
- ☐ Deafness
- ☐ Depression

Acronym

- ☐ MELAS: mitochondrial encephalopathy lactic acidosis and stroke-like episodes

KEARNS-SAYRE SYNDROME (KSS)

Ophthalmic features

- ☐ Progressive external ophthalmoplegia (PEO)
- ☐ Salt and pepper pigmentary retinopathy

Neurological features

- ☐ Myopathy
- ☐ Cerebellar ataxia

Endocrine features

- ☐ Growth hormone deficiency
- ☐ Hypothyroidism
- ☐ Diabetes mellitus
- ☐ Autoimmune thyroiditis
- ☐ Hypopituitarism
- ☐ Hypoparathyroidism

Cardiac features

- ☐ Ventricular tachycardia: including Torsade de pointes: pacemakers are often required

Cerebrospinal fluid (CSF) analysis

- ☐ High protein: this is usually >100 mg/dl
- ☐ High lactate

Magnetic resonance imaging (MRI): sites of lesions

- ☐ Subcortical white matter
- ☐ Thalamus
- ☐ Globus pallidus
- ☐ Brainstem

Magnetic resonance imaging (MRI): other features

- ☐ Cerebral atrophy
- ☐ Cerebellar atrophy

Treatment with coenzyme Q

- ☐ This may improve neurological and cardiac symptoms
- ☐ It may also reduce cerebrospinal fluid protein (CSF) lactate

DOI: 10.1201/9781003221258-105

LEBER HEREDITARY OPTIC NEUROPATHY (LHON): CLINICAL FEATURES

Genetic point mutations

- [ ] G11778A: this has the worst outcome
- [ ] T14484C: this has the best outcome
- [ ] G3460A

Genetics

- [ ] Only 50% of males with the mutation are affected
- [ ] Only 10% of females with the mutation are affected
- [ ] There is a positive maternal family history in 50–60% of cases

Onset features

- [ ] The onset age is in the first two decades
- [ ] The peak onset age is 15–30 years
- [ ] 95% of carriers manifest the disease by the age of 50 years

Central visual loss

- [ ] The onset is acute or subacute
- [ ] It is painless
- [ ] Visual loss is simultaneous in 25% of cases
- [ ] Bilateral involvement develops within months
- [ ] It results from degeneration of retinal ganglion cells
- [ ] Optic atrophy develops later
- [ ] 4% show recovery

Visual signs

- [ ] Temporal (papillomacular bundle) optic atrophy: this is pathognomonic
- [ ] Preserved pupillary reflexes
- [ ] Peripapillary telangiectasia
- [ ] Disc pseudo-oedema
- [ ] Retinal vascular tortuosity

Cardiac features

- [ ] Pre-excitation
- [ ] Wolf–Parkinson–White (WPW) syndrome
- [ ] Lown–Gannong–Levine (LGL) syndrome
- [ ] Atrioventricular block

Neurological features

- [ ] Tremor
- [ ] Peripheral neuropathy (PN)
- [ ] Charcot–Marie–Tooth disease (CMT)
- [ ] Myopathy
- [ ] Dystonia
- [ ] Multiple sclerosis (Harding syndrome)
- [ ] Overlap with MELAS
- [ ] Longitudinally extensive transverse myelitis (LETM): case report

LHON+

- [ ] Dystonia
- [ ] Ataxia
- [ ] Juvenile onset encephalopathy

MELAS: CLINICAL FEATURES

Stroke-like features

- [ ] There are multiple stroke-like events
- [ ] The onset is stuttering
- [ ] Episodes begin from ages 20–70 years

Headaches

- [ ] These are migraine-like
- [ ] There is associated aura
- [ ] They are more frequent with older onset age of MELAS
- [ ] They often occur at the time of stroke-like episodes

Cognitive and encephalopathic features

- [ ] Impaired consciousness
- [ ] Intermittent encephalopathy
- [ ] Premature dementia

Other features

- [ ] Seizures: these often occur at the time of stroke-like events
- [ ] Lactic acidosis
- [ ] Diabetes
- [ ] Parkinsonism: with orofacial dyskinesias and freezing of gait

Suggested expanded phenotype: MCARNE

- [ ] Mitochondrial Cerebellar Ataxia
- [ ] Renal failure
- [ ] Neuropathy
- [ ] Encephalopathy

Differential diagnosis

- [ ] Multiple system atrophy (MSA)

Acronym

- [ ] MELAS: mitochondrial encephalomyopathy lactic acidosis and stroke-like episodes

MERRF: CLINICAL AND LABORATORY FEATURES

Genetics: A8344G

- [ ] MERRF is usually caused by an A-G substitution in the tRNA gene of mitochondrial DNA
- [ ] It may also be a T-C or a G-A substitution
- [ ] The transmission is maternal

Neurological features

- [ ] Seizures: often photosensitive
- [ ] Myoclonus: stimulus sensitive
- [ ] Muscle weakness
- [ ] Pyramidal features
- [ ] Ataxia
- [ ] Neuropathy
- [ ] Deafness
- [ ] Optic atrophy

Systemic features

- [ ] Cardiomyopathy
- [ ] Pigmentary retinopathy
- [ ] Ophthalmoplegia
- [ ] Multiple lipomas
- [ ] Diabetes mellitus

Magnetic resonance imaging (MRI)

- [ ] Cerebral atrophy
- [ ] Basal ganglia calcification

Muscle biopsy

- [ ] Ragged red fibers (RRF) are present in over 90% of cases

Acronym

- [ ] MERRF: myoclonic epilepsy with ragged red fibers

MITOCHONDRIAL POLYMERASE GAMMA (POLG): PHENOTYPES

Progressive external ophthalmoplegia (PEO)

- [ ] Adult onset ptosis

Epilepsy: types

- [ ] Myoclonic epilepsy
- [ ] Focal motor or visual seizures
- [ ] Secondarily generalised seizures
- [ ] Refractory occipital lobe epilepsy (OLE)
- [ ] Status epilepticus (SE)
- [ ] Late-onset epileptic encephalopathy
- [ ] Epilepsia partialis continua (EPC)

SANDO

- [ ] Sensory Ataxia
- [ ] Neuropathy
- [ ] Dysarthria
- [ ] Ophthalmoplegia

Childhood-onset Alpers syndrome

- [ ] Intractable seizures
- [ ] Psychomotor regression
- [ ] Hepatopathy
- [ ] Lactic acidosis

Distal myopathy with cachexia

- [ ] Distal upper limb weakness
- [ ] Early ophthalmoplegia

Childhood-onset developmental syndrome

- [ ] Global developmental delay
- [ ] Hypotonia
- [ ] Faltering growth
- [ ] Epilepsy

SANO

- [ ] Sensory ataxia
- [ ] Neuropathy
- [ ] Ophthalmoparesis
- [ ] There is no dysarthria

Other phenotypes

- [ ] POLG ataxia (POG-A)
- [ ] Mitochondrial recessive ataxia syndrome (MIRAS)
- [ ] Spinocerebellar ataxia with epilepsy (SCAE)
- [ ] MERRF
- [ ] MELAS
- [ ] MNGIE-like phenotype

Acronyms

- [ ] MERRF: Myoclonic epilepsy with ragged red fibers
- [ ] MELAS: Mitochondrial encephalomyopathy, lactic acidosis, stroke-like episodes

Mitochondrial disorders management

MITOCHONDRIAL DISEASES: INVESTIGATIONS

Blood tests

- ☐ Lactate: especially after overnight fast
- ☐ Fasting glucose
- ☐ Creatinine kinase (CK)
- ☐ Calcium
- ☐ Alkaline phosphatase
- ☐ Urea and electrolyte
- ☐ Thyroid function tests (TFT)
- ☐ Acylcarnitine profiles: to exclude lipid disorders
- ☐ Fibroblast growth factor 21 (FGF21): this is a marker of mitochondrial disease
  - ○ It may reduce the need for muscle biopsy

Genetic tests

- ☐ Mitochondrial DNA (mtDNA) mutation screen
- ☐ Polymerase gamma (POLG) mutation screen: if mtDNA mutations are negative

Cardiorespiratory tests

- ☐ Electrocardiogram (ECG)
- ☐ Echocardiogram: if there are cardiac features
- ☐ Lying and standing forced vital capacity (FVC)

Urine analysis

- ☐ Dipstick: this gives an indication of renal disease
- ☐ Urinary organic and amino acids
- ☐ Urine mtDNA mutation screen

Cerebrospinal fluid (CSF)

- ☐ Protein: this is raised
- ☐ Lactate: this is raised: it is also raised following seizures and stroke

Electroencephalogram (EEG)

- ☐ Diffuse slowing: with encephalopathy
- ☐ Seizures

Brain imaging: indications

- ☐ Central nervous system signs
- ☐ Cognitive features
- ☐ Electroencephalogram (EEG) abnormalities

Muscle biopsy: histochemistry

- ☐ Gomori trichrome
- ☐ Succinate dehydrogenase (SDH)
- ☐ Cytochrome oxidase (COX): for ragged red fibers (RRF)

Muscle biopsy: other studies

- ☐ Respiratory chain studies
- ☐ Molecular genetic analysis of mitochondrial DNA
- ☐ Sequencing of mitochondrial genome (research)

Other investigations

- ☐ Electromyogram (EMG)

MITOCHONDRIAL DISEASES: SURVEILLANCE

Monitoring

- ☐ History and examination annually
- ☐ Electrocardiogram (ECG) annually
- ☐ Echocardiogram or cardiac magnetic resonance imaging (MRI): 3–5 yearly
- ☐ Fasting glucose annually
- ☐ Calcium every 1–2 years

Ophthalmology referral: indications

- ☐ Ptosis
- ☐ Optic atrophy
- ☐ Retinopathy
- ☐ Ophthalmoplegia

Other referrals

- ☐ Physiotherapy: for spasticity
- ☐ Chest physiotherapy: for respiratory features
- ☐ Speech therapy: for dysphagia

DOI: 10.1201/9781003221258-106

MITOCHONDRIAL DISEASES: SPECIFIC TREATMENTS

Metabolic treatments

- ☐ Ubiquinone (co-enzyme Q10) 100 mg tid
- ☐ L-carnitine
- ☐ Creatine monohydrate
- ☐ Alpha lipoic acid
- ☐ Vitamin C
- ☐ Vitamin K
- ☐ Folinic acid: for central folate deficiency in KSS
- ☐ Bicarbonate: for lactic acidosis
- ☐ Dichloroacetate: for lactic acidosis but it is neurotoxic
- ☐ Thiamine and riboflavin: for migraine

L-Arginine

- ☐ This reduces stroke-like episodes in MELAS
- ☐ It is given within 30 minutes of stroke
- ☐ It causes vasodilatation

Treatments of MNGIE

- ☐ Allogenic stem cell transplant
- ☐ Peritoneal dialysis

Other treatments

- ☐ Idebenone for LHON

Acronyms

- ☐ KSS: Kearn–Sayre syndrome
- ☐ MELAS: mitochondrial encephalomyopathy lactic acidosis and stroke-like episodes
- ☐ MERRF: myoclonic epilepsy with ragged red fibers
- ☐ LHON: Leber hereditary optic neuropathy

MITOCHONDRIAL DISEASES: SYMPTOMATIC TREATMENTS

Treatment of seizures

- ☐ Levetiracetam
- ☐ Lamotrigine
- ☐ Carbamazepine
- ☐ Clonazepam

Treatments of myoclonus in MERRF

- ☐ Piracetam
- ☐ Levetiracetam
- ☐ Clonazepam

Cardiac treatments

- ☐ Beta blockers: for cardiomegaly
- ☐ Angiotensin converting enzyme inhibitors (ACEI): for cardiomegaly
- ☐ Pacemakers: for conduction defects

Other treatments

- ☐ Exercise
- ☐ Parenteral nutrition
- ☐ Nocturnal respiratory support for myopathy
- ☐ Surgery: for ptosis and diplopia
- ☐ Hearing aids
- ☐ Cochlear implants

Drugs and activities to avoid

- ☐ Aminoglycosides: if there is a high risk of deafness such as A3243G MELAS mutation
- ☐ Valproate: it interferes with mitochondrial function
- ☐ Metformin: it can precipitate lactic acidosis
- ☐ Overexertion: to prevent rhabdomyolysis
- ☐ Dehydration: to prevent rhabdomyolysis

Acronyms

- ☐ MELAS: mitochondrial encephalomyopathy lactic acidosis and stroke-like episodes
- ☐ MERRF: myoclonic epilepsy with ragged red fibers

CHAPTER 18

Developmental disorders

Systemic developmental disorders

CEREBRAL PALSY (CP): CLINICAL FEATURES

Risk factor

- ☐ Maternal obesity

Types

- ☐ Spasticity (pyramidal): this accounts for 75% of cases
- ☐ Dyskinesia (extrapyramidal): athetoid, choreiform, and dystonic forms
- ☐ Ataxia
- ☐ Diplegia or quadriplegia
- ☐ Cerebellar
- ☐ Mixed

Visual features

- ☐ Strabismus
- ☐ Glaucoma
- ☐ Myopia

Neurological features

- ☐ Developmental delay
- ☐ Microcephaly
- ☐ Epilepsy
- ☐ Stroke
- ☐ Behavioural problems
- ☐ Cognitive impairment
- ☐ Irritability
- ☐ Fragmented sleep
- ☐ Congenital anomalies
- ☐ Hearing impairment

Feeding difficulties

- ☐ Swallowing problems
- ☐ Poor sucking
- ☐ Drooling
- ☐ Sandifer syndrome: dystonic dyspepsia due to reflux

Peripheral features

- ☐ Scissoring gait
- ☐ Persistent fisting
- ☐ Persistence of primitive reflexes
- ☐ Fidgeting and spontaneous movements in infants
- ☐ Toe walking
- ☐ Pain

Autonomic features

- ☐ Urinary incontinence
- ☐ Urinary urgency
- ☐ Constipation

Skeletal features

- ☐ Foot contractures
- ☐ Scoliosis

CEREBRAL PALSY (CP): MANAGEMENT

Neuroimaging

- ☐ Magnetic resonance imaging (MRI) is the preferred modality
- ☐ It is abnormal in >80% of cases

Electroencephalography (EEG)

- ☐ This is indicated for diagnosing epilepsy or epileptic syndromes
- ☐ It is not indicated for diagnosing aetiology of CP

Screening

- ☐ Learning disability
- ☐ Ophthalmologic impairments
- ☐ Hearing impairments
- ☐ Speech and language disorders
- ☐ Oromotor dysfunction
- ☐ Coagulopathies: this is a high risk for cerebral infarction in hemiplegic forms

Metabolic and genetic tests: indications

- ☐ Positive family history
- ☐ Episodic metabolic decompensation

Treatment of dystonia

- ☐ Baclofen
- ☐ Deep brain stimulation (DBS)
- ☐ Trihexyphenidyl is probably ineffective

Single level selective dorsal rhizotomy (SDR): for spasticity

- ☐ Laminectomy at the level of the conus medullaris
- ☐ This permanently reduces lower limb spasticity

Investigational treatments

- ☐ Stem cell therapy

DOI: 10.1201/9781003221258-108

AUTISM SPECTRUM DISORDERS (ASD): RISK FACTORS

PTEN gene mutation

- ☐ This is the main genetic risk factor
- ☐ It is part of the mTOR signaling pathway

Epilepsy

- ☐ 20% of people with autism have epilepsy
- ☐ There is possibly a shared aetiology
- ☐ The association peaks in early childhood and adolescence
- ☐ It usually manifests as infantile spasms, focal seizures, or Dravet syndrome

Other neurological risk factors

- ☐ Intellectual disability
- ☐ Tuberous sclerosis complex (TSC)
- ☐ Fragile X syndrome
- ☐ Catatonia
- ☐ Sturge–Weber syndrome

Other risk factors

- ☐ Low birth weight/prematurity
- ☐ Viral infections
- ☐ Antidepressant use in pregnancy
- ☐ Prenatal Valproate use

AUTISM SPECTRUM DISORDERS (ASD): CLINICAL FEATURES

Motor features

- ☐ Stereotypies
- ☐ Dyspraxia: this correlates with core autistic features
- ☐ Incoordination
- ☐ Abnormal saccades
- ☐ Gait disorders
- ☐ Tics

Cognitive features

- ☐ Impaired empathy (mind blindness): due to impaired theory of mind
- ☐ Systemising: the tendency to analyse inanimate systems
- ☐ Tendency for routines
- ☐ Repetitive behaviour
- ☐ Intellectual disability

Sleep-related features

- ☐ Difficulty falling asleep
- ☐ Prolonged night-time awakenings

Psychiatric features

- ☐ Aggression
- ☐ Anxiety
- ☐ Depression
- ☐ Attention deficit hyperactivity disorder (ADHD)
- ☐ Self-injurious behaviour
- ☐ Objectum sexuality: romantic attraction to inanimate objects

Gastrointestinal features

- ☐ Constipation
- ☐ Diarrhoea
- ☐ Food selectivity

Other features

- ☐ Visual and hearing impairments
- ☐ Epilepsy
- ☐ Hypermasculinised facial appearance

Differential diagnosis: childhood disintegrative disorder (CDD)

- ☐ This is late-onset regression
- ☐ The male prevalence is higher than in ASD
- ☐ There is more global and rapid regression
- ☐ Cognitive impairment is worse than in ASD
- ☐ There are more frequent seizures and psychosis
- ☐ There is a higher frequency of fear than in ASD
- ☐ The behaviours are more challenging than in ASD
- ☐ There is frequent loss of motor skills and continence: this is rare in ASD
- ☐ It has a worse prognosis than ASD

Intracranial developmental disorders

ARACHNOID CYSTS: FEATURES

Pathology

- ☐ They are congenital fluid-filled malformations

Genetic transmission of familial types

- ☐ X-linked dominant
- ☐ Autosomal recessive: on chromosome 6q
- ☐ De novo: in adults

Locations

- ☐ Sylvian
- ☐ Intraventricular
- ☐ Suprasellar
- ☐ Posterior fossa
- ☐ Spinal

Cognitive impairments

- ☐ Visuospatial
- ☐ Verbal attention
- ☐ Memory

Clinical features

- ☐ Macrocephaly in infants
- ☐ Headache
- ☐ Papilloedema: from raised intracranial pressure (ICP)
- ☐ Optic nerve compression
- ☐ Tinnitus
- ☐ Vertigo
- ☐ Weakness
- ☐ Hydrocephalus
- ☐ Scoliosis
- ☐ Visual loss
- ☐ Seizures
- ☐ Gait disturbance

Complications of cyst rupture

- ☐ Subdural haematoma (SDH)
- ☐ Subdural hygroma

Associated disorders

- ☐ Autosomal dominant polycystic kidney disease
- ☐ Cerebral aneurysms

Radiological differential diagnosis

- ☐ Cystic astrocytoma
- ☐ Cystic haemangioblastoma
- ☐ Hydatid cyst
- ☐ Abscesses
- ☐ Dermoid
- ☐ Dandy–Walker malformation
- ☐ Epidermoid: scalloped margins and bright on diffusion weighted imaging (DWI) and FLAIR sequences

ARACHNOID CYSTS: TREATMENT

Surgical indications

- ☐ Neural compression
- ☐ Hydrocephalus
- ☐ Refractory symptoms attributable to mass effect
- ☐ Large cysts
- ☐ Rupture
- ☐ Haemorrhage

Surgical treatments

- ☐ Endoscopic fenestration: this is the favoured option
- ☐ Microsurgical cyst excision
- ☐ Microsurgical cyst wall excision with fenestration
- ☐ Cysto-peritoneal shunting
- ☐ Stereotactic cysto-ventricular shunting
- ☐ Ventriculoperitoneal (VP) shunt
- ☐ Craniotomy
- ☐ Stereotactic aspiration

Complications of treatment

- ☐ Spasticity
- ☐ Hemiparesis
- ☐ Cerebrospinal fluid leak
- ☐ Hydrocephalus
- ☐ Subdural hygroma
- ☐ Postoperative cyst re-accumulation: this occurs in about 25% of cases

Precautions

- ☐ Participation in sports is not usually risky

DOI: 10.1201/9781003221258-109

DANDY–WALKER SYNDROME

Diagnostic features

- [ ] Large median posterior fossa cyst
- [ ] Abnormal cerebellar vermis
- [ ] Upwardly displaced tentorium
- [ ] Enlarged posterior fossa
- [ ] Antero-laterally displaced cerebellar hemispheres
- [ ] Normal brainstem
- [ ] 70–80% develop in the first year of life

Other cranial features

- [ ] Cataracts
- [ ] Intellectual disability
- [ ] Cleft palate

Systemic features

- [ ] Patent ductus arteriosus (PDA)
- [ ] Nephroblastoma
- [ ] Polycystic kidneys
- [ ] Visceral anomalies

Pettigrew syndrome (X-linked Dandy–Walker syndrome)

- [ ] Facial dysmorphism
- [ ] Intellectual disability
- [ ] Choreoathetosis

Radiological features

- [ ] Hydrocephalus
- [ ] Agenesis of the corpus callosum
- [ ] Occipital meningocele
- [ ] Aqueductal stenosis
- [ ] The tail sign: on foetal magnetic resonance imaging (MRI)

Treatment

- [ ] Ventriculoperitoneal (VP) shunt
- [ ] Cysto-peritoneal (CP) shunt
- [ ] Cysto-peritoneal and ventriculoperitoneal (CPVP) shunt
- [ ] Endoscopic third ventriculostomy (ETV)
- [ ] ETV with aqueductal stent placement
- [ ] ETV with fenestration of occluding membrane

AGENESIS OF THE CORPUS CALLOSUM: CLINICAL FEATURES

Anatomical associations

- [ ] Malformations of cortical development (MCD): especially grey matter heterotopia
- [ ] Absent or abnormal anterior commissure
- [ ] Absent or abnormal hippocampal commissure
- [ ] Abnormal ventricles
- [ ] Probst bundles: longitudinal callosal fascicles
- [ ] Inter-hemispheric cysts
- [ ] Inter-hemispheric lipomas

Abnormal systems

- [ ] Orbits
- [ ] Cerebellum
- [ ] Brainstem
- [ ] Olfactory system

Clinical associations

- [ ] Microcephaly
- [ ] Macrocephaly: less frequent than microcephaly
- [ ] Developmental delay
- [ ] Seizures
- [ ] Epicanthal folds
- [ ] Ocular hypertelorism
- [ ] Visual deficits
- [ ] Hearing impairment
- [ ] Congenital heart diseases
- [ ] Genitourinary abnormalities
- [ ] Isolated electroencephalogram (EEG) abnormalities

Spinal developmental disorders

CHIARI MALFORMATION: CLASSIFICATION

Classification of Chiari malformation

- ☐ Type 0: Mild herniation
- ☐ Type I: Tonsils 5mm below the foramen magnum
- ☐ Type II: Herniation of the vermis, the brainstem, and the fourth ventricle
- ☐ Type III: Occipital encephalocele
- ☐ Type IV: Cerebellar aplasia/hypoplasia

CHIARI MALFORMATION: CLINICAL FEATURES

Headaches: exacerbating manoeuvres

- ☐ Exertion
- ☐ Coughing
- ☐ Straining
- ☐ Head dependent position
- ☐ Neck extension

Lower brainstem and cerebellar features

- ☐ Dizziness
- ☐ Tinnitus
- ☐ Nystagmus
- ☐ Deafness
- ☐ Diplopia
- ☐ Dysphagia and dysarthria
- ☐ Vocal cord paralysis
- ☐ Tongue atrophy and fasciculations
- ☐ Absent gag reflex
- ☐ Trigeminal neuralgia
- ☐ Vertigo: positional or triggered by head movement

Features of raised intracranial pressure (ICP)

- ☐ Suboccipital headache
- ☐ Neck pain
- ☐ Visual obscurations
- ☐ Papilloedema
- ☐ Nausea and vomiting

Spinal cord features

- ☐ Acral sensory loss
- ☐ Spastic weakness
- ☐ Incontinence
- ☐ Impotence
- ☐ Syrinx features: suspended sensory loss and long tract signs

Sleep disorders

- ☐ Sleep disordered breathing
- ☐ Central sleep apnoea
- ☐ REM sleep behaviour disorder (RBD)

Other features

- ☐ Movement disorders: ataxia, tremor
- ☐ Memory difficulties
- ☐ Chronic fatigue
- ☐ Short neck
- ☐ Fasciculations
- ☐ Respiratory arrest at onset
- ☐ Postural tachycardia syndrome (POTS) with syncope
- ☐ Impaired activities of daily living

Clinical outcome measures

- ☐ Chicago Chiari Outcome Scale
- ☐ The Chiari Symptom Profile

DOI: 10.1201/9781003221258-110

SPINA BIFIDA: PATHOLOGY AND RISK FACTORS

Pathology

- ☐ Spina bifida is caused by a failure of fusion of the caudal neural tube
- ☐ Most cases are idiopathic

Types

- ☐ Spina bifida aperta: there is a visible external lesion
- ☐ Spina bifida occulta: there is no external lesion

Genetic risk factors

- ☐ Chromosomal abnormalities
- ☐ C677T Methyl tetrahydrofolate (MTHFR) gene mutation
- ☐ Family history of spina bifida or anencephaly
- ☐ Curranino syndrome

Maternal risk factors

- ☐ Folate deficiency in pregnancy
- ☐ Pre-gestational maternal diabetes mellitus
- ☐ Obese mothers
- ☐ Maternal gastric bypass surgery: this causes nutritional deficiency
- ☐ Maternal fever
- ☐ Valproate exposure
- ☐ Carbamazepine exposure

Possible risk factors

- ☐ Fumonisins (mycotoxins)
- ☐ Paternal exposure to Agent Orange
- ☐ Maternal exposure to pesticides

SPINA BIFIDA: CLINICAL FEATURES

Spinal cord features

- ☐ Paraparesis
- ☐ Urinary and faecal incontinence
- ☐ Lower limb deformities
- ☐ Sensory impairment
- ☐ Anal sphincter disturbance in severe cases

Skeletal abnormalities

- ☐ Kyphosis and scoliosis
- ☐ Long bone and feet deformities
- ☐ Hemivertebrae
- ☐ Defective ribs

Features of tethered cord

- ☐ Progressive spastic distal weakness
- ☐ Urinary symptoms
- ☐ Pain-localised or radicular

Local skin lesions

- ☐ Tuft of hair
- ☐ Nevus
- ☐ Dysplastic skin
- ☐ Angiomatous patches
- ☐ Lipoma
- ☐ Dermal sinus

Ocular abnormalities

- ☐ Anophthalmos
- ☐ Hypotelorism
- ☐ Microphthalmos
- ☐ Colobomata
- ☐ Lenticonus
- ☐ The optic nerves, retinal ganglion cells, and macula are preserved

Urogenital features

- ☐ Urinary tract reflux and hydronephrosis
- ☐ Genital anaesthesia
- ☐ Erectile dysfunction
- ☐ Cryptorchidism
- ☐ Bladder extrophy
- ☐ Hypospadias
- ☐ Unilateral renal agenesis
- ☐ Ureteropelvic junction obstruction
- ☐ Multicystic dysplastic kidney
- ☐ Horseshoe kidney

Other features

- ☐ Chiari malformation type II
- ☐ Hydrocephalus in 80% of cases
- ☐ Meningomyelocele
- ☐ Latex allergy

SPINA BIFIDA: COMPLICATIONS AND MANAGEMENT

Complications

- ☐ Pressure sores
- ☐ Scoliosis
- ☐ Neuropathic pain
- ☐ Epilepsy
- ☐ Urinary tract infections
- ☐ Spasticity
- ☐ Learning disability
- ☐ Increased risk-taking behaviours
- ☐ Chronic idiopathic headache
- ☐ Cerebrospinal fluid (CSF) leak
- ☐ Meningitis

Magnetic resonance imaging (MRI): features

- ☐ Neural abnormalities
- ☐ Hydrocephalus
- ☐ Chiari malformation

Screening for spina bifida

- ☐ Prenatal ultrasound screening: at 12, 22 and 32 weeks
- ☐ Maternal α fetoprotein (AFP) screening

Treatment

- ☐ Shunting for hydrocephalus
- ☐ Tethered cord release
- ☐ Spinal fusion for scoliosis

SYRINGOMYELIA

Classification

- ☐ Type I: with obstruction of foramen magnum
- ☐ Type II: no foramen magnum obstruction or idiopathic
- ☐ Type III: with other spinal cord disorders: tumours, trauma, arachnoiditis, myelomalacia
- ☐ Type IV: pure hydromyelia

Causes

- ☐ Chiari malformation
- ☐ Spinal cord tumours
- ☐ Trauma
- ☐ Arachnoiditis: post trauma or infection
- ☐ Idiopathic

Clinical features

- ☐ Urinary symptoms
- ☐ Thoracic dysaesthesia
- ☐ Spinal pain
- ☐ Gait difficulty
- ☐ Radicular pain
- ☐ Myelopathic features
- ☐ Horner's syndrome: unilateral or alternating
- ☐ Alternating oculosympathetic spasm
- ☐ Upper limb weakness and atrophy
- ☐ Upper limb pain and temperature loss
- ☐ Dystonia

Differential diagnosis

- ☐ Lepromatous leprosy
- ☐ Tangier disease
- ☐ Facial onset sensory and motor neuronopathy (FOSMN)

Treatment

- ☐ Conservative measures: preferred over surgery
- ☐ Laminectomy
- ☐ Lysis of adhesions
- ☐ Cranio-cervical decompression

CHAPTER 19

Allied neurological disorders

Neuro-ophthalmology

PTOSIS

Central neurological causes

- [ ] Oculomotor nerve palsy
- [ ] Horner's syndrome

Peripheral neurological causes

- [ ] Myasthenia gravis (MG)
- [ ] Myotonic dystrophy
- [ ] Limb girdle muscular dystrophy 1C (LGMD 1C)
- [ ] Oculopharyngeal muscular dystrophy (OPMD)
- [ ] Progressive external ophthalmoplegia (PEO)
- [ ] Localised myopathy of the levator palpabrae superioris

Congenital causes

- [ ] Isolated
- [ ] Congenital myasthenia
- [ ] Congenital Horner's syndrome
- [ ] Congenital oculomotor nerve palsy
- [ ] Anomalous synkinesis
- [ ] Blepharophimosis
- [ ] Anophthalmos (phthisis bulbi)

Structural causes

- [ ] Trauma
- [ ] Levator dehiscence
- [ ] Eyelid/orbital tumours
- [ ] Eyelid swelling
- [ ] Fibrosis of the extraocular muscles
- [ ] Sagging eyebrow
- [ ] Post-surgery

Medical conditions

- [ ] Envenomation
- [ ] Grave's disease
- [ ] Obstructive sleep apnoea
- [ ] Functional

Enhanced ptosis

- [ ] This is worsening of contralateral ptosis when the ipsilateral eyelid is manually held open
- [ ] It is typically caused by myasthenia gravis (MG)
- [ ] It may also be caused by mitochondrial diseases, Miller Fisher syndrome (MFS), and LEMS

Differential diagnosis of ptosis

- [ ] Blepharospasm
- [ ] Hemifacial spasm
- [ ] Apraxia of eyelid opening

Acronym

- [ ] LEMS: Lambert–Eaton myasthenic syndrome

ROSS SYNDROME

Clinical features

- [ ] Segmental anhidrosis
- [ ] Tonic pupils
- [ ] Hyporeflexia
- [ ] Facial flushing: from compensatory hyperhidrosis

Pathology

- [ ] It is a disorder of thermoregulation
- [ ] There is impaired heat production and heat dissipation
- [ ] This is due to loss of sweating
- [ ] There is also loss of cutaneous blood flow regulation
- [ ] There is degeneration of cholinergic sudomotor and cutaneous sensory nerves

Associations

- [ ] Horner's syndrome
- [ ] Cytomegalovirus (CMV)
- [ ] Sjogren's syndrome

Differential diagnosis

- [ ] Holmes Adie pupil: this shows no anhidrosis
- [ ] Harlequin syndrome: this has normal pupils

Treatment

- [ ] Botulinum toxin for hyperhidrosis

DOI: 10.1201/9781003221258-112

ARGYLL ROBERTSON PUPIL

Clinical features

- ☐ Small irregular pupil
- ☐ Poor reaction to light
- ☐ Brisk reaction to accommodation: light-near dissociation
- ☐ Iris atrophy

Causes

- ☐ Neurosyphilis: tabes dorsalis
- ☐ Dorsal midbrain lesions
- ☐ Neurosarcoidosis
- ☐ Ciliary nerve lymphoma
- ☐ Lymphocytic meningoradiculitis: Banwarth's syndrome

Differential diagnosis

- ☐ Holmes Adie syndrome (HAS)
- ☐ Spinocerebellar ataxia type 1 (SCA1)
- ☐ Oculomotor nerve regeneration
- ☐ Optic nerve diseases

HARLEQUIN SYNDROME

Clinical features

- ☐ Unilateral hypohidrosis
- ☐ Contralateral facial flushing and sweating on exposure to heat or exercise
- ☐ Abnormal pupillary hypersensitivity to Pilocarpine constriction
- ☐ Abnormal pupillary hypersensitivity to Phenylephrine dilatation

Possible associated features

- ☐ Horner's syndrome
- ☐ Ross syndrome

Pathology

- ☐ Dysfunction of the upper thoracic sympathetic chain

Neurological causes

- ☐ Idiopathic
- ☐ Congenital
- ☐ Brainstem stroke
- ☐ Carotid artery dissection
- ☐ Guillain–Barre syndrome (GBS)
- ☐ Syringomyelia
- ☐ Multiple sclerosis (MS)
- ☐ Autoimmune ganglionopathy
- ☐ Diabetic peripheral neuropathy

Iatrogenic causes

- ☐ Internal jugular vein catheterisation
- ☐ Mediastinal surgery
- ☐ Thyroidectomy
- ☐ Trans-sphenoidal pituitary surgery
- ☐ Epidural anaesthesia
- ☐ Thoracic paravertebral block

Neoplastic causes

- ☐ Mediastinal tumours
- ☐ Superior mediastinal neurinoma
- ☐ Spinal invasion of apical lung tumours

Vascular causes

- ☐ Elongated inferior thyroid artery
- ☐ Anterior radicular artery occlusion

Other causes

- ☐ Pure autonomic failure (Bradbury-Eggleston syndrome)
- ☐ Toxic goitre
- ☐ Upper thoracic trauma

Treatment

- ☐ Botulinum toxin
- ☐ Sympathectomy

HORNER'S SYNDROME

Central causes

- ☐ Idiopathic: this accounts for 40% of cases
- ☐ Cervical artery dissection (painful Horner's)
- ☐ Lateral medullary syndrome
- ☐ Tumours
- ☐ Haemorrhage
- ☐ Demyelination

Preganglionic causes

- ☐ Iatrogenic
- ☐ Apical lung tumours
- ☐ Thyroid cancer
- ☐ Mediastinal tumours

Postganglionic causes

- ☐ Iatrogenic
- ☐ Trauma
- ☐ Carotid dissection
- ☐ Carotid aneurysm
- ☐ Carotid-cavernous fistula
- ☐ Cavernous sinus thrombophlebitis
- ☐ Tolosa Hunt syndrome
- ☐ Skull base tumours
- ☐ Cervical syringomyelia
- ☐ Lyme neuroborreliosis

Clinical features: anhidrosis

- ☐ This is impaired facial sweating
- ☐ It is hemifacial if the lesion is proximal to the carotid bifurcation
- ☐ It involves the medial forehead if the lesion is distal to the carotid bifurcation
- ☐ There is no anhidrosis if the lesion is central

Clinical features: others

- ☐ Ptosis
- ☐ Miosis
- ☐ Anisocoria: this is worse in the dark
- ☐ Transient dilated conjunctival blood vessels
- ☐ Harlequin syndrome

Assessments

- ☐ Failure of the pupil to dilate with 4% cocaine
- ☐ Failure to dilate with 1% Hydroxyamphetamine: with postganglionic lesions

REVERSE HORNER'S SYNDROME

Pathogenesis

- ☐ This results from cervical sympathetic (Stellar) plexus dysfunction
- ☐ Its features are opposite of Horner's syndrome
- ☐ It may eventually result in Horner's syndrome

Iatrogenic causes

- ☐ Thoracostomy
- ☐ Thoracoplasty
- ☐ Neck surgery
- ☐ Thoracic sympathectomy
- ☐ Brachial plexus block
- ☐ Epidural anaesthesia
- ☐ Mandible tumour surgery
- ☐ Carotid injuries
- ☐ Jugular vein cannulation
- ☐ Parotidectomy

Other causes

- ☐ Trauma
- ☐ Cervical rib
- ☐ Tuberculosis
- ☐ Atypical pneumonia
- ☐ Thoracic aneurysms
- ☐ Rib and oesophageal tumours

Clinical features

- ☐ Mydriasis
- ☐ Wide palpebral fissures
- ☐ Exophthalmos
- ☐ Increased facial sweating
- ☐ Pale cold face
- ☐ Upper limb hyperhidrosis
- ☐ Hemifacial atrophy
- ☐ Eyelid retraction
- ☐ Headache
- ☐ Tremor

Treatment

- ☐ Upper thoracic sympathectomy

Synonym

- ☐ Pourfour du petit syndrome

Neurotology

DIZZINESS: CAUSES

Vestibular

- ☐ Benign paroxysmal positional vertigo (BPPV)
- ☐ Vestibular neuritis
- ☐ Meniere's disease
- ☐ Vestibular paroxysmia
- ☐ Bilateral vestibulopathy
- ☐ Motion sickness
- ☐ Mal de debarquement syndrome (MDDS)
- ☐ Otosclerosis

Neurological

- ☐ Migraine associated
- ☐ Stroke
- ☐ Posterior circulation TIA
- ☐ Cerebellar ataxia
- ☐ Multiple sclerosis (MS)
- ☐ Tumours
- ☐ Foramen magnum abnormalities

Cardiovascular

- ☐ Orthostatic hypotension
- ☐ Vasovagal
- ☐ Cardiogenic
- ☐ Carotid sinus syndrome
- ☐ Arrhythmias

Medical

- ☐ Anaemia
- ☐ Post-traumatic syndrome
- ☐ Hyperviscosity
- ☐ Infection
- ☐ Hypoglycaemia
- ☐ Drug intoxication
- ☐ Paget's disease

Functional

- ☐ Anxiety
- ☐ Hyperventilation
- ☐ Psychogenic

PERSISTENT POSTURAL PERCEPTUAL DIZZINESS (PPPD)

Pathology and epidemiology

- ☐ This is a chronic vestibular dysfunction
- ☐ It results from impaired multi-system sensory processing
- ☐ There is grey matter volume loss on MRI-voxel based morphometry
- ☐ It is more frequent in middle age and in women

Core features

- ☐ Dizziness
- ☐ Non-spinning vertigo
- ☐ Unsteadiness
- ☐ Visual hypersensitivity
- ☐ Fluctuating symptoms

Associated features

- ☐ Functional gait disorder
- ☐ Anxiety and fear of falling
- ☐ Avoidance behaviour
- ☐ Sleep disorders
- ☐ Hypercholesterolemia
- ☐ Migraine
- ☐ Carbohydrate metabolism disorders

Provoking factors and triggers

- ☐ Upright posture
- ☐ Visual stimuli
- ☐ Head or body movements
- ☐ Sleep deprivation
- ☐ Benign paroxysmal positional vertigo (BPPV)
- ☐ Vestibular neuronitis
- ☐ Vestibular migraine
- ☐ Traumatic brain injury (TBI)
- ☐ Whiplash injury
- ☐ Generalised anxiety and panic attacks
- ☐ Dysrhythmias
- ☐ Drug reactions

Diagnostic criteria

- ☐ Symptoms are present for most days and for at least three months
- ☐ Symptoms are worsened by upright posture and motion
- ☐ Symptoms cause significant distress and dysfunction
- ☐ There are no alternative causes

Treatment

- ☐ Vestibular rehabilitation
- ☐ Selective serotonin reuptake inhibitors (SSRI)
- ☐ Serotonin norepinephrine reuptake inhibitors (SNRI)
- ☐ Cognitive behaviour therapy (CBT)

DOI: 10.1201/9781003221258-113

Synonyms

- [ ] Phobic postural vertigo
- [ ] Space-motion discomfort
- [ ] Visual vertigo
- [ ] Chronic subjective dizziness

VERTIGO: MEDICAL CAUSES

Vestibular causes

- [ ] Meniere's disease: the episodes last 20 minutes to hours
- [ ] Benign paroxysmal peripheral vertigo (BPPV)
- [ ] Perilymph fistula
- [ ] Superior canal dehiscence
- [ ] Autoimmune inner ear disease
- [ ] Otosclerosis
- [ ] Vestibular paroxysmia (VP)

Neurological causes

- [ ] Vestibular migraine: the episodes last minutes to days
- [ ] Vertebrobasilar transient ischaemic attacks (TIAs): episodes last <1 hour
- [ ] Brainstem tumours
- [ ] Familial benign recurrent vertigo: related to migraine
- [ ] Episodic ataxia type 2 (EA2)
- [ ] Colloid cyst of the third ventricle

Systemic causes

- [ ] Orthostatic hypotension: the episodes last seconds to a few minutes
- [ ] Cardiac arrhythmias
- [ ] Takayasu arteritis
- [ ] Panic attacks: the episodes last minutes
- [ ] Drugs

POSTERIOR CANAL BPPV

Causes

- [ ] Idiopathic
- [ ] Traumatic brain injury (TBI)
- [ ] Labyrinthitis
- [ ] Meniere's disease

Clinical features

- [ ] Rotational vertigo
- [ ] Latency
- [ ] Adaptation
- [ ] Reversibility
- [ ] Fatigability

Risk factors

- [ ] Low vitamin D levels
- [ ] Dementia
- [ ] Fractures
- [ ] Ischaemic stroke

Co-morbidities

- [ ] Migraine
- [ ] Anxiety disorders
- [ ] Osteoporosis
- [ ] High serum uric acid level
- [ ] Menopause
- [ ] Hypertension
- [ ] Diabetes
- [ ] Depression

Provoking tests

- [ ] Hallpike test
- [ ] Supine roll provoking test: if Hallpike test is negative:
  - This tests for horizontal (lateral) canal BPPV

Evidenced treatments

- [ ] Particle repositioning manoeuvre (PRM)
- [ ] Semont manoeuvre
- [ ] Vitamin D and calcium supplementation

Insufficient-evidenced treatments

- [ ] Brandt-Daroff exercises
- [ ] Habituation exercises
- [ ] Self-administered particle repositioning manoeuvres (PRM)
- [ ] Self-administered Semont manoeuvre
- [ ] Surgical fenestration and occlusion of posterior canal
- [ ] Singular neurectomy

Non-evidenced treatments

- [ ] Mastoid vibration during PRM
- [ ] Restriction after PRM

Acronym

- [ ] BPPV: benign paroxysmal positional vertigo

HORIZONTAL CANAL BPPV

Demographic features

- [ ] This is the second most frequent cause of BPPV after posterior canal BPPV
- [ ] It accounts for about 20% of all BPPV
- [ ] Most cases are idiopathic

Secondary causes

- [ ] Trauma
- [ ] Surgery
- [ ] Bed rest
- [ ] Viral infections
- [ ] Canal switch during particle repositioning manoeuvre (PRM)

Diagnostic manoeuvres

- [ ] Head turn while supine: this changes the direction of nystagmus
- [ ] Supine head roll (Pagnini-McClure) manoeuvre
- [ ] Lampert (barbeque roll) manoeuvre
- [ ] Gufoni manoeuvre

Treatment: Vannucchi-Asprella (Liberatory) manoeuvre

- [ ] The patient is positioned supine with head up at 30°
- [ ] The head is then turned 30° to the affected side for 5 minutes
- [ ] It is then rapidly turned 180° to the other side for 5 minutes
- [ ] The patient then avoids lying down and shaking the head for 48 hours

Acronym

- [ ] BPPV: benign paroxysmal positional vertigo

TINNITUS: CAUSES

Neurological causes

- [ ] Head injury
- [ ] Whiplash
- [ ] Multiple sclerosis (MS)
- [ ] Vestibular schwannoma
- [ ] Cerebellopontine angle tumours
- [ ] Palatal myoclonus
- [ ] Lyme disease
- [ ] Meningitis
- [ ] Syphilis
- [ ] Idiopathic stapedial muscle spasm

Otological causes

- [ ] Noise-induced hearing loss
- [ ] Presbyacusis
- [ ] Otosclerosis
- [ ] Otitis
- [ ] Impacted cerumen
- [ ] Sudden deafness
- [ ] Meniere's disease
- [ ] Temporomandibular joint (TMJ) dysfunction
- [ ] Patulous Eustachian tube
- [ ] Vascular compression of the auditory nerve: this presents with typewriter tinnitus

Systemic causes

- [ ] Thyroid disorders
- [ ] Hyperlipidemia
- [ ] Vitamin B12 deficiency
- [ ] Anaemia
- [ ] Zinc deficiency
- [ ] Depression
- [ ] Anxiety
- [ ] Fibromyalgia
- [ ] Drugs

PULSATILE TINNITUS: CAUSES

Vascular fistulae

- [ ] Dural arteriovenous fistula (dAVF)
- [ ] Carotid-cavernous fistula
- [ ] Carotid-jugular fistula
- [ ] Superficial temporal artery arteriovenous fistula

Other vascular causes

- [ ] Cervical artery dissection
- [ ] Carotid atherosclerosis/stenosis
- [ ] Carotid fibromuscular dysplasia
- [ ] Arterial bruits: worse at night
- [ ] Venous hums: especially with hypertension
- [ ] Subclavian artery occlusion
- [ ] Arteriovenous shunts: after head injury or surgery
- [ ] Intracranial hypertension

Neoplastic causes

- [ ] Vascular tumours
- [ ] Glomus tumour

DOWNBEAT NYSTAGMUS

Classification

- ☐ Idiopathic
- ☐ Secondary

Idiopathic: types

- ☐ Pure
- ☐ Cerebellar
- ☐ Syndromic: with vestibulopathy, polyneuropathy, or ataxia

Secondary: causes

- ☐ Multiple system atrophy (MSA)
- ☐ Spinocerebellar ataxia (SCA)
- ☐ Sporadic adult onset ataxia
- ☐ Cerebellar ischaemia
- ☐ Posterior fossa vascular lesions
- ☐ Cranio-cervical abnormalities
- ☐ Vestibulo-cerebellar lesions
- ☐ Drug toxicity
- ☐ Episodic ataxia type 2 (EA2)

Clinical features

- ☐ It is poorly suppressed by visual fixation
- ☐ It may be worsened by head hanging position
- ☐ It shows a variable response to convergence: increased, reduced, or inverted
- ☐ It may be evoked by looking down and outwards

Functional magnetic resonance imaging (MRI)

- ☐ This shows focal vermal and lateral cerebellar atrophy in idiopathic cases

Treatment

- ☐ Clonazepam
- ☐ Baclofen
- ☐ Gabapentin
- ☐ 4-aminopyridine (4-AP)
- ☐ 3, 4-diaminopyridine (3,4 DAP)

Psychiatry

OTHELLO SYNDROME

Clinical features

- Delusion of jealousy or infidelity (delusional jealousy)
- Verbal hostility
- Homicidal acts

Neurodegenerative causes

- Dementia with Lewy bodies (DLB)
- Parkinson's disease (PD)
- Alzheimer's disease (AD)
- Behavioural variant frontotemporal dementia (bvFTD)

Focal cerebral causes

- Stroke
- Meningioma
- Intracranial haemorrhage
- Encephalomalacia
- Subdural haematoma (SDH)

Psychiatric causes

- Mood disorders
- Psychosis
- Delusional disorders

Drug-induced

- Alcohol
- Methamphetamine
- Valproate
- Dopamine agonists
- Amantadine
- Zonisamide

CAPGRAS SYNDROME: CLINICAL FEATURES

Pathology

- This is the delusion that a close person has been replaced by an impostor
- It results from impairment of the emotional and autonomic response to familiar faces
- It is caused by disconnection of brain areas
- It may be associated with other delusions
- The subject may offer justifications for the delusion

Disconnected areas

- The right temporal fusiform face recognition area
- The limbic system
- The right frontal cortex

People frequently presumed to be replaced

- Family member
- Close partner
- Care professional
- Friend

Variations of affected replaced people or places

- Strangers
- Multiple people
- The subject
- The subject's mirror image
- Non-humans, e.g. pets
- Inanimate objects

Associated hallucinations

- Somatosensory
- Olfactory
- Tactile

Synonyms

- Delusion de sosies
- Illusion of doubles

DOI: 10.1201/9781003221258-114

CAPGRAS SYNDROME: CAUSES

Psychoses

- ☐ Schizophreniform psychoses
- ☐ Major depression
- ☐ Schizophrenia
- ☐ Delusional disorders
- ☐ Bipolar disorder
- ☐ Schizoaffective disorders

Neurodegenerative diseases

- ☐ Dementia with Lewy bodies (DLB): most common
- ☐ Alzheimer's disease (AD)
- ☐ Frontotemporal dementia (FTD)
- ☐ Parkinson's disease (PD)

Neurological infections

- ☐ Neurosyphilis
- ☐ HIV infection

Other neurological causes

- ☐ Epilepsy
- ☐ Multiple sclerosis (MS)
- ☐ Stroke
- ☐ Watershed infarction
- ☐ Limbic encephalitis
- ☐ Migraine
- ☐ Head injury
- ☐ Tuberous sclerosis complex (TSC)

Toxic causes

- ☐ Methamphetamine
- ☐ Lithium
- ☐ Ketamine
- ☐ Morphine
- ☐ Diazepam

Metabolic causes

- ☐ Hypothyroidism
- ☐ Homocystinuria
- ☐ Critical illness

Other causes

- ☐ Electroconvulsive therapy (ECT)
- ☐ Pre-eclampsia
- ☐ Urinary tract infection

Synonyms

- ☐ Delusion de sosies
- ☐ Illusion of doubles

ATTENTION DEFICIT HYPERACTIVITY DISORDER (ADHD): CLINICAL FEATURES

Epidemiology

- ☐ ADHD occurs in 3–10% of children
- ☐ Childhood ADHD persists into adulthood in 10–60% of cases
- ☐ ADHD occurs in 4.5% of adults

Core clinical features

- ☐ Hyperactivity: this is less severe in adults
- ☐ Inattention: this is more evident in females
- ☐ Impulsivity
- ☐ Mood lability
- ☐ Temper
- ☐ Disorganisation
- ☐ Stress sensitivity: low frustration tolerance

Subtypes

- ☐ Predominantly inattentive
- ☐ Predominantly hyperactive-impulsive
- ☐ Combined

Manifestations

- ☐ Difficulty starting tasks
- ☐ Poor attention to details
- ☐ Impaired self-organisation
- ☐ Difficulty prioritising tasks
- ☐ Poor persistence in tasks requiring sustained mental effort
- ☐ Chaotic lifestyle
- ☐ Impaired academic performance
- ☐ Poor employment history
- ☐ Impaired relationships
- ☐ Impaired quality of life
- ☐ Impaired driving safety
- ☐ Accident-proneness
- ☐ Suicide risk

Adult ADHD rating scales

- ☐ Copeland Symptom Checklist for Adult ADHD
- ☐ Wender Utah Rating Scale
- ☐ Brown Adult ADHD Scale
- ☐ Pilot Adult ADHD Self-Report Scale (ASRS)

ATTENTION DEFICIT HYPERACTIVITY DISORDER (ADHD): RISK FACTORS AND COMORBIDITIES

Acquired risk factors

- [ ] Maternal smoking
- [ ] Maternal alcohol
- [ ] Low birth weight
- [ ] Prenatal brain injury

Genetic risk factors

- [ ] BAIAP2: brain-specific angiogenesis inhibitor 1-associated protein 2
- [ ] SLC6A3: dopamine transporter
- [ ] D4 dopamine receptor gene (DRD4 7) mutation

Psychiatric co-morbidities

- [ ] Anxiety
- [ ] Depression
- [ ] Bipolar disorder
- [ ] Substance use disorder
- [ ] Personality disorder
- [ ] Binge eating

Cognitive co-morbidities

- [ ] Poor short-term memory
- [ ] Executive dysfunction
- [ ] Impaired verbal learning

Neurological co-morbidities

- [ ] Epilepsy
- [ ] Hearing impairment
- [ ] Head injury
- [ ] Learning disability
- [ ] Neurofibromatosis
- [ ] Foetal alcohol syndrome
- [ ] Intellectual deficiency
- [ ] Tourette syndrome (TS)
- [ ] Restless legs syndrome (RLS)
- [ ] Cataplexy
- [ ] Disturbed sleep
- [ ] Insomnia

Medical co-morbidities

- [ ] Hyperthyroidism
- [ ] Hypothyroidism
- [ ] Sleep apnoea

Neurosurgery

POST-CONCUSSION SYNDROME (PCS)

Definitions related to concussion

- [ ] Concussion is acute trauma-induced altered mental function
- [ ] Concussion usually follows mild to moderate head injury
- [ ] Concussion symptoms usually last less than 24 hours
- [ ] Post-concussion syndrome is when symptoms persist for more than 3 months
- [ ] Post traumatic encephalopathy is when the symptoms become permanent

Risk factors

- [ ] Negative perceptions of mild traumatic brain injury
- [ ] Stress
- [ ] Anxiety
- [ ] Depression
- [ ] All-or-nothing behaviour

General features

- [ ] Headache
- [ ] Dizziness
- [ ] Nausea
- [ ] Irritability
- [ ] Restlessness

Neuropsychiatric features

- [ ] Blurred vision
- [ ] Diplopia
- [ ] Photophobia
- [ ] Amnesia
- [ ] Impaired attention and judgment
- [ ] Possible future risk of dementia
- [ ] Frustration
- [ ] Aggression
- [ ] Anxiety and depression

Other features

- [ ] Tinnitus
- [ ] Fatigue
- [ ] Slurred speech
- [ ] Noise sensitivity
- [ ] Sleep disturbance

Risk factors for progression

- [ ] Patient's positive perception of outcome
- [ ] Older age at injury
- [ ] Premorbid cerebral or physical disability
- [ ] Post-injury low self-esteem and stress

Treatment

- [ ] Cognitive behaviour therapy (CBT)
- [ ] Selective serotonin reuptake inhibitors (SSRIs): for depression
- [ ] Cholinesterase inhibitors: for memory and attention problems
- [ ] Methylphenidate: for mood and aggression
- [ ] Trazodone: for sleep disturbance
- [ ] Amantadine or Modafinil: for fatigue

DOI: 10.1201/9781003221258-115

NORMAL PRESSURE HYDROCEPHALUS (NPH): RISK FACTORS

Acquired risk factors

- ☐ Compensated congenital hydrocephalus
- ☐ Hypertension
- ☐ Hyperlipidemia
- ☐ Diabetes
- ☐ Obesity
- ☐ Psychosocial factors
- ☐ Hypertension
- ☐ Physical inactivity
- ☐ Cerebrovascular disease
- ☐ Peripheral vascular disease

Genetic risk factors

- ☐ ETINPH gene mutation: on chromosome 19q
  - ○ This causes familial NPH with familial essential tremor
- ☐ SFMBT1 gene mutation: on chromosome 3p
- ☐ Apolipoprotein E (ApoE) e3 allele on chromosome 19
- ☐ CFAP43 gene: encodes cilia- and flagella-associated protein
- ☐ Familial aggregation in some cases: probably autosomal dominant

NORMAL PRESSURE HYDROCEPHALUS (NPH): CLINICAL FEATURES

Onset features

- ☐ NPH starts in adulthood: after the age of 40 years
- ☐ It usually starts in the sixth to eighth decades

Diagnostic (Hakim) triad

- ☐ Gait impairment
- ☐ Urinary incontinence
- ☐ Dementia

Cognitive features

- ☐ Frontal subcortical impairment
- ☐ Inattention
- ☐ Executive dysfunction
- ☐ There is no agnosia, apraxia, or aphasia

Gait disturbance: types

- ☐ Apraxic
- ☐ Bradykinetic
- ☐ Magnetic: glue footed

Gait features

- ☐ Slow with reduced gait velocity
- ☐ Broad-based
- ☐ Short shuffling steps
- ☐ Reduced knee extension
- ☐ Reduced step height

Posture features

- ☐ Erect trunk
- ☐ Feet rotated outward
- ☐ Normal arm swing
- ☐ Difficulty turning on the longitudinal axis of the body

Urinary impairment

- ☐ There is urge incontinence
- ☐ This results from bladder hyperactivity

Associated features

- ☐ Falls
- ☐ Difficulty tandem walking
- ☐ Difficulty with stairs and slopes
- ☐ Lack of response to external cues
- ☐ The gait impairment may be intermittent

Co-morbid conditions

- ☐ Depression
- ☐ Apathy
- ☐ Alzheimer's disease (AD): in about 20% of shunt-treated cases
- ☐ Movement disorders: usually Parkinsonism
- ☐ Frontotemporal dementia (FTD)

NORMAL PRESSURE HYDROCEPHALUS (NPH): MRI FEATURES

MRI measurements

☐ Evans' index ≥0.3: this is the ratio of the width of the lateral ventricles to the width of the inner skull
☐ Callosal angle >40 degrees
☐ Mamillopontine distance <1cm

Ventricular features

☐ Temporal horn enlargement
☐ Convex third ventricle
☐ Thin, elevated corpus callosum
☐ Trans-ependymal flow
☐ Accentuated flow void in the Sylvian aqueduct
☐ Periventricular signal changes
☐ Periventricular oedema

Cortical features

☐ Flattening of the sulci
☐ High convexity tightness: this predicts response to shunting
☐ The choroidal-hippocampal fissures are normal or mildly abnormal
    ○ They are markedly abnormal in Alzheimer's disease (AD)

Pain management

COMPLEX REGIONAL PAIN SYNDROME (CRPS): TRIGGERS

Trauma

- ☐ Fractures: especially of the wrist
- ☐ Sprains
- ☐ Surgery
- ☐ Spinal cord injury
- ☐ Brachial plexus injury
- ☐ Brain injury

Neurological

- ☐ Multiple sclerosis (MS)
- ☐ Stroke
- ☐ Space occupying lesions

Medical

- ☐ Myocardial infarction (MI)
- ☐ Cardiac surgery
- ☐ Herpes zoster infection
- ☐ Migraine
- ☐ Asthma

Infective

- ☐ Parvovirus B19
- ☐ Campylobacter jejuni
- ☐ Lyme disease
- ☐ Rubella
- ☐ Hepatitis B virus (HBV)

Drugs

- ☐ Phenobarbitone
- ☐ Isoniazid (INH)
- ☐ Angiotensin converting enzyme inhibitors (ACEI): administered at the time of trauma

Other possible triggers

- ☐ Possible genetic predisposition
- ☐ Immobilisation
- ☐ Immunisation
- ☐ Electric shock
- ☐ Motor neurone disease (MND)
- ☐ Cancer
- ☐ Autoimmune diseases

COMPLEX REGIONAL PAIN SYNDROME (CRPS): CLINICAL FEATURES

Pain features

- ☐ Acutely painful, red, and swollen limb
- ☐ Allodynia
- ☐ Hyperpathia
- ☐ Proximal but not distal spread of symptoms

Motor features

- ☐ Muscle wasting and weakness
- ☐ Impaired motor control
- ☐ The limb may feel alien

Movement disorders

- ☐ Dystonia
- ☐ Myoclonus
- ☐ Tremor

Autonomic features

- ☐ Abnormal sweating
- ☐ Sphincter disturbance
- ☐ Skin changes
- ☐ Nail and hair changes

Other features

- ☐ Stiff limb
- ☐ Contractures
- ☐ Osteoporosis
- ☐ Perceptual disturbances
- ☐ 15% are uncontrolled after 5 years

Co-morbidities

- ☐ Migraine: this is 3.6 times more likely in CRPS
- ☐ Osteoporosis
- ☐ Asthma
- ☐ Pre-syncope and syncope: in 40% of cases

DOI: 10.1201/9781003221258-116

FACIAL PAIN: TYPICAL CAUSES

Ocular causes

- ☐ Optic neuritis
- ☐ Acute glaucoma
- ☐ Cavernous sinus lesions
- ☐ Ocular myositis
- ☐ Orbital inflammation/infection/deposits
- ☐ Tolosa Hunt syndrome (THS)

Facial nerve related

- ☐ Bell's palsy
- ☐ Ramsay Hunt syndrome (post herpetic neuralgia)

Facial neuralgias

- ☐ Trigeminal
- ☐ Glossopharyngeal
- ☐ Nervus intermedius (geniculate)
- ☐ Nasociliary: previously Charlin's neuralgia
- ☐ Sphenopalatine (Sluder's neuralgia)
- ☐ Supraorbital

Primary headaches

- ☐ Migraine: especially in the V2 facial nerve distribution
- ☐ Persistent idiopathic facial pain (PIFP)
- ☐ Idiopathic stabbing headache
- ☐ Cluster headache
- ☐ Paroxysmal hemicranias
- ☐ SUNCT

Vascular causes

- ☐ Giant cell arteritis (GCA)
- ☐ Internal carotid dissection and aneurysms
- ☐ Lateral medullary infarct-Wallenberg's syndrome
- ☐ Thalamic infarcts
- ☐ Aneurysms

Structural causes

- ☐ Rhinosinus abnormalities
- ☐ Temporomandibular joint (TMJ) disorders
- ☐ Nasopharyngeal carcinoma
- ☐ Dental, e.g. infection
- ☐ External compression headache, e.g. goggles

Acronym

- ☐ SUNCT: Short lasting unilateral neuralgiform headache with conjunctival injection and tearing

FACIAL PAIN: ATYPICAL CAUSES

Pourfour du Petit's syndrome

- ☐ This is caused by lesions in the first dorsal root or cervical sympathetic chain
- ☐ It results in oculosympathetic hyperactivity
- ☐ It presents with mydriasis, lid retraction, and exophthalmos
- ☐ There is associated hyperhidrosis

Referred facial pain: origins

- ☐ Carotid dissection
- ☐ Ischaemic heart disease (IHD)
- ☐ Laryngeal disease
- ☐ Lung tumours compressing the vagus nerve

Other atypical causes

- ☐ Trochlear headache
- ☐ Red ear syndrome
- ☐ Eagle syndrome (stylohyoid syndrome)
- ☐ Base of skull lesions
- ☐ Neck tongue syndrome
- ☐ Angina
- ☐ Psychosomatic

Neuroradiology

BILATERAL THALAMIC LESIONS

Toxic causes

- ☐ Carbon monoxide (CO)
- ☐ Cyanide
- ☐ Methanol

Metabolic causes

- ☐ Wernicke encephalopathy
- ☐ Hypoxia
- ☐ Hypo/hyperglycaemia
- ☐ Osmotic myelinolysis
- ☐ Wilson's disease
- ☐ Leigh disease
- ☐ Liver disease

Degenerative causes

- ☐ Huntington's disease (HD)
- ☐ Neurodegeneration with brain iron accumulation (NBIA)
- ☐ Creutzfeldt Jakob disease (CJD)
- ☐ Variant Creutzfeldt Jakob disease (vCJD)
- ☐ Fahr disease
- ☐ Neurofibromatosis type 1 (NF1)

Vascular causes

- ☐ Cerebral vein thrombosis (CVT)
- ☐ Artery of Percheron occlusion
- ☐ Cerebral hypoperfusion
- ☐ Posterior reversible encephalopathy syndrome (PRES)

Inflammatory and infective causes

- ☐ Fabry disease
- ☐ Behcet's disease
- ☐ Viral encephalitis
- ☐ Toxoplasmosis
- ☐ Acute necrotising encephalopathy (ANE)

Neoplastic causes

- ☐ Primary CNS lymphoma (PCNSL)
- ☐ Primary bilateral thalamic glioma (PBTG)

CEREBELLOPONTINE ANGLE (CPA) LESIONS

Vestibular schwannomas

- ☐ These account for 75–90% of CPA lesions
- ☐ They cause worse hearing loss than the other lesions
- ☐ Cerebellar signs and facial weakness are less frequent
- ☐ There is less frequent hydrocephalus than with meningioma
- ☐ They are less prone to recurrence
- ☐ They show spotty signal voids on high resolution MRI: more often than with meningiomas

Other tumours

- ☐ Brainstem glioma
- ☐ Chondroma
- ☐ Chondrosarcoma
- ☐ Chordoma
- ☐ Choroid plexus papilloma
- ☐ Chloroma
- ☐ Desmoplastic medulloblastoma
- ☐ Ependymoma
- ☐ Epidermoid
- ☐ Haemangioma
- ☐ Haemangiopericytoma
- ☐ Malignant triton tumour
- ☐ Melanoma
- ☐ Meningioma: this accounts for 10% of cases
- ☐ Metastases
- ☐ Paragangliomas (glomus jugulare tumours)
- ☐ Pinealoblastoma
- ☐ Rhabdoid tumour
- ☐ Subarachnoid spread of tumours

Non-tumour CPA lesions

- ☐ Aneurysm
- ☐ Arachnoid cyst
- ☐ Brain abscess
- ☐ Cholesteatoma
- ☐ Cholesterol granuloma
- ☐ Cavernoma
- ☐ Dermoid cyst
- ☐ Epidermoids
- ☐ Ganglionic hamartoma
- ☐ Lipoma

Uncommon lesions

- ☐ Craniopharyngioma
- ☐ Endolymphatic sac tumour
- ☐ Lymphoma
- ☐ Pituitary adenoma

DOI: 10.1201/9781003221258-117

ENHANCING MENINGEAL LESIONS

Extra-axial

- ☐ Meningioma
- ☐ Sarcoidosis
- ☐ Metastases

Leptomeningeal (pia-arachnoid)

- ☐ Meningitis
- ☐ Meningoencephalitis
- ☐ Moyamoya disease: this demonstrates the Ivy sign
- ☐ Meningeal carcinomatosis
- ☐ Angiitis

Linear pachymeningeal (dura-arachnoid)

- ☐ Post-operative
- ☐ Spontaneous intracranial hypotension (SIH)

Superficial gyral

- ☐ Reperfusion after cerebral ischaemia
- ☐ Healing phase of cerebral infarction
- ☐ Encephalitis

Nodular subcortical

- ☐ Haematogenous dissemination
- ☐ Metastases
- ☐ Septic emboli

Deeper lesions

- ☐ Abscesses
- ☐ Necrotic tumours
- ☐ Low-grade tumours
- ☐ Demyelinating lesions
- ☐ Primary central nervous system lymphoma (PCNSL)
- ☐ Ependymitis

Infective causes

- ☐ Viral
- ☐ Bacterial
- ☐ Fungal
- ☐ Tuberculosis (TB)

Other causes

- ☐ Rheumatoid arthritis
- ☐ Eosinophilic granuloma
- ☐ Neurosarcoidosis
- ☐ Cerebral vein thrombosis (CVT)
- ☐ Subarachnoid haemorrhage (SAH)
- ☐ Intrathecal chemotherapy (chemical meningitis)
- ☐ Trauma

Neuropharmacology

INTRAVENOUS IMMUNOGLOBULINS (IVIG): USE

Definite indications: Level A evidence

- [ ] Guillain–Barre syndrome (GBS)
- [ ] Chronic inflammatory demyelinating polyradiculoneuropathy (CIDP)
- [ ] Severe myasthenia gravis (MG)
- [ ] Multifocal motor neuropathy (MMN)
- [ ] Lambert–Eaton myasthenic syndrome (LEMS)
- [ ] Some paraneoplastic neuropathies

Conditional indications: second- or third-line treatments

- [ ] Dermatomyositis as second-line treatment (Level B evidence)
- [ ] Polymyositis as second-line treatment (Level C evidence)
- [ ] Relapsing-remitting multiple sclerosis (RRMS) (Level B evidence)

Conditions with insufficient evidence of benefit

- [ ] IgM paraproteinaemic peripheral neuropathy (PN)
- [ ] Inclusion body myositis (IBM)
- [ ] Diabetic radiculoplexus neuropathy
- [ ] Miller Fisher syndrome (MFS)
- [ ] Post-polio syndrome (PPS)
- [ ] Guillain–Barre syndrome (GBS) in children
- [ ] Stiff person syndrome (SPS)

Precautions

- [ ] Informed consent
- [ ] IgA levels for infusion reaction
- [ ] Document objective improvement

Monitoring tests

- [ ] Pre- and post-infusion renal and liver function tests
- [ ] IgM paraproteinaemia for cryoglobulins: risk of renal failure
- [ ] Hepatitis C virus (HCV) status at intervals, e.g. annually
  - ○ But not hepatitis B (HBV) or HIV
- [ ] Screen for vascular risk factors[1]
- [ ] A recent report suggests routine blood monitoring is not necessary

INTRAVENOUS IMMUNOGLOBULINS (IVIG): COMPLICATIONS

Thromboembolic stroke

- [ ] This occurs in 0.6% of cases
- [ ] It develops with the first infusion in 50% of cases: usually within 24 hours of infusion
- [ ] Many strokes are multifocal
- [ ] Almost all subjects have other stroke risk factors

Other major complications

- [ ] Aseptic meningitis
- [ ] Myocardial infarction (MI)
- [ ] Renal failure
- [ ] Thrombotic events

Other complications

- [ ] Headache
- [ ] Fever
- [ ] Hypertension
- [ ] Nausea
- [ ] Asthenia
- [ ] Arthralgia
- [ ] Anorexia
- [ ] Dizziness
- [ ] Malaise
- [ ] Transient hyperglycaemia
- [ ] Urticaria
- [ ] Acute loss of pigmented hair: case report

DOI: 10.1201/9781003221258-118

STEROID THERAPY

Main precautions

- ☐ Use the lowest dose necessary
- ☐ Administer as a daily dose if there is associated diabetes mellitus
- ☐ Protect the gut with proton pump inhibitors (PPIs)

Dietary precautions

- ☐ Low sodium
- ☐ Low carbohydrate
- ☐ High protein
- ☐ Avoid excess alcohol and smoking

Bone protection precautions

- ☐ Vitamin D
- ☐ Calcium
- ☐ Bisphosphonates
- ☐ Calcitonin: if with fracture or if bisphosphonates are not tolerated

Tuberculosis prophylaxis: indications

- ☐ Previous tuberculosis (TB)
- ☐ Positive PPD skin test

Pneumocystis jirovecii (carinii) prophylaxis

- ☐ Risk of infection is high with steroid dose >20 mg daily and if used for >4 weeks
- ☐ Steroids cause 90% of this infection in patients without HIV
- ☐ Prophylaxis is with Trimethoprim-sulfamethoxazole 160 mg/800 mg daily
- ☐ Other prophylactic agents are Atovaquone, Dapsone, and Pentamidine

Other precautions

- ☐ Thiazides and sodium restriction: if there is substantial hypercalciuria or hypertension
- ☐ Oral contraceptive pills (OCPs): if the patient is premenopausal with irregular menses
- ☐ Testosterone: for hypogonadal men

Indications for not restricting live vaccines on steroids

- ☐ When the treatment course is less than 2 weeks
- ☐ When using short lasting alternate day regime
- ☐ When administering topical, intra-articular, or soft tissue steroids
- ☐ When giving physiological replacement doses
- ☐ When the long-term daily dose is 10 mg or less

Monitoring tests on steroids

- ☐ Bone mass density (BMD): at baseline, then 6-monthly, then annually
- ☐ Blood pressure (BP): at each visit
- ☐ Regular eye examination: for glaucoma and cataracts
- ☐ Fasting blood glucose (FBS): periodically
- ☐ Potassium: periodically

Obstetric neurology

EPILEPSY: MANAGEMENT IN PREGNANCY

Pre-conception counselling

- ☐ Contraception
- ☐ Antiepileptic drug (AED) teratogenicity
- ☐ Breastfeeding

Pre-conception supplementation

- ☐ Folic acid 5 mg daily

Intra-partum management

- ☐ High resolution ultrasound scan at 18–20 weeks
- ☐ Vitamin K 20 mg daily from 36 weeks if on an enzyme-inducing AED

Post-partum management: if mother is on an enzyme-inducing AED

- ☐ Vitamin K1 20 mg daily orally for a week before delivery
  - ○ Alternatively, 10 mg parenterally during labour
- ☐ Vitamin K1 1 mg for the baby: on days 1 and 28
- ☐ Breastfeeding on AEDs is encouraged
- ☐ Osteoporosis assessments

ANTIEPILEPTIC DRUGS (AEDS) IN PREGNANCY

Guidelines for using contraceptives in epilepsy

- ☐ Intrauterine contraceptive devices (IUDs) have the lowest failure rate
- ☐ Progestin IUDs are probably safe and effective
- ☐ Avoid progesterone only contraceptive pills and implants
- ☐ Use depo or double dose oral contraceptives with enzyme-inducing AEDs
- ☐ Use additional barrier contraception with enzyme-inducing AEDs

Considerations for using Valproate in women with childbearing potential

- ☐ Valproate is contraindicated in women with child-bearing potential
- ☐ Use Valproate in these cases only if other drugs are ineffective
- ☐ Use the lowest effective dose of Valproate
- ☐ Regularly review for alternative treatments
- ☐ Lamotrigine and Carbamazepine are the safest alternatives to Valproate

Blood monitoring of AED levels in pregnancy: indications

- ☐ Lamotrigine
- ☐ Phenytoin
- ☐ Carbamazepine
- ☐ Levetiracetam
- ☐ Oxcarbazepine

DOI: 10.1201/9781003221258-119

CAUSES OF HEADACHES IN PREGNANCY

Preeclampsia: criteria

☐ The onset of headache was after 20 weeks of pregnancy
☐ The subject was normotensive before pregnancy
☐ There is hypertension with systolic BP >140mmHg or diastolic BP >90mmHg
☐ There is proteinuria of >0.3g in 24-hour urine collection

Migraine

☐ Migraine improves during pregnancy: this is probably due to rising oestrogen levels
☐ Migraine worsens in the postpartum period

Other primary headaches

☐ Tension-type headache (TTH)
☐ Cluster headaches (CH)

Meningitis

☐ This is usually with Streptococcus pneumoniae or Listeria monocytogenes
☐ Treat with third-generation cephalosporins, e.g. Cefotaxime or Ceftriaxone
☐ Add Ampicillin to cover for Listeria

Vasculopathies

☐ Reversible cerebral vasoconstriction syndrome (RCVS)
☐ Posterior reversible encephalopathy syndrome (PRES)
☐ Vasculitis

Other causes

☐ Cerebral vein thrombosis (CVT)
☐ Aneurysmal subarachnoid haemorrhage (SAH)
☐ Idiopathic intracranial hypertension (IIH)
☐ Pituitary tumours: adenomas and meningiomas
☐ Pituitary apoplexy
☐ Cerebral artery dissection (CAD)
☐ Carbon monoxide toxicity
☐ Post-dural puncture headache (PDPH)

Causes of acute post-partum headache

☐ Cerebral venous thrombosis (CVT)
☐ Cerebral angiopathy
☐ Cervical artery dissection (CAD)
☐ Intracerebral haemorrhage (ICH)
☐ Ischaemic stroke
☐ Meningitis
☐ Migraine
☐ Post-dural puncture headache (PDPH)
☐ Post-partum hypertension
☐ Post-partum preeclampsia and eclampsia
☐ Reversible cerebral vasoconstriction syndrome (RCVS)
☐ Pituitary apoplexy
☐ Subarachnoid haemorrhage (SAH)

MIGRAINE TREATMENT IN PREGNANCY

Antiemetics

☐ Metoclopramide is probably safe
☐ Domperidone is probably safe
☐ Ondansteron and Droperidol should be used with caution
☐ Prochlorperazine is contraindicated

Triptans

☐ These are usually contraindicated but they are probably not teratogenic
☐ Sumatriptan may be used with caution if absolutely indicated
☐ Do detailed foetal ultrasound if other triptans are used in the first trimester

Aspirin

☐ This should be avoided after 30 weeks
☐ It is used with caution in the first and second trimesters
☐ It causes premature closure of the ductus arteriosus
☐ It also causes bleeding and inhibits labour

Other analgesics

☐ Paracetamol is safe: it is preferable to Aspirin
☐ Non-steroidal anti-inflammatory drugs (NSAIDs) are generally contraindicated in pregnancy
　○ Avoid them after 30 weeks
☐ Tramadol and Codeine are safe in the third trimester
　○ Use with caution in earlier trimesters
☐ Propofol

Betablockers

☐ They are of choice for migraine prophylaxis in pregnancy
☐ They are not teratogenic
☐ They may reduce placental perfusion
☐ They should be avoided in the third trimester
☐ Propranolol is the safest option in pregnancy

Other prophylactic drugs

☐ Tricyclic antidepressants: they are safe for migraine and tension headache
　○ Reduce the dose in terminal pregnancy
☐ Botulinum toxin
☐ Magnesium
☐ Metoprolol
☐ Nerve blocks

Contraindicated drugs

☐ Valproate
☐ Dihydroergotamine (DHE)
☐ Caffeine
☐ ACE inhibitors
☐ Topiramate
☐ Prochlorperazine: this causes congenital heart defects and cleft palate

Relatively contraindicated steroids

☐ Dexamethasone in early pregnancy
☐ Ketorolac in the third trimester
☐ Prednisolone in the first trimester

STROKE IN PREGNANCY: CAUSES

Pregnancy-induced gestational hypertension: risk factors

- ☐ Chronic hypertension
- ☐ Obesity
- ☐ Age >40 years
- ☐ Previous preeclampsia or gestational hypertension
- ☐ Nulliparity
- ☐ Multiparity ≥3
- ☐ Multiple pregnancy
- ☐ Pre-existing vascular disease
- ☐ Collagen vascular disease
- ☐ Diabetes mellitus
- ☐ Renal disease

Preeclampsia and eclampsia: features

- ☐ Proteinuria
- ☐ Thrombocytopenia
- ☐ Renal impairment
- ☐ Abnormal liver function
- ☐ Pulmonary oedema

HELLP syndrome: features

- ☐ Haemolysis
- ☐ Elevated liver enzymes
- ☐ Low platelets

Hypercoagulable states

- ☐ Prothrombotic disorders in the third trimester
- ☐ Oestrogen-related hypercoagulability
- ☐ Antiphospholipid antibody syndrome
- ☐ Thrombotic thrombocytopaenic purpura (TTP)

Other causes of ischaemic stroke

- ☐ Cervical artery dissection (CAD)
- ☐ Cardioembolism from peripartum cardiomyopathy
- ☐ Reversible cerebral vasoconstriction syndrome (RCVS)
- ☐ Moyamoya disease
- ☐ Blood transfusion
- ☐ Amniotic fluid embolism (AFE)
- ☐ Acute blood loss
- ☐ Hyperemesis

Causes of subarachnoid haemorrhage (SAH)

- ☐ Cerebral aneurysms
- ☐ Arteriovenous malformations (AVMs)
- ☐ Disseminated intravascular coagulation (DIC)

Causes of intracerebral haemorrhage (ICH)

- ☐ Hypertension
- ☐ Cerebral vein thrombosis (CVT)

NEUROLOGICAL COMPLICATIONS OF LABOUR

Post-partum nerve injuries

- ☐ Lateral cutaneous nerve of the thigh
- ☐ Common peroneal nerve
- ☐ Obturator nerve
- ☐ Femoral nerve
- ☐ Sciatic nerve: with regional block
- ☐ Lumbosacral plexus

Transient neurological symptoms (TNS) with Caesarean delivery

- ☐ These occur in about 9% of cases
- ☐ They last 1–2 days
- ☐ They affect the buttocks or legs

Other neurological complications of labour

- ☐ Pre-eclampsia causing stroke in labour
- ☐ Persistent pain and sensory disturbance
- ☐ Epidural haematoma or abscess
- ☐ Meningitis
- ☐ Cauda equina syndrome (CES)
- ☐ Post-dural puncture headache (PDPH)

Functional neurology

FUNCTIONAL MOVEMENT DISORDERS: GENERAL FEATURES

Demographic features

- [ ] These account for about 3% of movement disorders
- [ ] About a fifth may develop after the age of 60 years

Types

- [ ] Tremor: this accounts for 50% of cases
- [ ] Dystonia
- [ ] Myoclonus
- [ ] Parkinsonism
- [ ] Gait disorders
- [ ] Facial movement disorders

Clinical features

- [ ] Abrupt onset
- [ ] Variability
- [ ] Distractibility
- [ ] Secondary gain
- [ ] Selective disabilities
- [ ] Fatigue
- [ ] Stimulus sensitivity
- [ ] Positive placebo effect
- [ ] Lack of response to treatment

The 'whack-a-mole' sign

- [ ] Movements re-emerge in other body parts when supressed in one part

The 'huffing and puffing' sign

- [ ] This is an effort associated sign
- [ ] It is seen with psychogenic gait disorders

Associations

- [ ] Previous psychogenic illnesses
- [ ] Childhood emotional or physical trauma
- [ ] Psychiatric illnesses: these are seen in about 50% of cases
- [ ] Organic diseases: these co-exist in 25% of cases

FUNCTIONAL DYSTONIA

General features

- [ ] This has a sudden onset
- [ ] There is usually a precipitating cause
- [ ] The progression is rapid
- [ ] It improves with suggestion
- [ ] It remits under sedation and anaesthesia

Functional generalised dystonia

- [ ] There is fixed posturing of the body part
- [ ] Lower limb involvement is very common: unlike in adult-onset organic dystonia
- [ ] There is paroxysmal worsening in some cases
- [ ] Pain is often prominent
- [ ] It is often associated with other psychogenic movement disorders

Functional blepharospasm

- [ ] The onset is abrupt
- [ ] It usually follows emotional stress
- [ ] It may be asymmetric or alternate between the eyes
- [ ] It has a fluctuating clinical course
- [ ] It may resolve with placebo or spontaneously
- [ ] The blink reflex recovery cycle is normal: unlike in organic blepharospasm

Functional dysphonia

- [ ] This is a disorder of voice quality, pitch, or loudness
- [ ] The onset is usually after an upper respiratory tract infection
- [ ] There are no structural or neurologic causes
- [ ] It is more frequent in women

DOI: 10.1201/9781003221258-120

FUNCTIONAL TREMOR

Demographic features

- [ ] This accounts for >50% of psychogenic movement disorders
- [ ] The mean onset age is 50 years
  - ○ This is a younger age than essential tremor
- [ ] There is a female preponderance: 70–75% of cases are women
- [ ] A family history of tremor is infrequent
- [ ] Litigation is involved in a fifth of cases
- [ ] It may develop after deep brain stimulation (DBS) for essential tremor

Course

- [ ] It is frequently sudden onset and non-progressive
- [ ] A precipitating event is frequent, e.g. work-related accident
- [ ] There may be spontaneous remissions
- [ ] The outcome is poor if it is prolonged (>1 year)
- [ ] Symptoms persist in up to 90% of cases

Characteristics

- [ ] It is usually bilateral
- [ ] It is complex and difficult to classify
- [ ] It has variable direction, amplitude, and frequency
- [ ] It is usually absent in the fingers, tongue, and face
- [ ] It worsens with attention
- [ ] There are no other neurologic signs
- [ ] It is unresponsive to anti-tremor drugs
- [ ] Patients overestimate the persistence of the tremor

Associated disorders

- [ ] Psychiatric disorders
- [ ] Pain
- [ ] Diffuse sensory deficits

Positive entrainment test

- [ ] This is sensitive and specific for functional tremor
- [ ] It is done by tapping the thumb and forefinger of the less or non-affected limb
- [ ] The examiner sets a tapping rhythm which the patient's tremor follows
- [ ] The examiner varies the rhythm which the patient's tremor adapts to

Positive co-activation test

- [ ] Weight (loading) increases the tremor's amplitude

Other positive tests

- [ ] Distractibility with alternate finger tapping
- [ ] Suggestibility with tuning fork
- [ ] Worsening with hyperventilation
- [ ] Response to suggestion
- [ ] Response to placebo
- [ ] Pause of tremor during contralateral ballistic movement

Treatment

- [ ] Tremor retrainment
- [ ] Botulinum toxin: this may improve psychogenic palatal tremor

FUNCTIONAL PARKINSONISM

General features

- [ ] This accounts for 1.5% of Parkinsonism
- [ ] It accounts for 10% of psychogenic movement disorders
- [ ] The gender ratio is equal
- [ ] The presentation is with one or more features of Parkinsonism
- [ ] The course is fluctuating with remissions
- [ ] It may improve spontaneously or to placebo
- [ ] It may improve with antidepressants
- [ ] There is early disability

Characteristics of tremor

- [ ] The tremor is at rest and on action
- [ ] It has a variable frequency and rhythm
- [ ] It persists through action
- [ ] The tremor spreads to other parts when the limb is restrained
- [ ] There is frequent leg involvement: unlike in organic Parkinsonism
- [ ] There is usually no finger tremor
- [ ] There is no re-emergent tremor
- [ ] The tremor demonstrates entrainment

Characteristics of rigidity

- [ ] There is voluntary resistance (Gegenhalten)
- [ ] There is no cogwheeling
- [ ] It is reduced with distraction or synkinesis

Characteristics of bradykinesia

- [ ] There is effortful reduced arm swing
- [ ] The arm is held tightly to the side or front of the body
- [ ] The rigidity does not improve with running: unlike in organic Parkinsonism
- [ ] There is no hypometria
- [ ] There is no decremental amplitude and speed on testing

Other features

- [ ] Absence of micrographia
- [ ] Absence of hypomimia
- [ ] Absence of hypophonia
- [ ] Stuttering or whispering speech
- [ ] Give-way weakness
- [ ] Normal dopamine transporter (DaT) scan

FUNCTIONAL SEIZURES

General features

- [ ] They arise from apparent sleep but EEG verifies wakefulness
- [ ] The onset is gradual with a waxing and waning course
- [ ] There is no tonic phase
- [ ] About 60% have stereotyped events
- [ ] They are prolonged events usually lasting more than 2 minutes
- [ ] Injury avoidance is characteristic
- [ ] There may be experiential avoidance
  - ○ This is the active avoidance of situations, places, thoughts, or feelings
- [ ] There is memory recall

Characteristic movements

- [ ] Swooning
- [ ] Pelvic thrusting
- [ ] Side-to-side body or head movements
- [ ] Asynchronous movements
- [ ] Flexion and extension
- [ ] Abduction and adduction
- [ ] Rotation
- [ ] Ictal stuttering: this is not seen in epilepsy

Panic symptoms

- [ ] Hyperventilation
- [ ] Palpitations and sweating
- [ ] Shortness of breath and a choking feeling
- [ ] Chest discomfort
- [ ] Dizziness and unsteadiness
- [ ] Derealisation and depersonalisation
- [ ] Paraesthesias
- [ ] Chills or hot flushes
- [ ] Feeling of wanting to get out of the situation
- [ ] Fear of going crazy, of losing control, or of dying

Eye features

- [ ] The eyes are shut during the episodes
- [ ] The patient resists forced eye opening
- [ ] The corneal reflex is normal
- [ ] There is impaired visual fixation: tested with the Henry and Woodruff sign or mirror

Cognitive features

- [ ] Catastrophising
- [ ] Perseverative negative thinking

Frequent co-morbidities

- [ ] Asthma
- [ ] Chronic pain
- [ ] Migraines
- [ ] Depression
- [ ] Sleep impairment

Synonyms

- [ ] Non-epileptic attack disorder (NEAD)
- [ ] Psychogenic non-epileptic seizures (PNES)

FUNCTIONAL HEMIPARESIS

Clinical features

- [ ] The hemiparesis has a non-pyramidal distribution
- [ ] It may show collapsing (give-way) weakness
- [ ] There is absence of pronator drift
- [ ] The gait is dragging
- [ ] The associated psychogenic pain is worse than in organic disease
- [ ] The functional disability is the same as with organic weakness

Distinctive clinical signs

- [ ] Hoover's sign
- [ ] The abduction finger sign
- [ ] The abductor sign
- [ ] The Spinal Injuries Centre test
- [ ] The co-contraction sign
- [ ] The arm drop test
- [ ] The Barré test: manoeuvre de la jambe
- [ ] Hysterical tongue spasm: spasme glosso-labié unilateral
- [ ] The platysma sign: signe du peaucier
- [ ] The Babinski trunk-thigh test
- [ ] The supine catch sign
- [ ] Inverse pyramidal leg weakness
- [ ] The elbow flex-ex sign: with unilateral arm weakness
- [ ] Drift without pronation sign

Co-morbid psychiatric disorders

- [ ] Major depression
- [ ] Generalised anxiety disorder
- [ ] Panic disorder
- [ ] Somatisation

Social impact

- [ ] There is a high level of physical and psychological morbidity
- [ ] The subjects are less likely to be in work than people with organic disease
- [ ] There is a similar frequency of receiving state benefits as organic disease
- [ ] There is no excess litigation or compensation-seeking

Predictors of good outcome

- [ ] Short duration of symptoms
- [ ] Early diagnosis
- [ ] Absence of personality disorder

CHAPTER 20

Systemic neurological disorders

Cardiac

ATRIAL FIBRILLATION (AF) AND STROKE RISK

Embolic stroke risk with AF

- [ ] AF increases ischemic stroke risk 5-fold
- [ ] AF is responsible for 20% of all strokes

Embolic stroke risk factors with AF

- [ ] Age >75 years
- [ ] Congestive cardiac failure (CCF)
- [ ] Hypertension
- [ ] Diabetes mellitus
- [ ] Smoking
- [ ] Structural heart disease
- [ ] Previous stroke or transient ischaemic attack (TIA)
- [ ] Rheumatic mitral stenosis
- [ ] Prosthetic heart valves: especially mechanical mitral valve

CHA2DS2-VASc stroke risk prediction items

- [ ] Congestive heart failure: 1 point
- [ ] Hypertension: 1 point
- [ ] Age ≥ 75 years: 1 point
- [ ] Diabetes mellitus: 1 point
- [ ] Stroke/TIA/thromboembolism: 2 points
- [ ] Vascular disease: myocardial infarction, peripheral arterial disease, aortic plaque: 1 point
- [ ] Age 65–74 years: 1 point
- [ ] Sex (female): 1 point

CHA2DS2-VASc risk estimation

- [ ] 0. Low risk: 1.2–3%
- [ ] 1. Intermediate risk: 2.8–4%
- [ ] ≥2. High risk: 5.9–18.2%: this requires anticoagulation

PATENT FORAMEN OVALE (PFO) AND MIGRAINE

Epidemiology of PFO and migraine

- [ ] PFO is present in 30% of the population
- [ ] There is probably no association between migraine and isolated PFO
- [ ] Migraine is associated with PFO if accompanied by atrial septal aneurysm (ASA)
- [ ] There is possibly an increased frequency of PFO in migraine with aura
- [ ] Migraineurs may have larger PFOs than non-migraineurs

Drug treatment

- [ ] Consider Aspirin as first choice

Preventive measures

- [ ] Smoking cessation
- [ ] Avoid combined oral contraceptive pills (OCPs)
- [ ] Treat hypertension, diabetes, and raised cholesterol
- [ ] Assess prothrombotic risks like MTHFR polymorphisms

Benefit of PFO closure

- [ ] Closure is not advised for isolated PFO
- [ ] There is no evidence of benefit in migraine

Indications for PFO closure

- [ ] Associated atrial septal aneurysm (ASA)
- [ ] Associated thrombophilia
- [ ] Associated peripheral venous thrombosis

Complications of PFO closure

- [ ] Cardiac tamponade
- [ ] Pulmonary embolism
- [ ] Atrial fibrillation
- [ ] Bleeding

DOI: 10.1201/9781003221258-122

PATENT FORAMEN OVALE (PFO) AND STROKE: CLINICAL ASPECTS

Epidemiology of PFO and stroke

- [ ] PFO is present in 30% of the population
- [ ] PFO is detected in >50% of young cryptogenic stroke
- [ ] PFO is detected in about 80% of people with migraine who develop stroke
- [ ] PFO is prevalent in older people with cryptogenic stroke
- [ ] People >60 years accounted for 60% of cases in one review

Predictors of stroke with PFO

- [ ] PFO associated with atrial septal aneurysm (ASA)
- [ ] PFO with large right-to-left shunt

Predictors of recurrent stroke with PFO

- [ ] Migraine with aura
- [ ] Large spontaneous right-to-left shunt
- [ ] Thrombophilia

Medical treatment

- [ ] Antiplatelets are the usual first line medical therapy for stroke with PFO
- [ ] There is insufficient evidence of benefit from anticoagulation
- [ ] Consider anticoagulation if there is an associated venous source of embolism
- [ ] Use inferior vena cava filter if anticoagulation is not feasible in this situation

PATENT FORAMEN OVALE (PFO) AND STROKE: PFO CLOSURE

Benefits for PFO closure

- [ ] Many systematic reviews report that PFO closure reduces the risk of recurrent stroke
- [ ] The risk reduction has been calculated at 58%
- [ ] The outcomes are better if PFO closure is combined with antiplatelet therapy
- [ ] The highest benefit of PFO closure is in men and in people with large PFOs

Precautions before PFO closure

- [ ] Assess each patient's anatomical PFO risk
- [ ] Asses clinical risk of recurrent stroke
- [ ] Assess bleeding risk
- [ ] Assess risk of atrial fibrillation (AF)
- [ ] Exclude vascular risk factors
- [ ] Utilise shared decision-making

PFO closure techniques

- [ ] Transcatheter
- [ ] AMPLATZER PFO Occluder

Risks of PFO closure

- [ ] Atrial fibrillation (AF): especially in the first month after closure
- [ ] Atrial flutter
- [ ] Pulmonary embolism

Device-related PFO closure adverse events

- [ ] Vascular complications
- [ ] Conduction abnormalities
- [ ] Device dislocation
- [ ] Device thrombosis
- [ ] Air embolism
- [ ] Cardiac tamponade
- [ ] Cardiac perforation

Syncope

SYNCOPE: CLASSIFICATION

Cardiac syncope: types

- ☐ Arrhythmias
- ☐ Heart block
- ☐ Aortic stenosis
- ☐ Myocardial infarction (MI)
- ☐ Cardiac ischaemia

Reflex syncope: types

- ☐ Neurocardiogenic (vasovagal)
- ☐ Carotid sinus hypersensitivity
- ☐ Situational

Situational syncope: causes

- ☐ Straining, e.g. micturition and defaecation
- ☐ Warm environment
- ☐ Warm bath
- ☐ Low salt diet
- ☐ Prolonged recumbency
- ☐ Alcohol
- ☐ Vigorous exercise
- ☐ Dehydration
- ☐ Large meals (postprandial hypotension)

Drug-induced syncope: causes

- ☐ Alpha receptor blockers
- ☐ Angiotensin converting enzyme inhibitors (ACEI)
- ☐ Beta blockers
- ☐ Bromocriptine
- ☐ Calcium channel blockers
- ☐ Diuretics
- ☐ Ethanol
- ☐ Ganglionic blockers
- ☐ Hydralazine
- ☐ Monoamine oxidase inhibitors (MAOI)
- ☐ Nitrates
- ☐ Opiates
- ☐ Phenothiazines
- ☐ Sildenafil
- ☐ Tricyclics

Other forms of syncope

- ☐ Exertional syncope
- ☐ Deglutition syncope

NEUROCARDIOGENIC SYNCOPE

Clinical features

- ☐ There is little or no prodrome in a third of cases
- ☐ It may occur without a provoking factor
- ☐ It may occur with relatively insignificant falls in blood pressure
- ☐ The blood pressure decline may be gradual: over 10–15 minutes
- ☐ The blackout may be rapid
- ☐ Amnesia for loss of consciousness: this occurs in 28% of people who faint on tilt table testing

Triggers

- ☐ Fear of bodily injury
- ☐ Pain
- ☐ Venepuncture
- ☐ Prolonged standing
- ☐ Exposure to heat
- ☐ Exertion
- ☐ Coughing
- ☐ Swallowing
- ☐ Straining

Differential diagnosis

- ☐ Carotid hypersensitivity
- ☐ Situational syncope

Synonym

- ☐ Vasovagal syncope

DOI: 10.1201/9781003221258-123

SYNCOPE: DIFFERENTIAL DIAGNOSIS

Neurological differentials

- [ ] Seizures
- [ ] Transient ischaemic attacks (TIAs): carotid and vertebrobasilar
- [ ] Intracerebral haemorrhage (ICH)
- [ ] Subarachnoid haemorrhage (SAH)
- [ ] Cataplexy
- [ ] Falls without loss of consciousness
- [ ] Coma

Medical differentials

- [ ] Hypoglycaemia
- [ ] Hypoxia
- [ ] Hyperventilation with hypocapnia
- [ ] Intoxication

Cardiovascular differentials

- [ ] Cardiac arrest
- [ ] Subclavian steal syndrome
- [ ] Psychogenic pseudosyncope

SYNCOPE: DIFFERENTIAL DIAGNOSIS FROM SEIZURES

Prodromal predictors of syncope

- [ ] Light-headedness
- [ ] Nausea
- [ ] Palpitations

Ictal predictors of syncope

- [ ] Loss of tone is present in all cases of syncope: this is only seen in some seizures
- [ ] Fewer than 10 myoclonic jerks accompany syncope: there are >20 in seizures
  - This is the 10/20 rule
- [ ] Myoclonic jerks are less rhythmic in syncope than in seizures
- [ ] There is no lateral tongue biting in syncope unlike in seizures
- [ ] There is no consistent head-turn to one side in syncope

Post-ictal predictors of syncope

- [ ] Feeling of coming out of a dream

Therapeutic predictors of syncope

- [ ] Poor response to antiepileptic drugs (AEDs)
- [ ] Worsening on starting AEDs
- [ ] Phenytoin and Carbamazepine may induce bradycardia in syncope

Electroencephalogram (EEG) predictors of syncope

- [ ] This is often non-diagnostic

SYNCOPE: PREVENTIVE MANOEUVRES

Adequate fluid intake

- ☐ This prevents presyncope on tilt table in healthy subjects
- ☐ It works by increasing peripheral vascular resistance: not by increasing blood volume
- ☐ The drink should be taken just before engaging in syncope-precipitating activities

Preventative postures

- ☐ Sitting on the floor with the head between drawn-up knees
- ☐ Squatting on haunches
- ☐ Lying down
- ☐ Lying supine with the legs elevated
- ☐ Rising slowly
- ☐ Shaving sitting down
- ☐ Crossing the legs
- ☐ Putting a leg on a chair
- ☐ Head-up tilt sleeping at >10 degrees
- ☐ Forearm tensing
- ☐ Hand clenching
- ☐ Leg crossing and leg muscle tensing
- ☐ Elevating heels to contract calf muscles

Other preventative measures

- ☐ Education on avoiding predisposing situations
- ☐ Salt supplementation
- ☐ Tilt training: standing against a wall with the feet 20cm from the wall for 40 minutes every day
- ☐ Abdominal binders
- ☐ Waist-high elastic support stockings
- ☐ Moderate exercise
- ☐ Biofeedback therapy: for psychogenic syncope
- ☐ Cognitive behaviour therapy (CBT): for anxiety, depression, and fear of syncope

SYNCOPE: INTERVENTIONAL TREATMENTS

Midodrine: first line

- ☐ The dose is 2.5–15 mg 2–4 hourly
- ☐ There is a risk of supine hypertension
- ☐ It should not be taken within 5 hours of bedtime
- ☐ Users should not rest or sleep supine but recumbent
- ☐ It may cause piloerection, scalp itching, and urinary retention
- ☐ Use with caution in heart and renal failure

Droxidopa: first line

- ☐ The dose is 100 mg tid: maximum is 600 mg tid
- ☐ It increases circulating norepinephrine levels
- ☐ It should be avoided within 5 hours of bedtime: to prevent supine hypertension
- ☐ It may cause headache, dizziness, nausea, and fatigue

Fludrocortisone: second line

- ☐ The dose is 0.1–0.2 mg/day: maximum 1mg/day
- ☐ It increases renal water and sodium absorption
- ☐ It also increases vascular resistance
- ☐ It may cause supine hypertension
- ☐ It may also cause hypokalemia and oedema
- ☐ Use with caution in congestive heart failure

Pyridostigmine

- ☐ The dose is 30–60 mg 1–3 times daily
- ☐ It may be more effective in combination with Midodrine
- ☐ It does not cause supine hypertension
- ☐ It may cause abdominal cramps, diarrhoea, and sialorrhoea
- ☐ It may also cause excessive sweating and urinary incontinence

Other drugs to consider

- ☐ Desmopressin: in nocturnal polyuria
- ☐ Octreotide: in postprandial hypotension
- ☐ Erythropoeitin: in anaemia
- ☐ Metoprolol: especially in older patients
- ☐ Clonidine
- ☐ Yohimbine
- ☐ Ephedrine sulphate
- ☐ Fluoexetine
- ☐ Paroxetine
- ☐ Pseudoephedrine

Pacemaker: indications

- ☐ Cardioinhibitory carotid sinus syncope
- ☐ Frequent cardioinhibitory reflex syncope in people >40 years
- ☐ Frequent unpredictable syncope on tilt testing
- ☐ Syncope that has failed other treatments
- ☐ Syncope with no pre-warning

Respiratory

NEUROMUSCULAR RESPIRATORY DYSFUNCTION: CAUSES

Anterior horn cell (AHC) disorders

- ☐ Motor neurone disease (MND)
- ☐ Poliomyelitis and post-polio syndrome (PPS)
- ☐ Spinal muscular atrophy (SMA)
- ☐ Kennedy disease: X-linked spinal and bulbar muscular atrophy (SBMA)
- ☐ Paralytic rabies

Peripheral nerve disorders

- ☐ Guillain–Barre syndrome (GBS)
- ☐ Chronic inflammatory demyelinating polyneuropathy (CIDP)
- ☐ Critical illness polyneuropathy (CIPN)
- ☐ Diaphragmatic paralysis
- ☐ Charcot–Marie–Tooth disease (CMT)
- ☐ Brachial plexopathy
- ☐ Phrenic neuropathy
- ☐ Acute intermittent porphyria (AIP)

Neuromuscular junction (NMJ) disorders

- ☐ Myasthenia gravis (MG)
- ☐ Lambert–Eaton myasthenic syndrome (LEMS)
- ☐ Botulism
- ☐ Curare poisoning

Muscle diseases

- ☐ Polymyositis and dermatomyositis
- ☐ Muscular dystrophies
- ☐ Mitochondrial encephalomyopathies
- ☐ Acid maltase deficiency
- ☐ Congenital myopathy

Toxins

- ☐ Organophosphates
- ☐ Thallium
- ☐ Arsenic
- ☐ Lead
- ☐ Gold
- ☐ Lithium
- ☐ Botulism
- ☐ Diphtheria
- ☐ Scorpion and snake bites
- ☐ Seafood poisoning: fish, shellfish, crab
- ☐ Tick paralysis

Other causes

- ☐ Vincristine
- ☐ Antibiotics
- ☐ Anticholinesterases
- ☐ Lymphoma
- ☐ Vasculitis
- ☐ Hereditary tyrosinaemia

PULMONARY ARTERIOVENOUS MALFORMATION (PAVM)

Genetic mutations

- ☐ Endoglin gene mutations: on chromosome 9
- ☐ Activin receptor-like kinase 1 gene mutations: on chromosome 12

Cardiorespiratory features

- ☐ Symptoms often start in the 4th to 6th decade
- ☐ Exertional dyspnoea and hypoxaemia
- ☐ Orthodeoxia (orthostatic hypoxaemia): because most PAVMs are basal
- ☐ Platypnoea: dyspnoea that improves on reclining
- ☐ Myocardial infarction
- ☐ High output cardiac failure
- ☐ Pulmonary hypertension
- ☐ Digital clubbing
- ☐ Chest bruit
- ☐ Coexisting hereditary haemorrhagic telangiectasia (HHT)

Neurological presentations

- ☐ Migraine
- ☐ TIAs and stroke: from paradoxical embolism
- ☐ Brain abscess
- ☐ Seizures

Systemic features

- ☐ Cyanosis
- ☐ Polycythaemia
- ☐ Osteomyelitis

100% oxygen screening test

- ☐ 100% oxygen is given for 20 minutes
- ☐ Shunt fraction is >5%

Investigations

- ☐ Chest X-Ray: this shows rounded lesions with band shaped shadows
- ☐ Contrast echocardiogram: to assess right to left shunt
- ☐ Chest contrast computed tomography (CT): if echocardiogram is positive
- ☐ Digital subtraction angiography (DSA)
- ☐ Pulmonary angiography: if non-invasive tests are strongly suggestive

Treatment

- ☐ Embolotherapy
- ☐ Antibiotics before surgical or dental procedures

DOI: 10.1201/9781003221258-124

HEREDITARY HAEMORRHAGIC TELANGIECTASIA (HHT)

Genetic types

- ☐ HHT type 1: ENG gene mutations
- ☐ HHT type 2: ACVRL1 gene mutations
- ☐ HHT overlap: SMAD4 gene mutations

Curacao diagnostic criteria

- ☐ Autosomal dominant transmission
- ☐ Recurrent epistaxis
- ☐ Mucocutaneous telangiectasias
- ☐ Visceral arteriovenous malformations (AVMs)
- ☐ HHT in a first degree relative
- ☐ Definite diagnosis: if ≥3 features are present
- ☐ Possible diagnosis: if 2 features are present

Arteriovenous malformations (AVMs): epidemiology

- ☐ HHT accounts for almost all multiple AVMs
- ☐ It accounts for 65% of solitary pulmonary AVMs

Arteriovenous malformations (AVMs): sites

- ☐ Cerebral in 20%
- ☐ Pulmonary in 50%
- ☐ Hepatic in 60%

Telangiectasias (dilated blood vessels): sites

- ☐ Nasal mucosa
- ☐ Lips
- ☐ Conjunctiva
- ☐ Gastrointestinal tract

Haemorrhagic features

- ☐ Epistaxis: this occurs in 90% of cases
- ☐ Gastrointestinal bleeding
- ☐ Conjunctival bleeding: this may result in bloody tears
- ☐ Chronic anaemia

Cerebral features

- ☐ Headache
- ☐ Seizures
- ☐ Ischaemic stroke: this results from vascular steal
- ☐ Haemorrhage
- ☐ Cerebral abscesses

Pulmonary features

- ☐ Dyspnoea
- ☐ Haemorrhage
- ☐ Embolisation

Brain magnetic resonance imaging (MRI)

- ☐ There are basal ganglia T1 hyperintensities in about a quarter of cases

Synonym

- ☐ Rendu-Osler-Weber disease

Rheumatology

ANTIPHOSPHOLIPID SYNDROME (APS): NEUROLOGICAL FEATURES

Demographic features

- [ ] The mean onset age is 42 years
- [ ] Males are more often older at onset
- [ ] Males have more epilepsy and thrombosis
- [ ] Females have more migraine and arthritis
- [ ] Younger onset patients (<15 years) have more chorea and jugular thrombosis
- [ ] Older onset patients (>50 years) have more stroke and angina
- [ ] Catastrophic APS occurs in about 0.8% of cases

Vascular features

- [ ] Transient ischaemic attack (TIA)
- [ ] Stroke
- [ ] Acute ischaemic encephalopathy
- [ ] Cerebral vein thrombosis (CVT)

Neuroinflammatory features

- [ ] Optic neuropathy
- [ ] Transverse myelitis (TM)

Cognitive features

- [ ] Multi infarct dementia
- [ ] Transient global amnesia (TGA)

Movement disorders

- [ ] Dystonia
- [ ] Parkinsonism
- [ ] Hemiballism
- [ ] Chorea
- [ ] Cerebellar ataxia

Psychiatric features

- [ ] Depression
- [ ] Psychosis
- [ ] Behavioural disorders

Peripheral neurological features

- [ ] Sensorineural deafness
- [ ] Peripheral neuropathy (PN)
- [ ] Guillain–Barre syndrome (GBS)

Other features

- [ ] Epilepsy
- [ ] Migraine: this is especially in teenage-onset patients
- [ ] Idiopathic intracranial hypertension (IIH)

ANTIPHOSPHOLIPID SYNDROME (APS): SYSTEMIC FEATURES

Underlying disorders

- [ ] Primary APS
- [ ] Systemic lupus erythematosus (SLE)
- [ ] Lupus-like syndrome
- [ ] Primary Sjogren's syndrome
- [ ] Rheumatoid arthritis (RA)
- [ ] Systemic sclerosis (SS)
- [ ] Systemic vasculitis
- [ ] Dermatomyositis

Thromboembolic features

- [ ] Deep vein thrombosis (DVT)
- [ ] Superficial thrombophlebitis
- [ ] Pulmonary embolism (PE)

Haematological features

- [ ] Haemolytic anaemia
- [ ] Thrombocytopaenia

Dermatological features

- [ ] Livido reticularis
- [ ] Skin ulcers
- [ ] Pseudovasculitic skin lesions

Obstetric features

- [ ] Preeclampsia/eclampsia
- [ ] Abruptio placenta
- [ ] Premature birth
- [ ] Foetal loss

Vascular features

- [ ] Myocardial infarction (MI)
- [ ] Digital gangrene

DOI: 10.1201/9781003221258-125

SYSTEMIC LUPUS ERYTHEMATOSUS (SLE): NEUROLOGICAL FEATURES

Inflammatory and immune

- ☐ Chorea: this is the initial presentation in most cases
- ☐ Lupus myelitis
- ☐ Aseptic meningitis
- ☐ Stiff person syndrome (SPS)

Psychiatric

- ☐ Anxiety
- ☐ Mood disorders
- ☐ Psychosis

Peripheral

- ☐ Cranial neuropathies
- ☐ Mononeuritis multiplex
- ☐ Mononeuropathy
- ☐ Small fiber neuropathy

Other features

- ☐ Headache
- ☐ Seizures
- ☐ Acute confusional state
- ☐ Cerebrovascular disease
- ☐ Cognitive dysfunction

RHEUMATOID MENINGITIS

Epidemiology

- ☐ This usually develops in long-standing rheumatoid arthritis (RA)
- ☐ It may be the presenting feature of RA
- ☐ It may be triggered by Adalimumab

Features of rheumatoid meningitis

- ☐ Stroke-like episodes
- ☐ Seizures
- ☐ Recurrent headaches
- ☐ Altered mental state
- ☐ Behavioural changes
- ☐ Cognitive decline
- ☐ Cranial neuropathies
- ☐ Parkinsonism

Features of rheumatoid pachymeningitis

- ☐ Seizures
- ☐ Focal neurological deficits
- ☐ Optic neuropathy
- ☐ Optic atrophy
- ☐ Deafness
- ☐ Painful ophthalmoplegia

Autoimmune tests

- ☐ Rheumatoid factor
- ☐ Anti-cyclic citrullinated peptide antibody

Magnetic resonance imaging (MRI) brain: features

- ☐ Leptomeningeal enhancement
- ☐ Periventricular white matter disease

Cerebrospinal fluid (CSF) analysis

- ☐ Raised white cell count

Brain biopsy: features

- ☐ Cortical lymphocytic vasculitis
- ☐ Patchy lymphoplasmacytic infiltration of dural small vessels
- ☐ Rheumatoid nodules

Treatment

- ☐ Steroids
- ☐ Cyclophosphamide
- ☐ Methotrexate

Treatment of rheumatoid pachymeningitis

- ☐ Immunosuppression
- ☐ Surgical decompression

SJOGREN'S SYNDROME: NEUROLOGICAL FEATURES

Demographic features

- ☐ Neurological features occur in 20% of cases
- ☐ These precede the diagnosis of Sjogren's syndrome in about 80–90% of cases
- ☐ Central nervous system (CNS) involvement occurs in more than 50% of cases
- ☐ Peripheral nerves are involved in >60% of cases

Variant presentations

- ☐ Relapsing-remitting multiple sclerosis (RRMS)-like presentation
- ☐ Primary progressive multiple sclerosis (PPMS)-like presentation
- ☐ Motor neuron disease (MND)-like presentation

Central features

- ☐ Encephalopathy: this runs an acute and recurrent course
- ☐ Seizures
- ☐ Aseptic meningitis
- ☐ Cognitive impairment
- ☐ Dementia
- ☐ Psychiatric disorders
- ☐ Myelopathy: this may be acute or chronic
- ☐ Cerebellar ataxia

Dorsal root ganglionopathy (DRG)

- ☐ This is usually a small fiber neuropathy with neuronal loss
- ☐ It presents with an unusual pattern of burning pain
- ☐ It is non-length dependent
- ☐ It involves the face, trunk, and proximal extremities
- ☐ Magnetic resonance neurography (MRN) may help in the diagnosis

Cranial mononeuropathies

- ☐ Trigeminal
- ☐ Facial
- ☐ Vestibulocochlear
- ☐ Optic

Peripheral neuropathy (PN): types

- ☐ Symmetric axonal sensorimotor polyneuropathy (PN)
- ☐ Sensory ataxic neuropathy
- ☐ Painful sensory neuropathy without sensory ataxia
- ☐ Multiple mononeuropathy
- ☐ Autonomic neuropathy

Other features

- ☐ Myositis

SYSTEMIC SCLEROSIS (SS): NEUROLOGICAL FEATURES

Central neurological features

- ☐ Headache
- ☐ Cognitive impairment
- ☐ Chorea
- ☐ Seizures
- ☐ Superficial siderosis: case report
- ☐ Compressive myelopathy: this is secondary to spinal calcinosis
- ☐ Acute cerebral vasculopathy: this is due to vasospasm

Psychiatric features

- ☐ Anxiety
- ☐ Depression

Peripheral neuropathy (PN)

- ☐ It is a non-length dependent neuropathy
- ☐ Large and small nerve fibers are affected
- ☐ It may be the presenting feature of systemic sclerosis
- ☐ There is associated autonomic neuropathy

Mononeuropathies

- ☐ Carpal tunnel syndrome (CTS)
- ☐ Mononeuropathy multiplex

Cranial neuropathies

- ☐ Trigeminal sensory neuropathy: this may be the presenting feature
- ☐ Trigeminal neuralgia (TN): this may be bilateral
- ☐ Glossopharyngeal
- ☐ Facial
- ☐ Vestibulochochlear

Myopathies

- ☐ Inclusion body myositis (IBM)
- ☐ Myopathy

Other features

- ☐ Autonomic neuropathy
- ☐ Brachial plexopathy

Synonym

- ☐ Scleroderma

Endocrine

THYROTOXICOSIS

Ophthalmological features

- [ ] Exophthalmic ophthalmoplegia
- [ ] Optic nerve lesions
- [ ] Retinopathy

Cerebral features

- [ ] Thyrotoxic crisis
- [ ] Encephalopathy
- [ ] Choreoathetosis
- [ ] Coma

Psychiatric features

- [ ] Psychosis
- [ ] Anxiety
- [ ] Depression

Vascular features

- [ ] Ischaemic stroke
- [ ] Cardioembolic stroke: from atrial fibrillation (AF)
- [ ] Reversible intracranial stenosis: this is similar to moyamoya disease
- [ ] Cerebral vein thrombosis (CVT)

Other features

- [ ] Proximal myopathy
- [ ] Cardiac syncope

Autoimmune neurological associations

- [ ] Myasthenia gravis (MG)
- [ ] Periodic paralysis

HYPOTHYROIDISM

Central neurological features

- [ ] Cognitive impairment
- [ ] Dementia
- [ ] Cerebellar dysfunction
- [ ] Epilepsy
- [ ] Coma
- [ ] Deafness
- [ ] Stroke: with autoimmune thyroiditis

Peripheral neuropathy

- [ ] Axonal peripheral neuropathy (PN)
- [ ] Carpal tunnel syndrome (CTS)

Muscle features

- [ ] Myopathy
- [ ] Pseudomyotonia
- [ ] Muscular hypertrophy
- [ ] Raised creatinine kinase (CK)
- [ ] Woltman's sign: this is delayed relaxation of the reflexes
  - It is also seen with pregnancy, anorexia nervosa, diabetes, and old age

Muscle syndromes

- [ ] Hoffman's syndrome
  - Subjects present with muscle hypertrophy, myoedema, and pain
- [ ] Kocher-Debre-Semelaigne syndrome
  - Affected subjects have a dysmorphic appearance
  - They present with painless muscle swellings

Psychiatric features

- [ ] Anxiety
- [ ] Depression
- [ ] Psychosis

DOI: 10.1201/9781003221258-126

DIABETIC NEUROPATHY: TYPES

Diabetic peripheral neuropathy types

- ☐ Sensorimotor polyneuropathy
- ☐ Autonomic neuropathy
- ☐ Polyneuropathy associated with glucose intolerance
- ☐ Acute painful diabetic neuropathy with weight loss
- ☐ Hypoglycaemic (hyperinsulinaemic) neuropathy
- ☐ Polyneuropathy after ketoacidosis
- ☐ Chronic inflammatory demyelinating polyneuropathy (CIDP)

Diabetic cranial neuropathy

- ☐ Abducens
- ☐ Oculomotor
- ☐ Trochlear
- ☐ Trigeminal

Diabetic mononeuropathy

- ☐ Median: carpal tunnel syndrome (CTS)
- ☐ Ulnar
- ☐ Peroneal
- ☐ Lateral femoral cutaneous: meralgia paraesthetica

Diabetic radiculopathy

- ☐ Diabetic thoracic radiculopathy
  - ○ This is symmetric and multi-dermatomal
  - ○ It results in abdominal wall weakness
- ☐ Diabetic lumbosacral radiculoplexus neuropathy
- ☐ Diabetic cervical radiculoplexus neuropathy: this is worse distally

Insulin neuritis

- ☐ This is treatment-induced neuropathy of diabetes
- ☐ It is a small fiber neuropathy
- ☐ It is acute onset
- ☐ It develops within 8 weeks of rapid correction of hyperglycaemia

Haematology

SICKLE CELL DISEASE (SCD): NEUROLOGICAL FEATURES

Stroke: types

- ☐ Ischaemic: these account for 75% of strokes in SCD
- ☐ Intracerebral haemorrhage (ICH)
- ☐ Subarachnoid haemorrhage (SAH)

Other haemorrhages

- ☐ Intraventricular (IVH)
- ☐ Subdural (SDH)
- ☐ Extradural

Acute painful crisis

- ☐ This results from vaso-occlusive crises
- ☐ Rapid treatment with opioids is indicated

Chronic pain

- ☐ This is pain occurring on most days for at least 6 months
- ☐ The pain is worse with palpation or movement
- ☐ It is associated with a reduced range of movement in the affected area

Other neurological features

- ☐ Cerebral aneurysms
- ☐ Headache
- ☐ Febrile seizures
- ☐ Central nervous system vasculopathy
- ☐ Cognitive impairment
- ☐ Sensory neuropathy
- ☐ Paraplegia
- ☐ Cerebral fat embolism (CFE)

HODGKIN'S LYMPHOMA: NEUROLOGICAL FEATURES

Parenchymal features

- ☐ Transient ischaemic attacks (TIAs)
- ☐ Stroke
- ☐ Cardioembolism: from cardiomyopathy
- ☐ Cranial nerve palsies
- ☐ Headache
- ☐ Weakness
- ☐ Papilloedema
- ☐ Seizures
- ☐ Cavernous sinus syndrome

Leptomeningeal features

- ☐ Cerebrospinal fluid (CSF) eosinophilia: this occurs frequently
- ☐ Reed-Sternberg cells may be seen in the CSF

Paraneoplastic features

- ☐ Paraneoplastic cerebellar degeneration: due to anti-Tr and anti mGLuR1 antibodies
- ☐ Limbic encephalitis: due to anti NMDAR antibodies
- ☐ Guillain–Barre syndrome (GBS)
- ☐ Chorea
- ☐ Ataxia
- ☐ Stiff person syndrome (SPS)
- ☐ Myasthenia gravis
- ☐ Central nervous system (CNS) vasculitis

Radiotherapy-related features

- ☐ Dropped head syndrome
- ☐ Premature carotid atherosclerosis
- ☐ Brachial plexopathy

Chemotherapy-related features

- ☐ Toxic peripheral neuropathy (PN)

Other affected sites

- ☐ Dural
- ☐ Epidural spinal cord
- ☐ Corpus callosum
- ☐ Pituitary

DOI: 10.1201/9781003221258-127

NON-HODGKIN'S LYMPHOMA (NHL): NEUROLOGICAL FEATURES

Guillain–Barre syndrome (GBS)

☐ GBS is the typical clinical presentation of NHL
☐ GBS may also result from Rituximab and Vincristine therapy

Spinal cord features

☐ Spinal cord compression
☐ Cauda equina compression

Peripheral nerve features

☐ IgM anti-MAG neuropathy
☐ Paraneoplastic peripheral neuropathy (PN)
☐ Pure sensory ganglionopathy

Neurolymphomatosis

☐ This is invasion of nerves by aggressive NHL
☐ It is usually caused by diffuse large cell B cell lymphoma (DLCBL)
☐ It may occur in the setting of Waldenstrom's macroglobulinaemia
☐ It presents with painful radiculopathy, plexopathy, or neuropathy
☐ It affects multiple cranial and peripheral nerves

Other features

☐ Meningeal infiltration

Nutritional

SUBACUTE COMBINED DEGENERATION (SCD)

Causes

- [ ] Pernicious anaemia
- [ ] Cobalamin C disease
- [ ] Nitrous oxide inhalation and anaesthesia
- [ ] Tripterygium glycoside: treatment for glomerulonephritis
- [ ] Vegan diet
- [ ] Crohn's disease
- [ ] Common variable immunodeficiency syndrome (CVID)
- [ ] Gastric cancer
- [ ] Gastric resection

Clinical features

- [ ] Dysaesthesias
- [ ] Gait disorder
- [ ] Spastic paraparesis
- [ ] Impaired vibration
- [ ] Impaired joint position sense
- [ ] Lhermitte's phenomenon
- [ ] Hydrocephalus: case report

Associated features of B12 deficiency

- [ ] Axonal or demyelinating peripheral neuropathy
- [ ] Cognitive impairment
- [ ] Neuropsychiatric features, e.g. depression
- [ ] Optic atrophy
- [ ] Spinal myoclonus
- [ ] Pancytopaenia

Magnetic resonance imaging (MRI): features

- [ ] Inverted V sign: this is symmetrical high signal in the dorsal columns
  - ○ It may also involve the anterior columns
- [ ] Syringomyelia: case reports
- [ ] The MRI may be normal

Differential diagnosis

- [ ] Copper deficiency myelopathy

Treatment

- [ ] Cobalamin

ALCOHOL SYNDROMES: CLASSIFICATION

Direct alcohol effects

- [ ] Acute intoxication
- [ ] Alcohol withdrawal syndrome
- [ ] Delirium tremens
- [ ] Wernicke encephalopathy
- [ ] Korsakoff syndrome
- [ ] Alcohol hangover
- [ ] Alcoholic blackouts
- [ ] Alcoholic grayouts
- [ ] Alcoholic amblyopia
- [ ] Alcoholic myelopathy

Alcohol-related movement disorders

- [ ] Chorea
- [ ] Orolingual dyskinesia
- [ ] Akathisia
- [ ] Cerebellar ataxia
- [ ] Asterixis: from hepatic failure

Alcohol withdrawal-related movement disorders

- [ ] Alcohol tremor
- [ ] Transient Parkinsonism: this also occurs with heavy drinking
- [ ] Transient dyskinesias: this is also seen with heavy alcohol abuse

Metabolic syndromes

- [ ] Hepatic encephalopathy
- [ ] Effects of hypoglycaemia
- [ ] Foetal alcohol syndrome
- [ ] Alcoholic pellagra encephalopathy
- [ ] Acquired hepatocerebral degeneration: with bilateral globus pallidus lesions

Degenerative and demyelinating syndromes

- [ ] Osmotic demyelination disorder (ODD)
- [ ] Extra pontine myelinolysis
- [ ] Marchiafava-Bignami syndrome: demyelination and necrosis of the corpus callosum
- [ ] Neurodegenerative dementia
- [ ] Alcoholic cerebellar degeneration

Other alcohol syndromes

- [ ] Peripheral neuropathy (PN): motor, sensory, and autonomic
- [ ] Optic neuropathy occasionally
- [ ] Cerebellar cognitive affective disorders
- [ ] Haemorrhagic strokes
- [ ] Subacute encephalopathy with seizures in alcoholics (SESA)
- [ ] Traumatic brain injury (TBI)

DOI: 10.1201/9781003221258-128

Alcohol-triggered neurological disorders

- [ ] Paroxysmal non kinesigenic dyskinesia (PNKD)
- [ ] Ocular neuromyotonia
- [ ] Migraine
- [ ] Cluster headaches (CH)
- [ ] Porphyria

BARIATRIC SURGERY: NEUROLOGICAL SYNDROMES

Peripheral neuropathies

- [ ] Acute post-gastric surgery (APGARS) neuropathy: burning feet
- [ ] Isolated neuropathy
- [ ] Isolated myeloneuropathy
- [ ] Axonal Guillain–Barre syndrome (GBS)-like syndrome
- [ ] Optic neuropathy
- [ ] Radiculoplexopathy

Mononeuropathies

- [ ] Carpal tunnel syndrome (CTS)
- [ ] Meralgia paraesthetica

Stretch and traumatic injuries

- [ ] Brachial plexus
- [ ] Ulnar nerve
- [ ] Compression injuries

Other neurological syndromes

- [ ] Encephalopathy
- [ ] Myelopathy
- [ ] Myopathy
- [ ] Gastroparesis
- [ ] Excess vagal simulation
- [ ] Wernicke-Korsakoff syndrome

Prevention

- [ ] Thiamine 100 mg daily in the first year after surgery
- [ ] Monitor blood 6-monthly for other nutritional deficiencies

GLUTEN SENSITIVITY NEUROLOGY

Movement disorders

- [ ] Cerebellar ataxia
- [ ] Progressive ataxia with palatal tremor (PAPT)
- [ ] Stimulus sensitive foot myoclonus
- [ ] Myoclonus ataxia

Gobbi syndrome

- [ ] Coeliac disease, epilepsy, and cerebral calcifications (CEC)
- [ ] It presents with occipital epilepsy: this is usually drug-resistant
- [ ] There are associated cerebral calcifications
- [ ] It is most frequent in Italy, Spain, and Argentina

Other epilepsy syndromes

- [ ] Childhood partial epilepsy with occipital paroxysms
- [ ] Fixation off sensitivity (FOS)
- [ ] Temporal lobe epilepsy (TLE) with hippocampal sclerosis

Other central neurological features

- [ ] Visual impairment: with cerebral calcifications
- [ ] Headaches
- [ ] Dementia
- [ ] Myelopathy
- [ ] Stiff person syndrome (SPS)

Psychiatric features

- [ ] Gluten psychosis
- [ ] Depression

Peripheral neurological features

- [ ] Neuromyotonia
- [ ] Myopathy
- [ ] Inclusion body myositis (IBM)
- [ ] Peripheral neuropathy (PN)

Restless legs syndrome (RLS)

- [ ] This is present in about a third of cases
- [ ] It is possibly due to iron deficiency

Magnetic resonance imaging (MRI) features

- [ ] White matter abnormalities
- [ ] Reduced cerebellar volume
- [ ] Cerebral calcifications

Disputed gluten sensitivity syndromes

- [ ] Ataxia
- [ ] Peripheral neuropathy (PN)
- [ ] Central nervous system (CNS) demyelination

Synonym

- [ ] Coeliac disease

Renal

URAEMIC ENCEPHALOPATHY

Cognitive features

- [ ] Fluctuating cognition
- [ ] Impaired concentration

Frontal lobe dysfunction

- [ ] Paratonia
- [ ] Grasp reflex
- [ ] Palmomental reflex

Movement disorders

- [ ] Multifocal myoclonus
- [ ] Asterixis
- [ ] Tremor
- [ ] Clumsiness

Neuropsychiatric features

- [ ] Apathy
- [ ] Delirium
- [ ] Hallucinations
- [ ] Emotional lability
- [ ] Depression
- [ ] Anxiety
- [ ] Suicide

Pyramidal features

- [ ] Alternating hemiparesis
- [ ] Spasticity
- [ ] Sleep inversion

Other features

- [ ] Fatigue
- [ ] Meningism
- [ ] Seizures
- [ ] Coma

Electroencephalogram (EEG)

- [ ] Triphasic waves
- [ ] Slowing of alpha rhythm
- [ ] Excess of delta and theta waves

RENAL DIALYSIS: NEUROLOGICAL COMPLICATIONS

Vascular complications

- [ ] Intracerebral haemorrhage (ICH)
- [ ] Cerebral vein thrombosis (CVT)
- [ ] Anterior ischaemic optic neuropathy (AION
- [ ] Posterior reversible encephalopathy syndrome (PRES)

Sleep impairments

- [ ] Insomnia
- [ ] Excessive daytime sleepiness (EDS)
- [ ] Sleep apnoea

Peripheral complications

- [ ] Nerve injury: this is secondary to vascular access
- [ ] Carpal tunnel syndrome (CTS): this is due to β2 microglobulin amyloidosis
- [ ] Peripheral neuropathy (PN)

Wernicke's encephalopathy: risk factors

- [ ] Anorexia
- [ ] Vomiting
- [ ] Intravenous alimentation
- [ ] Glucose loading
- [ ] Infections

Other neurological complications of dialysis

- [ ] Dialysis disequilibrium syndrome: this occurs in early dialysis sessions
- [ ] Dialysis dementia: this is due to aluminium overload
- [ ] Osmotic demyelination disorder (ODD): pontine and extrapontine
- [ ] Restless legs syndrome (RLS)
- [ ] Papilloedema
- [ ] Cognitive impairment
- [ ] Drug toxicity
- [ ] Hypotension
- [ ] Haemodialysis headache

Imaging features

- [ ] White matter changes
- [ ] Cerebral atrophy

DOI: 10.1201/9781003221258-129

Vasculitis

VASCULITIS: CLASSIFICATION

Large vessel vasculitis

- [ ] Giant cell arteritis (GCA)
- [ ] Takayasu's arteritis

Medium vessel vasculitis

- [ ] Polyarteritis nodosa (PAN)
- [ ] Kawasaki's disease

Small vessel vasculitis: ANCA associated (AAV)

- [ ] Granulomatosis with polyangiitis (GPA)
- [ ] Eosinophilic granulomatosis with polyangiitis (EGPA)
- [ ] Microscopic polyangiitis

Small vessel vasculitis: others

- [ ] Henoch Schonlein purpura (HSP)
- [ ] Hypersensitivity vasculitis (leukocytoclastic vasculitis)
- [ ] Cryoglobulinaemic vasculitis

Variable vessel vasculitis

- [ ] Behcet's disease
- [ ] Cogan's disease

Single organ vasculitis

- [ ] Cutaneous leukocytoclastic angiitis
- [ ] Cutaneous arteritis
- [ ] Primary central nervous system vasculitis
- [ ] Isolated aortitis

Vasculitis with systemic diseases

- [ ] Lupus
- [ ] Rheumatoid
- [ ] Sarcoid

Vasculitis with probable aetiology

- [ ] Hepatitis B virus (HBV)
- [ ] Hepatitis C virus (HCV)
- [ ] Syphilis
- [ ] Drug-induced
- [ ] Cancer-related

Other primary vasculitis syndromes

- [ ] Relapsing polychondritis
- [ ] Eales' disease

VASCULITIS: MANIFESTATIONS

Systemic symptoms

- [ ] Fever
- [ ] Weight loss
- [ ] Weakness
- [ ] Malaise
- [ ] Arthralgia and myalgia

Features of large vessel vasculitis

- [ ] Temporal headache
- [ ] Blindness
- [ ] Claudication: jaw and limb
- [ ] Absent pulses
- [ ] Unequal limb blood pressures
- [ ] Arterial bruits
- [ ] Aortic dilatation
- [ ] Aneurysms

Features of medium vessel vasculitis

- [ ] Ulcers and necrotic lesions
- [ ] Nail fold infarcts
- [ ] Nail crusting
- [ ] Livido reticularis
- [ ] Nodules
- [ ] Digital gangrene
- [ ] Abdominal pain
- [ ] Gastrointestinal bleeding
- [ ] Intestinal perforation
- [ ] Infarction: gut, kidneys, liver, spleen, pancreas
- [ ] Angina
- [ ] Acute myocardial infarction (AMI)
- [ ] Coronary artery aneurysms
- [ ] Ischaemic cardiomyopathy
- [ ] Necrotic lung lesions
- [ ] Epistaxis
- [ ] Sinusitis
- [ ] Deafness
- [ ] Stridor
- [ ] Microaneurysms
- [ ] Mononeuritis multiplex

Features of small vessel vasculitis

- [ ] Palpable purpura
- [ ] Ecchymoses
- [ ] Vesicles and bullae
- [ ] Splinter haemorrhages
- [ ] Uveitis
- [ ] Episcleritis
- [ ] Renal function impairment with haematuria and proteinuria
- [ ] Red cell casts
- [ ] Pulmonary haemorrhage

DOI: 10.1201/9781003221258-130

GIANT CELL ARTERITIS (GCA): CLINICAL FEATURES

Phenotypes

- [ ] Cranial arteritis
- [ ] Polymyalgia rheumatica (PMR)
- [ ] Large vessel vasculitis
- [ ] Systemic inflammatory disease
- [ ] Arteritic anterior ischaemic optic neuropathy (AAION)

Systemic features

- [ ] Scalp pain and tenderness: sudden onset
- [ ] Temporal artery abnormality: tender, thick, and reduced pulsation
- [ ] Fever: this may present as pyrexia of unknown origin (PUO)
- [ ] Weight loss
- [ ] Polymyalgia rheumatica (PMR)
- [ ] Intermittent claudication: jaw, tongue, limbs
- [ ] Increased risk of venous thromboembolism (VTE)
- [ ] Cough
- [ ] Aortic aneurysms
- [ ] Carotidynia

Ophthalmological features

- [ ] Amaurosis fugax
- [ ] Blindness with pale discs
- [ ] Blurred vision
- [ ] Diplopia
- [ ] Anisocoria
- [ ] Visual field defects
- [ ] Cough-induced transient blindness
- [ ] Arteritic anterior ischeamic optic neuropathy (AION)
- [ ] Central retinal artery occlusion (CRAO)
- [ ] Cilioretinal artery occlusion

Neurological features

- [ ] Headache
- [ ] Multiple cranial nerve palsies
- [ ] Hearing loss
- [ ] Stroke
- [ ] Guillain–Barre syndrome (GBS)
- [ ] Mononeuritis multiplex

Differential diagnosis

- [ ] Herpes zoster
- [ ] Migraine
- [ ] Transient ischaemic attack (TIA)
- [ ] Cluster headache (CH)
- [ ] Temporo-mandibular joint (TMJ) pain
- [ ] Pterygoid myositis
- [ ] Other causes of systemic vasculitis

Synonym

- [ ] Temporal arteritis

Surgery

NEUROLOGICAL COMPLICATIONS OF CARDIAC SURGERY

Stroke: risk factors

- ☐ Age >75 years
- ☐ Chronic renal insufficiency
- ☐ Recent myocardial infarction
- ☐ Previous stroke
- ☐ Carotid artery disease
- ☐ Hypertension
- ☐ Diabetes mellitus
- ☐ Moderate to severe left ventricular dysfunction
- ☐ Low cardiac output syndrome
- ☐ Atrial fibrillation (AF)

Stroke: risk prediction

- ☐ The highest risk is in the early post-operative period
- ☐ The CHADS2 score accurately predicts stroke risk
- ☐ The risk persists for 2 years

Encephalopathy: causes

- ☐ Microemboli
- ☐ Hypoperfusion
- ☐ Postoperative atrial fibrillation

Miscellaneous complications

- ☐ Cerebral fat embolism (CFE)
- ☐ Post-operative cognitive dysfunction (POCD)
- ☐ Dementia

NEUROLOGICAL COMPLICATIONS OF ORGAN TRANSPLANTATION

Demographic features

- ☐ Neurological complications develop in about a third of transplant recipients
- ☐ These are most frequent following liver transplantation

Causes and risk factors

- ☐ Opportunistic infections
- ☐ Immunosuppressive drug neurotoxicity
- ☐ Metabolic derangements
- ☐ Electrolyte abnormalities
- ☐ Underlying infections

Vascular complications

- ☐ Posterior reversible encephalopathy syndrome (PRES)
- ☐ Intracranial haemorrhage (ICH)
- ☐ Stroke

Neoplastic complications

- ☐ Post-transplantation lymphoproliferative disorder (PTLD)
- ☐ Lymphoma

Post-transplant autoimmune encephalitis

- ☐ Anti-NMDAR psychosis and orofacial dyskinesia
- ☐ Anti-AMPAR limbic encephalitis

Other neurological complications

- ☐ Seizures
- ☐ Metabolic encephalopathy
- ☐ Opportunistic infections
- ☐ Immune reconstitution inflammatory syndrome (IRIS)
- ☐ Drug neurotoxicity

Calcineurin-inhibitor neurotoxicity: features

- ☐ Posterior reversible encephalopathy syndrome (PRES)
- ☐ Optic neuropathy
- ☐ Tumefactive demyelination
- ☐ Osmotic demyelination disorder (ODD)
- ☐ Psychiatric features: akinetic mutism, catatonia, delusions, fugue-like states, mood changes
- ☐ Movement disorders: tremor, ataxia, and dystonia-Parkinsonism
- ☐ Peripheral neuropathy (PN)
- ☐ Peroneal neuropathy
- ☐ Brachial plexopathy
- ☐ Insomnia
- ☐ Headache: this may be acute onset
- ☐ Seizures: these may present as status epilepticus
- ☐ Cortical blindness

DOI: 10.1201/9781003221258-131

Magnetic resonance imaging (MRI): features

☐ Posterior reversible leukoencephalopathy syndrome (PRES)
☐ Osmotic demyelination disorders (ODD)
☐ Intracerebral haemorrhage (ICH)
☐ Abscesses
☐ Tumours

Neurochecklists complete index of online topics

DOI: 10.1201/9781003221258-132

BH. EPILEPSY MANAGEMENT

BH1. Epilepsy general management
BH2. Antiepileptic drugs (AEDs): management guidelines
BH3. Antiepileptic drugs (AEDs): major types
BH4. Antiepileptic drugs (AEDs): other types
BH5. Epilepsy interventional treatments
BH6. Epilepsy outcome

C. SLEEP DISORDERS

CA. SLEEP DISORDERS: GENERAL ASPECTS

CA1. Sleep disorders: classification and differentials
CA2. Sleep investigations

CB. PRIMARY SLEEP DISORDERS

CB1. Narcolepsy
CB2. Insomnia
CB3. Hypersomnia
CB4. Circadian rhythm sleep disorders (CRSD)

CC. REM SLEEP PARASOMNIAS

CC1. REM sleep behaviour disorder (RBD)
CC2. Anti IgLON5 antibody syndrome
CC3. Other REM sleep parasomnias

CD. OTHER SLEEP DISORDERS

CD1. Non-REM sleep parasmonias
CD2. Kleine-Levin syndrome (KLS)
CD3. Sleep violence
CD4. Sleep and neurological disorders

E. NEUROINFLAMMATORY AND AUTOIMMUNE DISORDERS

EA. MULTIPLE SCLEROSIS (MS)

EA1. Relapsing remitting multiple sclerosis (RRMS)
EA2. Primary progressive multiple sclerosis (PPMS)
EA3. Clinically isolated syndromes (CIS)
EA4. Multiple sclerosis (MS): investigations
EA5. Multiple sclerosis (MS): general treatments
EA6. Multiple sclerosis (MS): treatments guidelines
EA7. Multiple sclerosis (MS) treatments agents

EB. NEUROMYELITIS OPTICA (NMO)

EB1. Neuromyelitis optica (NMO): clinical aspects
EB2. Neuromyelitis optica (NMO): management

EC. NEUROSARCOIDOSIS

EC1. Neurosarcoidosis: clinical aspects
EC2. Neurosarcoidosis: management

ED. OTHER NEUROINFLAMMATORY DISORDERS

ED1. Acute disseminated encephalomyelitis (ADEM)
ED2. Behcet's syndrome
ED3. CLIPPERS
ED4. Anti MOG antibody disorders
ED5. Progressive multifocal leukoencephalopathy (PML)
ED6. Biotidinase deficiency
ED7. Miscellaneous neuroinflammatory disorders

EE. AUTOIMMUNE ENCEPHALITIS

EE1. Anti LGI1 VGKC autoimmune encephalitis
EE2. Anti CASPR2 VGKC autoimmune encephalitis
EE3. Anti NMDAR autoimmune encephalitis
EE4. Anti-glycine receptor syndrome
EE5. Anti GFAP autoimmune encephalitis
EE6. Anti DPPX autoimmune encephalitis
EE7. IgG4-related disease
EE8. Other autoimmune encephalitis

EF. PERIPHERAL AUTOIMMUNE DISORDERS

EF1. Neuromyotonia
EF2. Stiff person syndrome (SPS)
EF3. Peripheral nerve hyperexcitability (PNH)

F. INFECTIONS

FA. VIRAL INFECTIONS

FA1. Viral meningitis
FA2. Viral encephalitis
FA3. Viral myelitis
FA4. HIV
FA5. Tropical spastic paraparesis (TSP)
FA6. Hepatitis infections
FA7. Influenza
FA8. Rabies
FA9. Zika virus infection (ZIKV)
FA10. Ebola virus disease (EVD)
FA11. Coronavirus SARS-CoV-2
FA12. Varicella zoster virus (VZV)
FA13. Dengue virus (DENV)
FA14. West Nile virus (WNV)
FA15. Subacute sclerosing pan-encephalitis (SSPE)
FA16. Herpes simplex virus 2 (HSV2)
FA17. Japanese encephalitis virus (JEV)
FA18. Chikungunya virus (CHIK)
FA19. Miscellaneous viral infections

FB. BACTERIAL INFECTIONS

FB1. Bacterial meningitis
FB2. Tuberculosis (TB)
FB3. Lyme neuroborreliosis
FB4. Neurosyphilis
FB5. Neurobrucellosis
FB6. Leprosy
FB7. Whipple's disease
FB8. Tetanus
FB9. Botulism
FB10. Listeria
FB11. Miscellaneous bacterial infections

FC. PARASITIC INFECTIONS

FC1a. Parasitic infections: classification and general features
FC2. Cerebral malaria
FC3. Neurocysticercosis
FC4. Neuroschistosomiasis
FC5. Onchocerciasis
FC6. Trypanosomiasis
FC7. Toxoplasmosis
FC8. Primary amoebic meningoencephalitis (PAM)
FC9. Cerebral echinoccosis (hydatid disease)
FC10. Toxocariasis
FC11. Neurosparganosis
FC12. Neurognathostomiasis
FC13. Neuroangiostrongyliasis

FD. FUNGAL INFECTIONS

FD1. Fungal infections: classification and general features
FD2. Crypotcoccal meningitis
FD3. Histoplasmosis
FD4. Aspergillosis
FD5. Coccidiodomycosis

H. VASCULAR DISORDERS

HA. ISCHAEMIC STROKE

HA1. Transient ischaemic attacks (TIA)
HA2. Ischaemic stroke risk factors
HA3. Ischaemic stroke: clinical features
HA4. Ischaemic stroke: complications
HA5. Ischaemic stroke variants
HA6. Posterior circulation stroke
HA7. Stroke in the young
HA8. Embolic and cryptogenic stroke
HA9. Spinal cord infarction (SCI)
HA10. Ischaemic stroke imaging
HA11. Ischaemic stroke acute treatment
HA12. Ischaemic stroke medical management
HA13. Carotid artery treatments

HB. HAEMORRHAGIC STROKE

HB1. Intracerebral haemorrhage (ICH)
HB2. Anticoagulant-induced intracerebral haemorrhage (ICH)
HB3. Subarachnoid haemorrhage (SAH)

HC. VASCULAR MALFORMATIONS

HC1. Cerebral aneurysms
HC2. Arteriovenous malformations (AVM)
HC3. Cerebral cavernous malformations (cavernomas)
HC4. Dural arteriovenous fistula (DAVF)
HC5. Cerebrofaical arteriovenous metameric
    syndrome (CAMS)

HD. VASCULOPATHIES

HD1. Cervical artery dissection (CAD)
HD2. Cerebral amyloid angiopathy (CAA)
HD3. Reversible cerebral vasoconstriction syndrome (RCVS)
HD4. Primary angiitis of the central nervous system (PACNS)
HD5. CADASIL and CARASIL
HD6. Collagen 4 (COL4) mutation
HD7. Intracranial arterial dolichoectasia (IADE)
HD8. Carotidynia
HD9. Retinal vasculopathy with cerebral
    leukoencephalopathy (RVCL)
HD10. Miscellaneous vasculopathies

HE. VENOUS DISRODERS

HE1. Cerebral vein thrombosis (CVT)
HE2. Cavernous sinus related syndromes
HE3. Vein of Galen aneurysmal malformation (VGAM)

HF. SMALL VESSEL DISORDERS

HF1. Small vessel disease (SVD)
HF2. Cerebral microbleeds
HM4. Susac syndrome

HG. MISCELLANEOUS VASCULAR DISORDERS

HG1. Superficial siderosis (SS)
HG2. Moyamoya disease

I. CRANIAL NERVE DISORDERS

IA. OPTIC NERVE

IA1. Optic neuropathy
IA2. Optic neuritis
IA3. Ischaemic optic neuropathy
IA4. Optic atrophy

IB. TRIGEMINAL NERVE

IB1. Trigeminal neuropathy
IB2. Trigeminal neuralgia (TN)
IB3. Numb chin syndrome (NCS)
IB4. Other trigeminal nerve disorders

IC. FACIAL NERVE

IC1. Facial nerve palsy
IC2. Bell's palsy
IC3. Parry Romberg syndrome (PRS)
IC4. Miscellaneous facial nerve disorders

ID. VAGUS NERVE

ID1. Vagus nerve palsy
ID2. Dysphonia

IE. VESTIBULOCHOCHLEAR NERVE

IE1. Vestibulochochlear nerve dysfunction
IE2. Acute vestibular neuronitis

IF. OTHER CRANIAL NERVES

IF1. Olfactory nerve
IF2. Oculomotor nerve
IF3. Trochlear nerve
IF4. Abducens nerve
IF5. Glossopharyngeal nerve
IF6. Accessory nerve
IF7. Hypoglossal nerve

IG. CRANIAL NERVE ASSOCIATED DISORDERS

IG1. Taste dysfunction
IG2. Ophthalmoplegia
IG3. Congenital cranial dysinnervation disorders (CCDD)

L. ROOTS AND PLEXUS DISORDERS

LA. RADICULAR DISORDERS

LA1. Radiculopathy
LA2. Thoracic outlet syndrome (TOS)

LB. PLEXUS DISORDERS

LB1. Brachial plexopathy
LB2. Brachial neuralgia
LB3. Lumbosacral plexopathy

M. PERIPHERAL NERVE DISORDERS

MA. NEUROPATHY CAUSES AND CLINICAL ASSESSMENTS

MA1. Neuropathy causes by dominant features
MA2. Neuropathy causes by associated features
MA3. Neuropathy assessment

MB. AXONAL NEUROPATHY

MB1. Chronic idiopathic axonal polyneuropathy (CIAP)
MB2. Small fiber neuropathy
MB3. Autonomic neuropathy
MB4. Drug-induced and toxic neuropathy
MB5. Chemotherapy-induced neuropathy
MB6. Vasculitic neuropathy
MB7. Sensory neuronopathy
MB8. Electrical and lightening injuries
MB9. Miscellaneous axonal neuropathies

MC. ACQUIRED DEMYELINATING NEUROPATHIES

MC1. Demyelinating neuropathy: general aspects
MC2. Guillain–Barre syndrome (GBS)
MC3. Miller Fisher syndrome (MFS)
MC4. Bickerstaff brainstem encephalitis (BBE)
MC5. CIDP
MC6. Multifocal motor neuropathy (MMN)

MD. CHARCOT–MARIE–TOOTH DISEASE (CMT)

MD1. Charcot–Marie–Tooth disease (CMT): general aspects
MD2. Charcot–Marie–Tooth disease type 1 (CMT1)
MD3. Charcot–Marie–Tooth disease type 2 (CMT2)
MD4. Charcot–Marie–Tooth disease type 4 (CMT4)
MD5. Charcot–Marie–Tooth disease type X (CMTX)
MD6. Charcot–Marie–Tooth disease (CMT): other types

ME. OTHER HEREDITARY NEUROPATHIES

ME1. Hereditary sensory and autonomic neuropathy (HSAN)
ME2. Familial amyloid polyneuropathy (FAP)
ME3. HNPP
ME4. Distal hereditary motor neuropathy (dHMN)
ME5. Erythromelalgia
ME6. Miscellaneous hereditary neuropathies

MF. PARAPROTEINAEMIC NEUROPATHIES

MF1. Paraproteinaemic neuropathy
MF2. POEMS syndrome
MF3. Systemic amyloid neuropathy

MG. MONONEUROPATHIES

MG1. Median nerve
MG2. Ulnar nerve
MG3. Radial nerve
MG4. Femoral nerve
MG5. Sciatic nerve
MG6. Peroneal nerve
MG7. Tibial nerve
MG8. Long thoracic nerve
MG9. Greater auricular

O. MUSCLE DISORDERS

OA. MUSCLE SYMPTOMS AND SIGNS

OA1. Muscle weakness
OA2. Muscle atrophy
OA3. Muscle hypertrophy
OA4. Muscle signs
OA5. Gait disorders and falls
OA6. Neurological fatigue

OB. INFLAMMATORY MYOPATHIES

OB1. Inflammatory myopathy: classification and differentials
OB2. Inflammatory myopathy antibodies
OB3. Dermatomyositis
OB4. Immune mediated necrotising myopathy (IMNM)
OB5. Inclusion body myositis (IBM)
OB6. Focal myositis (FM)
OB7. Other inflammatory myopathies
OB8. Cancer associated myositis (CAM)
OB9. Inflammatory myopathy: management

OC. GLYCOGEN STORAGE DISEASES (GSD)

OC1. Pompe disease (GSD type II)
OC2. Cori disease (GSD type III)
OC3. McArdle's disease (GSD type V)
OC4. Other glycogen storage diseases

OD. LIPID STORAGE MYOPATHIES

OD1. Carnitine palmitoyl transferase (CPT II) deficiency
OD2. Multiple acyl-CoA dehydrogenase deficiency (MADD)
OD3. Neutral lipid storage disease
OD4. Other lipid storage myopathies

OE. MUSCLE CHANNELOPATHIES

OE1. Neurological channelopathies: general aspects
OE2. Hypokalaemic periodic paralysis
OE3. Hyperkalaemic periodic paralysis
OE4. Thyrotoxic periodic paralysis
OE5. Secondary periodic paralysis
OE6. Muscle hyperexcitability syndromes
OE7. Ryanodine receptor type 1 (RYR1) muscle disorders
OE8. Non-dystrophic myotonias

OF. CONGENITAL MYOPATHIES

OF1. Congenital myopathy classification
OF2. Core myopathy
OF3. Nemaline myopathy
OF4. Centronuclear myopathy (CNM)
OF5. Other congenital myopathies

OG. OTHER MYOPATHY SYNDROMES

OG1. Myofibrillar myopathy (MFM)
OG2. Distal myopathies
OG3. Myosinopathies
OG4. Autophagic vacuolar myopathy
OG5. Multisystem proteinopathy
OG6. Amyloid myopathy
OG7. Compartment syndrome
OG8. Miscellaneous myopathies

OH. DRUG-INDUCED MYOPATHIES

OH1. Drug-induced myopathies: classification
OH2. Statin myopathy
OH3. Steroid myopathy
OH4. Immune checkpoint inhibitors (ICI) toxicity

OI. CRAMPS AND RHABDOMYOLYSIS

OI1. Cramp disorders
OI2. Rhabdomyolysis

OJ. MUSCULAR DYSTROPHY

OJ1. Muscular dystrophy classes
OJ2. Duchenne muscular dystrophy (DMD)
OJ3. Becker muscular dystrophy (BMD)
OJ4. Facioscapulohumeral muscular dystrophy (FSHD)
OJ5. Limb girdle muscular dystrophy type 1 (LGMD1)
OJ6. Limb girdle muscular dystrophy type 2 (LGMD2)
OJ7. Limb girdle muscular dystrophy (LGMD): key features and management
OJ8. Emery–Dreifuss muscular dystrophy (EDMD)
OJ9. Myotonic dystrophy type 1
OJ10. Myotonic dystrophy type 2
OJ11. Congenital muscular dystrophy (CMD)
OJ12. Oculopharyngeal muscular dystrophy (OPMD)
OJ13. Scapuloperoneal muscular dystrophy

OK. MUSCLE INVESTIGATIONS

OK1. Creatinine kinase (CK)
OK2. Muscle imaging
OK3. Electromyogram (EMG)
OK4. Other muscle investigations

R. MITOCHONDRIAL DISORDERS

RA. MITOCHONDRIAL DISORDERS: FEATURES AND PHENOTYPES

RA1. Mitochondrial diseases: clinical features
RA2. Mitochondrial diseases: phenotypes

RB. NEUROLOGICAL MITOCHONDRIAL DISORDERS

RB1. CPEO AND KSS
RB2. Leber hereditary optic neuropathy (LHON)
RB3. Mitochondrial optic atrophy syndromes
RB4. MELAS
RB5. MERRF
RB6. POLG

RC. OTHER MITOCHONDRIAL DISORDERS

RC1. MNGIE
RC2. Leigh syndrome
RC3. Mitochondrial tRNAse syndromes
RC4. Miscellaneous mitochondrial disorders

RD. MITOCHONDRIAL DISEASES MANAGEMENT

RD1. Mitochondrial diseases: investigations and surveillance
RD2. Mitochondrial diseases: treatment

S. DEVELOPMENTAL DISORDERS

SA. SYSTEMIC DEVELOPMENTAL DISORDERS

SA1. Cerebral palsy
SA2. Autism spectrum disorders (ASD)

SB. INTRACRANIAL DEVELOPMENTAL DISORDERS

SB1. Malformations of cortical development (MCD)
SB2. Arachnoid cysts
SB3. Cerebral hemiatrophy
SB4. Posterior fossa developmental disorders

SC. CORPUS CALLOSUM DISORDERS

SC1. Agenesis of the corpus callosum
SC2. Other corpus callosum disorders

SD. CRANIAL DEVELOPMENTAL DISORDERS

SD1. Microcephaly
SD2. Macrocephaly: classification
SD3. Macrocephaly syndromes
SD4. Cranial sutural disorders

SE. SPINAL DEVELOPMENTAL DISORDERS

SE1. Chiari malformation
SE2. Spina bifida
SE3. Other spinal developmental disorders

SF. CILIOPATHIES

SF1. Ciliopathies classification
SF2. Oral-facial-digital syndrome (OFDS)
SF3. Meckel Gruber syndrome (MGS)

SG. NEUROCHRISTOPATHIES

SG1. Neurocristopathies: pathology and classification
SG2. Waardenburg syndrome
SG3. Treacher Collins syndrome (TCS)

SH. RASOPATHIES

SH1. Rasopathies classification
SH2. Rasopathy syndromes

SI. OTHER DEVELOPMENTAL DISORDERS

SI1. Tubilinopathies
SI2. Poland syndrome
SI3. Telomere biology disorders (TBD)
SI4. Synaesthesia

T. ALLIED NEUROLOGICAL DISORDERS

TA. NEUROPHTHALMOLOGY

TA1. Pupillary disorders
TA2. Horner's syndrome
TA3. Retinal disorders
TA4. Retinal vascular disorders
TA5. Visual hallucinations
TA6. Miscellaneous neuro-ophthalmology symptoms
TA7. Miscellaneous neuro-ophthalmology disorders

TB. NEUROTOLOGY

TB1. Dizziness
TB2. Vertigo
TB3. Tinnitus
TB5. Nystagmus
TB6. Mal de debarquement syndrome (MDDS)
TB7. Vestibular paroxysmia (VP)
TB8. Miscellaneous neurotology syndromes

TC. PSYCHIATRY

TC1. Delusions
TC2. Delusional misidentification: major syndromes
TC3. Attention deficit hyperactivity disorder (ADHD)
TC4. Miscellaneous psychiatry disorders

TD. NEUROSURGERY

TD1. Traumatic brain injury (TBI)
TD2. Sport-related concussion (SRC)
TD3. Normal pressure hydrocephalus (NPH)
TD4. Miscellaneous neurosurgical disorders

TE. PAIN MANAGEMENT

TE1. Complex regional pain syndrome (CRPS)
TE2. Facial pain
TE3. Neuropathic pain
TE4. Back pain
TE5. Burning mouth syndrome
TE6. Neuropathic itch
TE7. Miscellaneous pain disorders

TF. NEURORADIOLOGY

TF1. White matter lesions (WML)
TF2. Cerebral calcification
TF3. Neuroradiological lesions by location
TF4. Neuroradiological signs
TF5. Radiation necrosis
TF6. Perivascular spaces (PVS)
TF7. Toxic metabolic disorders imaging
TF8. Gadolinium-based contrast agents (GBCA)
TF9. Miscellaneous neuroradiology

TG. NEUROGENETICS

TG1. Genetic counselling
TG2. Chromosomal disorders
TG3. Trinucleotide repeat disorders
TG4. X-linked mental retardation disorders

TH. NEUROPHARMACOLOGY

TH1. Intravenous immunoglobulins (IVIg)
TH2. Immunosuppressants
TH3. Warfarin
TH4. New oral anticoagulants (NOACs)
TH5. Anticoagulants and surgery
TH6. Vaccinations
TH7. Miscellaneous neurological therapies

TI. OBSTETRIC NEUROLOGY

TI1. Pregnancy and preeclampsia
TI2. Pregnancy and epilepsy
TI3. Pregnancy and headaches
TI4. Pregnancy and stroke
TI5. Pregnancy and myasthenia gravis (MG)
TI6. Pregnancy and multiple sclerosis (MS)
TI7. Pregnancy and arteriovenous malformations (AVMs)
TI8. Pregnancy and other neurological disorders

TJ. FUNCTIONAL NEUROLOGY

TJ1. Functional neurological disorders (FND): general aspects
TJ2. Functional physical disorders
TJ3. Functional movement disorders
TJ4. Functional seizures
TJ5. Functional cognitive impairment

TK. NEUROTOXICITY

TK1. Snake bite toxicity
TK2. Spider and scorpion toxicity
TK3. Seafood toxicity
TK4. Tick paralysis

TL. OTHER ALLIED NEUROLOGY

TL1. Autonomic dysfunction
TL2. Radiotherapy
TL3. Neuro-aneasthesia
TL4. Palliative neurology

TM. NEUROLOGY GUIDANCE

TM1. Neurology evidence base
TM2. Neurology patient support